Shoulder Surgery

Edited by
Ian Bayley and Lipmann Kessel

Foreword by Sir Henry Osmond-Clarke

With 199 Figures

Springer-Verlag
Berlin Heidelberg New York 1982

Ian Bayley, FRCS,

Consultant Orthopaedic Surgeon,
The Royal National Orthopaedic Hospital,
234 Great Portland Street, London, W1N 6AD, UK.

Lipmann Kessel, MBE, MC, FRCS,

Professor Emeritus and Acting Director of Clinical Studies,
Institute of Orthopaedics,
The Royal National Orthopaedic Hospital,
234 Great Portland Street, London W1N 6AD, UK.

Proceedings of the Inaugural International
Conference on Surgery of the Shoulder.
Institute of Orthopaedics, University of London,
September 1980.

ISBN-13:978-1-4471-1316-4 e-ISBN-13:978-1-4471-1314-0
DOI: 10.1007/978-1-4471-1314-0

Library of Congress Cataloging in Publication Data
Main entry under title: Shoulder Surgery. Papers from the Conference on Surgery of the Shoulder held in 1980 under the aegis of the Institute of Orthopaedics and the University of London. Includes bibliographical references and index. 1. Shoulder — Surgery — Congresses. 2. Shoulder Joint — Surgery — Congresses. I. Bayley, Ian, 1942- . II. Kessel, Lipmann. III. Conference on Surgery of the Shoulder (1980: London, England). IV. University of London. Institute of Orthopaedics. [DNLM: 1. Shoulder — Surgery — Congresses. 2. Shoulder Joint — Surgery — Congresses. WE 810 S5595 1980]
RD557.5.S55 617'.572059 81-18325
ISBN-13:978-1-4471-1316-4 (U.S.) AACR2

Softcover reprint of the hardcover 1st edition 1982

Typeset by Photo-Graphics, Stockland, Honiton, Devon

2128/3916 543210

Foreword

It is interesting to observe the evolution of medical education over the years. The massive textbooks of the past have almost disappeared except as works of library reference. In their place we now find an increasing number of publications which explore the detail of particular specialities and sub-specialities. Once the young surgeon has acquired his basic knowledge of surgery in general (as it is now called), postgraduate education, whilst seeking to maintain the general scientific and humanistic principles of surgery, is forced to provide specialised reference works in a whole variety of fields, amongst which the postgraduate will choose his own future interest. This tendency emphasises the importance of the Conference on Surgery of the Shoulder organised by Professor Kessel and his colleagues. This first international gathering of surgeons and others in related disciplines who are interested in the disorders of the shoulder was self-funded under the aegis of the Institute of Orthopaedics and University of London, and it is to be hoped that other Universities, hospitals and medical foundations will give maximal financial and moral support for further ventures of this kind. This volume places on record the concepts and practices of those interested in the injury and disease of the shoulder joint, and thus becomes a reflection of our knowledge in this field in the second half of the twentieth century.

London, August 1981

Sir Henry Osmond-Clarke,
KCVO, CBE, FRCS, FRCSI

Preface

Some time early in 1980 when the idea was conceived of organising a conference on surgery of the shoulder, we were not aware that it was to become the Inaugural International conference, since none such had previously taken place. In the event, the response was almost overwhelming. 99% of those approached immediately agreed to participate, and only a few were unable to do so on account of previous commitments. We tried to gather together 'everybody who was anybody' in the world of shoulder surgery, and to a considerable extent we were successful beyond our most optimistic dreams.

Although we had half an idea that the proceedings of the Conference might be recorded, it was not until Springer made a forthright and unambiguous offer to publish, that our ambition became a reality.

The tranlation, editing and publication of conference proceedings presents unusual problems. There are both positive and negative qualities in such a publication. Its virtues lie in the breadth of ideas arising from the variety of approach from many different centres in the world, as well as a refreshing immediacy. Its deficiencies lie in the variation of styles in which the charm of the spoken word cannot always be conveyed into a written text. It is for this reason that the editors have inevitably been responsible for a certain amount of *gleichschaltung*, possibly to the discomfiture of some of the original authors, but hopefully easing the reader's task.

The publication attempts to be an up to date account of concepts and techniques concerned with most of the surgical problems of the shoulder. It does not pretend to be a comprehensive account of shoulder disorders. The choice of subject is, however, by no means arbitrary and is based on the conceptual developments of shoulder disorder during the past decade. For example, although the surgical anatomy and treatment of recurrent dislocation of the shoulder which so excited past generations is now a well understood routine problem, we have only recently begun to recognise that it is only one facet of a spectrum of shoulder instability. The analysis of the aetiology of shoulder pain until recently included in a ragbag diagnosis of 'bursitis', is now becoming increasingly refined and more accurately understood by the concept of the painful arc syndromes. Prosthetic replacement of the shoulder is so recently on the scene that it must inevitably find a place in this volume. The 'frozen shoulder' remains an enigma whose understanding can only be advanced by a full exchange of ideas from many different centres. Only those aspects of trauma to the shoulder girdle have been included when there is some contention regarding the traumatic anatomy and management: the standard range of fractures and dislocations are more properly treated in an appropriate textbook.

In 1961 F. Campbell Golding entitled his Makenzie-Davidson Memorial Lecture to the British Institute of Radiology: "The Shoulder – The Forgotten Joint". Hopefully the 1980 International Conference, followed by the publication of its proceedings, will do something to redress this balance. A fellowship of surgeons concerned with the shoulder has been created and preliminary arrangements for the next gathing in Toronto in 1983 is already underway.

London, August 1981 Ian Bayley and Lipmann Kessel

Contents

Section IV. The Frozen Shoulder

Section V. Rheumatoid Arthritis and Prosthetic Replacement

Conference Faculty

Dr. James E. Bateman — Toronto, Canada
Mr. J. Crawford Adams — London, England
Professor J. Debeyre — Paris, France
Professor A.F. DePalma — Fort Lauderdale, USA
Professor Lipmann Kessel — London, England
Mr. A.W.F. Lettin — London, England
Dr. Bo J. Lundberg — Gävle, Sweden
Professor M. Martini — Douera, Algeria
Dr. Jan A. Pahle — Oslo, Norway
Mr. Brian F. Reeves — Leeds, Englnad
Dr. Carter R. Rowe — Boston, USA
Professor J.T. Scales — London, England

Conference Secretary: Mr. J.I.L. Bayley — London, England

Contributors

Christian Akermark, MD,
Department of Orthopaedic Surgery,
Huddinge University Hospital,
141 86 Huddinge, Sweden.

B.E. Albrektsson, MD,
Department of Orthopaedic Surgery,
East Hospital,
S-416 85 Göteborg, Sweden.

Assistant Professor Carlos A. de Anquin,
University of Cordoba (R. Argentina),
Av. Malbran 980, Cordoba 5009
R. Argentina.

Professor Carlos E. de Anquin,
Chief Orthopaedic Department,
University of Cordoba (R. Argentina),
Av. Malbran 980, Cordoba, 5009
R. Argentina.

Professeur Agrege A. Apoil,
Centre de Chirurgie Orthopedique,
Hopital Saint Antoine,
814, rue du faubourg,
St. Antoine 75012, Paris, France.

G.P. Arden, FRCS,
Consultant Orthopaedic Surgeon,
Heatherwood Hospital,
Ascot, Berks.

N.J. Barton, FRCS,
Consultant Orthopaedic Surgeon,
Nottingham University Hospital and Harlow
Wood Orthopaedic Hospital, Mansfield.

J.I.L. Bayley, FRCS,
Institute of Orthopaedics,
Royal National Orthopaedic Hospital,
234 Great Portland Street, London, W1N 6AD.

F. Howard Beddow, MB, MChOrth,
FRCSE,
Consultant Orthopaedic Surgeon,
Royal Liverpool Hospital, Liverpool L7 8XP.
(and part time Clinical Lecturer, University of Liverpool)

A. Benjamin, FRCS,
Consultant Orthopaedic and Traumatic Surgeon,
West Hertfordshire Hospital,
Hemel Hempstead, Herts.

Eberhart Berg, MD,
Department of Surgery,
Ludvika Hospital, Sweden.

Georg Bergmann, Dipl-Ing,
Biomechanics Laboratory,
Orthopädische Klinkik und Poliklinik der
Freien Universität Berlin,
Clayallee 229, D-1000 Berlin 33, Germany.

N. Blackburn, FRCS,
Senior Orthopaedic Registrar,
Heatherwood Hospital, Ascot, Berks.

Dr. A. Boudjemaa,
Service de Chirurgie Orthopedique et
Traumatologique,
Centre Hospitals Universitaire de Douera,
Blida, Algeria.

S.A. Copeland, MB, BS, FRCS,
Consultant Orthopaedic Surgeon,
Royal Berkshire Hospital,
London Road, Reading, Berks. RG1 5AN.

James F. Crossan, BSc, MB, FRCS,
Consultant Orthopaedic Surgeon,
Victoria Infirmary, Glasgow G42 9TY.

Professeur Agrege Paul Dautry,
Hopital — école de la Croix-Rouge,
8 place de l'abbe
G. Henocque 75013 Paris, France.

Anthony F. DePalma, MD,
Emeritus Professor of Orthopaedic Surgery,
Thomas Jefferson Medical College,
Emeritus Professor of Orthopaedic Surgery,
New Jersey College of Medicine and Dentistry,
Chief of Orthopaedic Surgery,
North Ridge General Hospital,
Fort Lauderdale, Florida, U.S.A.

M.A. Elloy, BSc(Eng), PhD, CEng, MIMechE,
Bio-Engineering Unit,
University of Liverpool, Liverpool.

Professor P.M. Grammont,
Hopital du Bocage,
10 Bd. de Lattre de Tassigny,
21034 Dijon Cedex France.

Anthony G. Gristina, MD,
Bowman Gray School of Medicine,
Winston-Salem, North Carolina, U.S.A.

Bengt Gustafsson, MD,
Department of Orthopaedic Surgery,
Huddinge University Hospital,
141 86 Huddinge, Sweden.

Dr. Joseph Hardy,
Centre de Chirurgie Orthopedique,
Hopital Saint Antoine,
184 rue du faubourg,
St. Antoine 75012, Paris, France.

Peter Herberts, MD, PhD,
Associate Professor, Department of
Orthopaedic Surgery,
East Hospital,
S-416 85 Göteborg, Sweden.

D. Hirschowitz, FRCS,
Consultant Orthopaedic Surgeon,
West Hertfordshire Hospital,
Hemel Hempstead, Herts.

Lennart Hovelius, MD,
Department of Orthopaedic Surgery,
Gävle Hospital,
S-801 17 Gävle, Sweden.

Dr. F. Johnson, PhD,
Department of Surgery,
Medical School, Nottingham NG7 2UH.

J.R. Johnson, FRCS,
Senior Registrar in Orthopaedics,
Royal National Orthopaedic Hospital,
234 Great Portland Street, London, W1N 6AD

Lipmann Kessel, MBE, MC, FRCS,
Professor of Orthopaedics,
Institute of Orthopaedics,
Royal National Orthopaedic Hospital,
234 Great Portland Street, London, W1N 6AD.

Dr. Philippe Koechlin,
Centre de Chirurgie Orthopedique,
Hopital Saint Antoine,
184 rue du faubourg,
St. Antoine 75012, Paris, France.

Prof. Dr. Reinhard Kölbel, MSc(Biomechanics),
Biomechanics Laboratory,
Orthopädische Klinik und Poliklinik der
Freien Universität Berlin,
Clayallee 229, D-1000 Berlin 33, Germany.

L. Körner, MD, PhD,
Department of Orthopaedic Surgery,
East Hospital,
S-416 85 Göteborg, Sweden.

Harry H. Kretzler, Jr, MD,
1501 North 200th,
Seattle, Washington 98133, U.S.A.

C.R. Lamm,
Department of Diagnostic Radiology,
East Hospital,
S-416 85 Göteborg, Sweden.

Dr. U. Laumann,
Orthopädische Universitätsklinik Münster,
Hüfferstrasse 27,
4400 Münster, Germany.

Dr. G. Lelaurin,
Clinique Val Fleuri,
Rue Heritan, 71000 Macon, France.

Alan W.F. Lettin, MS, MB, BSc, FRCS,
Consultant Orthopaedic Surgeon,
St. Bartholomew's Hospital and
Royal National Orthopaedic Hospital,
London.

Anthony Leyshon, FRCS,
Senior Surgical Officer,
The Royal National Orthopaedic Hospital,
Brockley Hill, Stanmore, Middlesex.

B.J. Lundberg, MD,
Department of Orthopaedic Surgery,
Gävle Hospital,
S-801 17 Gävle, Sweden.

David L. MacIntosh, MD, CM, FRCS(C),
Associate Professor (retired),
Department of Surgery,
University of Toronto,
Toronto, Ontario, Canada.

Professor M. Martini,
Service de Chirurgie Orthopedique et
Traumatologique,
Centre Hospitals Universitaire de Douera,
Blida, Algeria.

Charles S. Neer III, MD, FACS,
Professor of Clinical Orthopaedic Surgery,
College of Physicians and Surgeons,
Columbia University,
New York, U.S.A.

M.W.J. Older, MB, BS, BDS, FRCS,
Consultant Orthopaedic Surgeon,
Royal Surrey County Hospital,
Guildford, Surrey.

Dr. D. Patte,
Clinique Medico Chirurgicale 'Les Fontaines',
54 Bd. Aristide Briand,
F-77000 Melun Cedex, France.

Dr. Claes J. Petersson,
Department of Orthopaedic Surgery,
Malmö General Hospital (University of Lund),
S-214 01 Malmö, Sweden.

Antonius Rohlmann, Dipl.-Ing,
Biomechanics Laboratory,
Orthopädische Klinik und Poliklinik der
Freien Universität Berlin,
Clayallee 229, D-1000 Berlin 33, Germany.

Professor R.L. Samilson, MD,
Clinical Professor of Orthopaedic Surgery,
University of California School of Medicine,
San Francisco, California, U.S.A.
(also Chairman, Residency Review Committee
for Orthopaedic Surgery. Member American
Board of Orthopaedic Surgery)

Daniel J. Scott, Jr, MD,
1331 Union Avenue,
Memphis, Tennessee 38104, U.S.A.

Dr. Kauko A. Solonen,
Orthopaedic Hospital of the Invalid
Foundation,
Tenholantie 10
00280 Helsinki 28, Finland.

Dennis J. Stoker, FRCP, FRCR,
Consultant Radiologist,
Royal National Orthopaedic and St. George's
Hospitals, London.
Director of Radiological Studies, Institute of
Orthopaedics, University of London.

Henrik Svend-Hansen, MD,
Department of Orthopaedic Surgery,
GU 4054, Rigshospitalet,
University Hospital,
2100 Copenhagen, Denmark.

J. Thorling, MD,
Department of Orthopaedic Surgery,
University of Linköping, Sweden.

Ramsay Vallance, MB, ChB, FRCS, FRCR,
DMRD,
Consultant Radiologist,
Gartnavel General Hospital,
Great Western Road, Glasgow.

W.A. Wallace, FRCS. Ed,
Department of Surgery,
Medical School, Nottingham NG7 2UH.

Michael Watson, MA, MRCP, FRCS,
Consultant Orthopaedic Surgeon,
Guy's Hospital, London, SE1 9RT
(also 92 Harley Street, London, W.1.)

Lawrence X. Webb, MD,
Bowman Gray School of Medicine,
Winston-Salem, North Carolina, U.S.A.

R. Peter Welsh, MB, ChB, FRCS(C),
Assistant Professor, Orthopaedic Surgery,
University of Toronto,
Toronto, Ontario, Canada.

A.M. Wiley, MBE, MCh, FRCS, FRCS(C),
Associate Professor of Surgery (Orthopaedics),
University of Toronto and Toronto Western
Hospital, Toronto, Canada.

Torsten Wredmark, MD,
Department of Orthopaedic Surgery,
Huddinge University Hospital,
141 86 Huddinge, Sweden.

Bruce T. Yoneda, MD, BSc,
Clinical Fellow, Division of Orthopedic Surgery,
Hospital for Sick Children,
Toronto, Ontario, Canada.

B.E. Zachrisson, MD, PhD,
Associate Professor,
Department of Diagnostic Radiology,
East Hospital,
S-416 85 Göteborg, Sweden.

Codman – His Influence on the Development of Surgery of the Shoulder

Carter R. Rowe

This is a very happy occasion for me, and an honour which could be given to a number of the contributors to this symposium. I am very appreciative and grateful. Ian Bayley, Honorary Secretary of the Inaugural International Conference in the Surgery of the Shoulder, wrote to me stating that the Organising Comittee had decided to include a designated lecture as part of the conference, and that the name which came to mind was Codman. He also inquired who around Boston was old enough to remember Codman and yet young enough to speak for an hour! I replied that only a very few were left to meet these criteria. Perhaps, as I had had the privilege of meeting Dr Codman and as both of us had paced the halls of the same hospital, the Massachusetts General, for many, many years, and as I was still alive and able to speak for some part of an hour, by the kind process of elimination, it fell to me to give the lecture. However, there is one of our colleagues with us today, a student of Codman's life, who has written the preface to the reprint of Codman's book, *The Shoulder,* I speak of Dr Anthony DePalma.

May we first express our gratitude to Professor Lipmann Kessel for the concept of an international meeting of surgeons interested in the shoulder and to Mr Ian Bayley for his extraordinary organisational ability in gathering us up from all parts of the globe to meet together and discuss the many problems of the shoulder.

With the convening of our meeting it is appropriate that we honour, with an eponymous lecture, one who has influenced every surgeon interested in the shoulder and who single handed shocked the medical profession out of the nineteenth century and into the twentieth; from the time-honoured custom of being satisfied with one's unchallenged surgical results to a new idea of follow-up evaluation in which the surgeon and the hospital must account for their results.

The choice of Dr Codman by Professor Kessel and his committee is timely and shows keen insight. Although many surgeons have contributed to surgery of the shoulder, no investigator has revealed the shoulder in its entirety as has Codman. My instruction concerning this lecture was "to deal with Codman himself—and his influence on the development of surgery of the shoulder". This assignment has been made quite easy, for few authors have revealed themselves as clearly and completely as Codman has in his classic book, *The Shoulder.*

One has only to read even a portion of his book to appreciate the uniqueness of Ernest Amory Codman. The reader will quickly realise that he has been introduced to a man of intellect, courage, conviction, controversy and irrepressible honesty, in fact at times too much honesty for his own good. Codman, who stood 6 feet 2 inches, a true Bostonian "carved from stubborn New England granite", was born on the 30th of December 1869 and died on the 23rd of November 1940. He graduated from Harvard College, where he was, as he stated, "a conventional enough Boston-Harvard boy", and entered Harvard Medical School in 1891 at the age of 22. For his third year, he visited various clinics in London, Paris, Berlin, Vienna and Cairo, an experience which enabled him to pass his third-year examinations and obtain his medical degree. His professional life was spent fighting for an idea, for necessary changes in the practice of medicine of his day, and in revealing the problems of the shoulder to the medical profession.

Students of Codman's life and works will list three diverse contributions to medicine.

The first was the End-Result Idea, which he described as "merely the common sense notion, that every hospital should follow every patient it treats, long enough to determine whether or not the treatment has been successful, and then to inquire, 'If not, why not?', with a view of preventing failures in the future". This was an

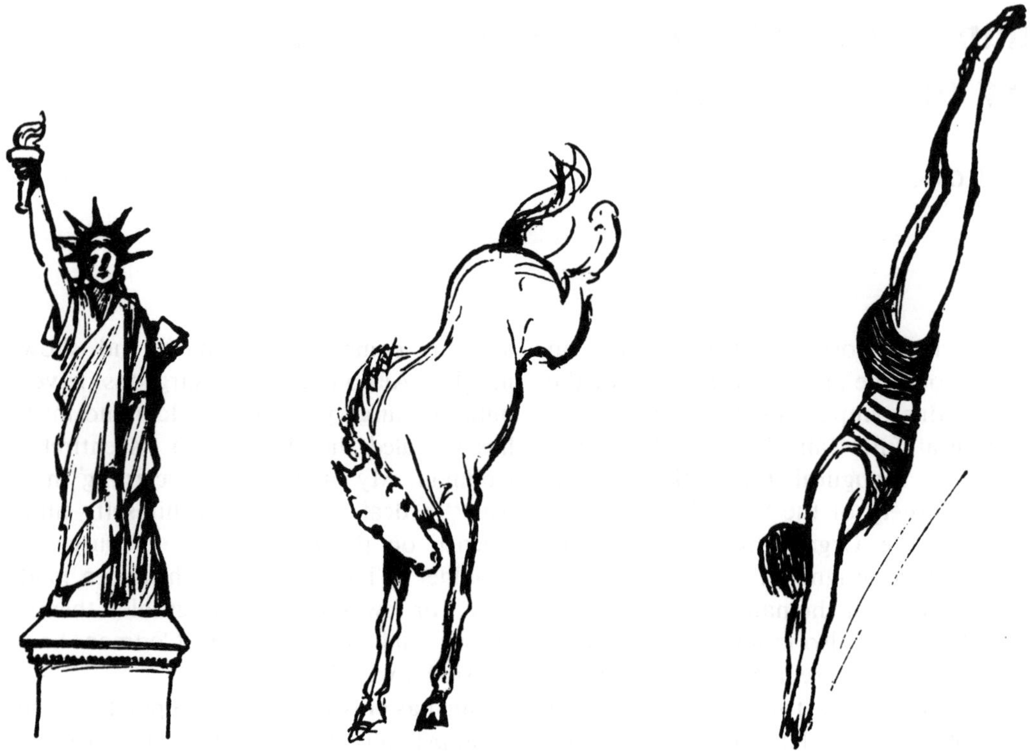

Fig. 1. Sketches by Dr Codman's cousin Lady Carter and Mr Philip Hale add to the individuality of *The Shoulder*

entirely new idea, and a rather electrifying one at that: how could an eminent surgeon in his right mind question his own results or indeed those of another surgeon? This was heresy, yet, as we know, it has become the accepted and unquestioned basis for clinical practice and research today.

The second major accomplishment was the establishment of the Registry of Bone Sarcoma, which was the first step doctors had taken to classify, evaluate, and follow-up the results of treatment of bone sarcoma. This set the stage, we might say, for the study of all tumours.

His third legacy was the publication of his book, *The Shoulder,* which was the first book limited to the shoulder and one in which one finds, in addition to its scientific content, the author's philosophy of life, his professional and social views, his hobbies— a book which every medical student and every surgeon interested in the shoulder should read, and reread (Fig. 1). In the author's words in the preface of his book— and this is very revealing of Codman:

Let him try his sense of humor, heavy as it may be, let him ride his hobbies, relate to his favorite anecdotes, tell his life history, or otherwise endeavor to please himself. Despite these amusements if you must, but do not forget that they are normal pleasures of the average man, especially if he is over sixty. No one is obliged to read a preface, but in it the author should introduce himself to the reader and give him a glimpse of his own personality, amusements, and intellectual processes.

What a delightful introduction, with a touch of fantasy and a sprinkling of egoism!

Although I had seen Dr Codman from afar as a student, I first met him when I was an orthopaedic resident at the Massachusetts General Hospital in 1937. He had been called in to see a patient with osteosarcoma of the shoulder and it was my lot to present the patient to Dr Codman. I remember him as a quiet, gentle person, with steady, penetrating eyes. One quickly sensed integrity, intelligence, and confidence. His faithful Irish setter always accompanied him when he visited the hospital, settling down quietly in the corner of the patient's room while he interviewed and examined the patient. Dr Codman had a good sense of humour and a nimbleness of mind, much as did Sir Robert Jones, and enjoyed putting it to use. Henry Marble, one of our pioneer hand surgeons, tells the story that early in his career when he assisted Dr Codman he received a message one day that Dr Codman wished to see him at noon of the coming Wednesday, "to pick a bone with you".

Knowing that Dr Codman was a very exacting person, he wondered what had gone wrong? What had he done, or had not done correctly? At noon on the Wednesday, Henry appeared at Dr Codman's office, rather worried and showing it. Dr Codman's secretary asked Henry to be seated, indicating that Dr Codman would see him in a few minutes. Soon she reappeared and ushered Henry into Dr Codman's office, where, in the centre of the room, a table was set, and two plump partridges, freshly cooked, were ready for lunch. "Henry, I shot these birds a few days ago, and thought you would enjoy picking a bone with me today". "That", Henry added with a smile, "was a very enjoyable bird!" Sir Harry Platt remembers Dr Codman, "He was somewhat eccentric, but a very interesting person — he did indeed leave us something".

I am certain that the majority of those of us in this room have read parts of or all of his book, *The Shoulder,* published in 1934 by Thomas Todd, Boston. It was out of print for many years, but has been republished by G. Miller & Co., Medical Publishers, Brooklyn, New York, with an excellent introduction by Dr Anthony DePalma.

Codman actually became interested in the shoulder when he spent his third year at Medical School travelling in Europe. "It was in Vienna", he wrote, "that my attention was first attracted to the subdeltoid bursa, because it was mentioned in a little book by Dr. E. Albert in 1893. I had never heard the bursa spoken of at home by my teachers." After completing his second year of surgical houseship at the MGH, he became an Assistant in Anatomy at Harvard Medical School, where he had the opportunity to dissect the subacromial bursa and study its pathology. Although the shoulder interested him very much, his primary interest, at that time, was his End-Result Idea. His work on the shoulder would have to wait. Referring to the medical practice of his day, he explained, "I am not a reformer on a principle, but merely because I am naturally disgusted with humbug, hypocrisy, smugness and cupidity." He sought to bring surgeons to attest to their operative results, and we will touch on this only to reveal Dr Codman in action.

A classic cartoon (Fig. 2) displayed at the closing of a meeting at which he had presided on Hospital Efficiency at the Boston Medical Library, January 6, 1915 caused quite an uproar. It shows an ostrich, representing the rich Back Bay

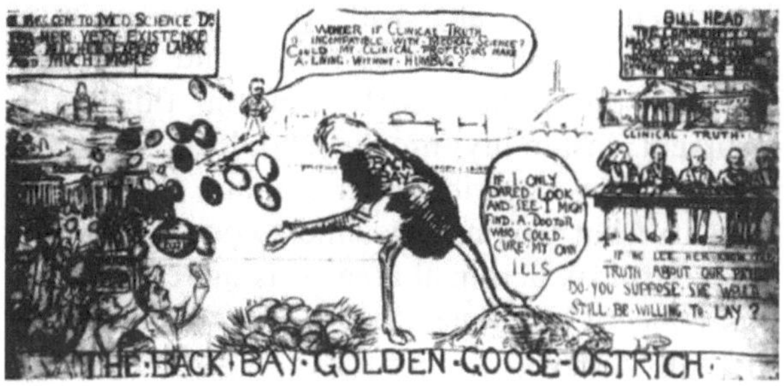

Fig. 2. The Back Bay Golden Goose

patient, with her head in the sand, devouring humbug and kicking out golden eggs to the professors. President Lowell of Harvard stands on the Cambridge Bridge, wondering if the professors could support themselves on their salaries, without the golden eggs. On the right, the Board of Trustees of the MGH is deliberating whether the Back Bay ostrich actually would continue kicking out her golden eggs if she knew by the End-Result System how many mistakes the professors were making. This cartoon jolted the local medical profession and resulted in his temporary separation from the Massachusetts General Hospital and the Massachusetts Medical Society and in the founding of his own hospital on Beacon Hill to demonstrate the effectiveness of his follow-up system. Through the freedom of his own hospital, he continued his fight for the End-Result System, which actually played a part in initiating the formation of the American College of Surgeons in 1913, but that would require another chapter in itself.

With his absence from Boston during World War One Dr Codman's hospital fell into financial difficulties and had to be closed. As he was in good graces again at the MGH, he accepted a special assignment on the shoulder which, in time, resulted in the publication of *The Shoulder* in 1934.

What were Codman's specific contributions on the shoulder, and what has been his influence on the development of shoulder surgery since then? When one mentions Codman, or his book, the subacromial bursa first comes to mind. This part of the body had received little attention before Codman became interested in it, studied its anatomy, and researched its clinical problems.

The painful bursa was Codman's only lead to account for the many puzzling problems under the acromion. The first section of this symposium is concerned specifically with the "painful arc" syndrome of the shoulder, the second with ruptures of the rotator cuff, and the third with recurrent instability of the shoulder. Each of these sections contributes in obvious and hidden ways to what Codman was most concerned with: the painful subacromial area. It is quite clear that this concern continues to challenge orthopaedic surgeons today.

Codman demonstrated in 1902 that calcific deposits, another major cause of shoulder pain and disability, were located in the substance of the rotator cuff rather than in the subacromial bursa and that by careful atraumatic surgery the deposits could be removed with complete relief to the patient. He also pointed out that absorption of the calcium left a weak area in the tendon which predisposed to its eventual rupture. When the calcium was surgically removed, the tendon should be repaired at the same time. His first publication on removal of calcium from the tendon was in 1904.

Dr Paul Norton recalls that in the early 1930s, when he was in charge of teaching third year medical students orthopaedics at the MGH, he frequently asked Dr Codman to lecture to them on the shoulder. Dr Norton wrote:

> His lectures were always pertinent, and he drew upon a wealth of personal observations to support the points of discussion. These lectures often resulted in quasi-heated debates between Dr Codman and myself, because for several years I had been needling calcium deposits in the rotator cuff. Old E.A. simply would have no part of it.

Dr Codman later gave Paul a copy of his book inscribed "Dear Doctor Norton, may your interest in sore shoulders continue, until you can correct every error in this book – Sincerely, E.A. Codman". I can see the twinkle in Dr Codman's eye when he wrote this.

His chapter on adhesive capsulitis, or "frozen shoulder", is indeed ahead of its time and should be read by every enthusiastic orthopaedic resident or young orthopaedic surgeon, who, it seems, must learn through experience. Dr Codman reveals his learning processes over the years and admits that he went through stages of forceful manipulations under anaesthesia, of opening the bursal areas surgically, and breaking up the adhesions. An interesting observation was made by him on one occasion when operating on a patient with a frozen shoulder, he inserted his finger into the bursal area and upon manipulation of the shoulder felt the tearing of the subscapularis muscle. Following this experience, he advised gradual rather than forceful stretching of the adhesions and wrote "I do not always give an anesthetic and break up the adhesions, as I used to do many years ago, nor do I open the bursa and break them up with my fingers, as I did for a period". We have all had to learn that the idiopathic "frozen shoulder" is a self-limited condition and that the majority of patients will become pain-free with full range of motion within a year or 18 months. Our problem has been: how can we shorten the painful period effectively and atraumatically? This syndrome remains a puzzling one and another challenge to our therapeutic approaches. For years Dr Julius Neviaser studied and wrote on this subject in America and his experience would have made a valuable contribution to the section on frozen shoulder.

Ruptures of the rotator cuff, primarily the supraspinatus tendon, were another consuming interest of Codman. He demonstrated that this lesion could be easily diagnosed and is credited with being the first surgeon to report the beneficial results of surgical repair of the rotator cuff in his paper "Complete Rupturing of the Supraspinatus Tendon. Operative Treatment with Report of Successful Cases" (*Boston Medical and Surgical Journal,* May 1911). For years, Dr Codman tried to convince his surgical colleagues that one of the principal causes of the lame shoulder was rupture of the rotator cuff. In some frustration, he wrote:

> A dog may bark up a tree for a long time before anyone comes to see what is up in the branches. For 20 years I bayed, but not continuously, about the importance of rupture of the supraspinatus and I owe a debt to Dr Philip Wilson, the first prominent surgeon, to take time enough to study the evidence that there was something at which to bay.

Dr Codman introduced the transacromial sabre approach to the rotator cuff and suggested that the greater tuberosity could be sacrificed to serve as a fresh bony attachment for the rotator cuff. He agreed with Dr Wilson that fascia could be used to reinforce complete ruptures. These principles have been researched and perfected by the late Harrison McLaughlin of New York, by the present very effective use of fascia reconstruction by Dr James Bateman of Toronto, and by the ingenious techniques of the contributors to the section on rotator cuff ruptures. Codman also researched the microcirculation of the rotator cuff, particularly of the "critical zone" of the tendon, which has lead to further investigation and recent contributions by Dr Ian McNab of Toronto, Canada.

Codman's observation of the anatomy, motions, and pathomechanics of the shoulder remains one of the most significant contributions to reconstructive surgery of the shoulder. His basic principles have stood the test of time and stand as the framework for the introduction and development of shoulder replacement prosthetic advances, which have been so imaginatively developed by Neer, Kessel, MacNab, Beddow, Scales, Post, Gristina, to name a few.

Perhaps one of Codman's most interesting and unique studies relative to shoulder motion and function is his *pivotal paradox,* demonstrating the loss of rotation of the glenohumeral joint as it moves from the side of the body to full elevation. "Certainly none of the authors who have written on dislocations and fractures in this region seems aware of the fact that in complete elevation of the arm almost no rotation can occur and that the extent of rotation diminishes as the arm is elevated". Thus, in full elevation of the shoulder, the rotator muscles have little if any, active function and are essentially neutralised. Sir Astley Cooper observed in 1825 that it was easier to reduce an anterior dislocation of the shoulder with the arm in full elevation than at the side of the body. Codman's pivotal paradox explains this: with the arm at the side of the body, the muscles are in spasm with full strength, which has to be overcome by the surgeon during reduction of the shoulder, whereas, in full elevation, there is loss of the ability to rotate and therefore little resistance by the muscles to prevent reduction. Codman's pivotal paradox thus resolves the overhead reduction technique of White (1764), LaMothe (1785), and Milch (1938). There are many other interesting aspects of the pivotal paradox phenomenon including the "envelope of motion", or the 90° of rotation which takes place when the shoulder is moved, but not rotated, from one plane to another. For instance, in moving the arm from the neutral position at the side of the body in the coronal plane to 90° of abduction, then to the sagittal plane, and down to the side of the body, the shoulder has rotated 90°. Or, if the arm is placed in 90° of external rotation at the side of the body, raised in abduction to full elevation and brought down to the side of the body, it is in 90° of internal rotation, having rotated 180° without intentional rotation by the patient.

Dr Codman also clearly demonstrated the four-part fracture of the humeral head, the pattern of which has been accepted today unchanged by Neer of New York and others, who continue to study the fracture and perfect techniques of open reduction and internal fixation. There has been no change since Codman's original classification. Codman; however, advised closed treatment for the majority of shoulder fractures with emphasis on his classic pendulum exercises for safe and early motion of the shoulder. Open reduction was resorted to only for severely displaced fractures. This sound advice remains in all orthopaedic textbooks today.

Concerning injuries of the acromioclavicular joint he wisely observed "employees are apt to find their shoulders too sore to permit labor, if compensation is paid". Has there been any change in man's situational reactions since then?

The Registry of Bone Sarcoma will stand as a timeless contribution to oncologists and orthopaedic surgeons. In his words, "My dream was that this one disease could be used as an example of the inadequacy of our present methods, and that some day the records would serve to demonstrate the value of the End-Result System". The Registry of Bone Sarcoma continues today in every large hospital and teaching centre. Is there a surgeon who does not remember Codman's triangle of bone sarcoma?

The philosopher, as pointed out in the *MGH News* in 1972, wonders with good reason how many times the wheel was invented or fire discovered. Now a wheel of new composition has rolled into view on the front pages of the medical world. *The Problem Oriented Medical Record,* an information sheet which dovetails with new computerised teaching techniques and recoverable information and medical histories. This organised storage of clinical information can be available on every patient. Rather than replacing the doctor, it has given him control and use of the mass of retrievable information available today. Is this not a reaffirmation of the End-Result System introduced by Dr Codman seventy years ago? The rediscovered wheel will have slow acceptance, as many of us are slow to try new methods, but every indication is that in one form or another it will be an important aspect of patient care and follow-up study in the future.

What Dr Codman fought for as a young surgeon in the early days of this century lives on as a pattern of safe and thorough patient care. Throughout life, Codman was a rational iconoclast, a realist and a dreamer, who enjoyed life. In his words, "I believe Don Quixote had a good time, and I have had mine too. What if we have occasionally attacked windmills? There was the joy of battle". He added "I may well admit that I have averaged at least 30 days a year in hunting and fishing in 36 states of the Union, in England, Scotland, Ireland, in Ontario, New Brunswick, Nova Scotia, Quebec, Cape Breton, in Egypt and the Yucatan— yet, I have never hit 10 ruffled grouse in succession". Codman concludes in the epilogue of his book, a proper introduction to this lecture, "Honors, except for those I have thrust on myself are conspicuously absent in my chart, but I am able to enjoy the hypothesis that I may receive some from a more receptive generation".

With the establishment of the Codman Lecture by our budding International Group concerned with the shoulder may we prove to be the "more receptive generation" and duly honor one of the great surgeons of our past, a man whose legacy we are so fortunate to inherit— Ernest Amory Codman, scholar, reformer, surgeon and delightful human being.

Section I. Painful Arc Syndromes

Moderator—Mr. J. Crawford Adams

I.1. Classification of the Painful Arc Syndromes

Michael S. Watson

The subacromial painful arc syndrome is common. A good deal of time is lost from work and many sleepless nights are endured because of it. The characteristic features are severe pain during *part* of the active excursion of the shoulder associated with full painless passive movement. Night pain is often severe. The pain is usually felt in the region of the deltoid muscle. However, radiation down the arm is not uncommon, and occasionally pain is felt in the epaulette region. The radiological examination often shows degenerative changes in the acromioclavicular joint and of the greater tuberosity. There may be calcific patches in the rotator cuff. None of these changes, however, is specific, and the shoulder may be reported as radiologically normal. Many patients suffer for some weeks and then the pain abates spontaneously. Others continue to be severely incapacitated for months or even years.

The surgeon's dilemma is in knowing which patients are likely to resolve and which are likely to become chronic when he first sees them. In either case inappropriate treatment may be offered if he makes the wrong decision: the naturally resolving condition needs no treatment and the severe chronic condition needs energetic early treatment.

We have shown that it is possible to predict the outcome of the painful arc syndrome at the first consultation in most cases. The differentiation between the resolving form and the refractory form depends almost entirely on the site of the lesion responsible for the symptoms. The site can be accurately localised by careful palpation, active and passive movement, and radiographs. It can be confirmed by an injection of local anaesthetic.

Identification

Time spent in palpating the shoulder is not wasted. There is always a small area over one of the tuberosities which is much more tender than the rest of the shoulder. It is sometimes necessary to adduct the shoulder fully before the tender area near the greater tuberosity is uncovered. Similarly it may be necessary to rotate the humerus while palpating the head and to identify the lesser and greater tuberosities.

The Anterior Form

Lesser tuberosity tenderness is usually associated with pain on abduction and on external rotation. The radiograph is frequently normal, although a small proportion of cases have degenerative changes in the acromioclavicular joint. Injection of local anaesthetic in and around the lesser tuberosity relieves the symptoms and abolishes the signs. A single injection of long-acting local steroid preparation into the same area usually results in resolution.

The Superior Form

Similar in number to the first group of patients is another group with tenderness in and around the greater tuberosity. Most have pain on abduction only. Almost all have acromioclavicular joint degeneration with loss of parallelism of the joint space, incongruity, sclerosis and osteophytosis. There are more men in this group than in the others, and more manual workers. Local anaesthetic confirms the localisation, but local steroid preparations rarely help. Indeed it is suspected that local steroids induce rupture of the supraspinatus tendon: several cases of this type of the painful arc syndrome have been seen to progress to rupture of the supraspinatus tendon, and all have had local steroid injections. When severe, symptoms may be relieved most reliably by surgical decompression in these cases. Through a deltoid-preserving incision the outer centimetre of the clavicle is excised and the projecting osteophytes are removed from both sides of the joint. The coracoacromial and the coracohumeral ligaments are then divided, fully exposing the rotator cuff. Rehabilitation is rapid and usually complete within a few weeks. The small number of patients with the refractory form of the anterior type usually have acromioclavicular degeneration, and they respond to similar surgical decompression.

The Posterior Form

A third group of similar size to the other two is composed of patients with pain arising from an area in the rotator cuff deep to the angle of the acromion. The average age is younger than that in the other groups, and many say that the onset of the pain followed a vigorous game of squash, tennis or badminton. The pain is made worse by internal rotation and by abduction. The radiograph is normal. These patients appear to have an acute traumatic lesion of the cuff, for they all subside within a few weeks of onset. Most have local steroids injected, but the role of these drugs in this form of the painful arc syndrome is doubtful.

Pathology

The refractory superior and anterior forms have been studied at operation. The outer end of the clavicle is expanded by osteophytes. The surrounding capsule is also swollen. The immediately subjacent coracoacromial and coracohumeral ligaments are displaced downwards and distort the underlying supraspinatus and subscapularis tendons. Where the tendons impinge against the distorted ligaments during abduction and rotation a degenerative lesion is formed. In the supraspinatus tendon and the long head of the biceps tendon this degeneration takes the form of thinning and fraying. The subscapularis tendon is swollen and red when it is affected. In some cases the supraspinatus tendon and the long head of the biceps tendon are found to be ruptured, but rupture of the subscapularis tendon has not been seen in this context.

The aetiology of the refractory form of the condition therefore appears to be as follows. For one reason or another the acromioclavicular joint becomes degenerate. There may be congenital incongruity or there may have been a previous injury to the joint causing acquired incongruity. Whatever the cause, the degenerate joint enlarges and distorts the surrounding coracoacromial and coracohumeral ligaments which bulge downwards. The anterior elements of the rotator cuff impinge against these bulging ligaments on abduction and rotation and are damaged by repeated minor trauma. The inflammatory reaction thus induced causes swelling and further trauma. The ischaemic nature of the supraspinatus tendon at this point impedes healing, and alteration of the collagen results, leading to eventual rupture. In the immediate neighbourhood the similarly damaged subscapularis tendon is more vascular, and although it becomes inflamed it does not atrophy or rupture.

I.2. The Role of Coracoacromial Arch Impingement as a Cause of Attrition of the Rotator Cuff

Robert L. Samilson

There are essentially four factors contributing to attritional changes in the rotator cuff of the shoulder. Phylogenetic changes have imposed certain biomechanical demands which are difficult to meet. Biochemical and structural ageing of tendon is a factor. The vascular anatomy of the rotator cuff contributes to attrition. Finally, and perhaps most importantly, impingement of the "critical area" of the rotator cuff beneath the coracoacromial arch is a consideration. This paper deals briefly with the first three of these factors and will concentrate on impingement.

Phylogeny

Inman has described the phylogenetic changes which have occurred about the shoulder girdle. As phylogeny proceeds, the deltoid muscle mass assumes ever increasing importance. Its size increases, and this is reflected in a progressively larger acromion and in distal migration of the deltoid tubercle on the humeral shaft. The supraspinatus, on the other hand, assumes decreasing anatomical prominence, as evidenced by an evolutionary decrease in the relative size of the supraspinous fossa as compared to the infraspinous fossa of the scapula. Furthermore, the scapula assumes a more vertical (rather than horizontal) position, as well as a more sagittal one. This occurs in conjunction with a change in shape of the chest wall. At the same time, the biceps mechanism changes. There is medial migration of the biceps groove, and as the scapula migrates dorsally on the rib cage, the long head of biceps takes a 90° turn from its origin to reach the biceps groove.

These phylogenetic changes impose functional alterations which may be important in the production of attrition. As phylogeny proceeds, the main force-couple in shoulder elevation changes from supraspinatus-biceps (the supraspinatus acting as humeral head depressor) in earlier development to infraspinatus-deltoid (the infraspinatus acting as humeral head depressor) in man. The angulation which the biceps must take in reaching the biceps groove and the decreasing muscle mass of supraspinatus may contribute to attritional changes in these structures.

Biochemical and Structural Ageing of Tendon

Brewer [3]has identified the following changes of a progressive nature, related to chronological age in autopsy specimens:

(1) osteitis of the greater tuberosity, cystic degeneration and irregularity of the cortical margin; (2) degenerative sulcus between the greater tuberosity and the articular surface; (3) disruption of the integrity of the attachment of the tendon to the bone by Sharpey's fibers; (4) loss of cellularity, loss of staining quality and fragmentation of the tendon; (5) diminution of the vascularity of the tendon and (6) diminution of fibrocartilage.

Morphological and biochemical age changes in tendon are described by Ippolito and associates [10]. Cellular changes with ageing include a decrease in tenoblasts, thinning of the size of tenocytes and decrease in cytoplasmic organelles. Matrix changes consist of irregular size of collagen fibres, increase in volume of extracellular matrix, increased diameter of some collagen fibres with decrease in size of newly formed fibres, and decrease in elastic fibres. Biochemical data indicate decrease in acid mucopolysaccharide and water content.

Blood Supply of Rotator Cuff

Rathbun and McNab [21] have studied the microvascular pattern of the rotator cuff.

Previously, Lindblom [15], Moseley [16], Rothman and Parke [22], and others identified a "critical zone" of relatively decreased blood supply in the supraspinatus tendon and in the long head of the biceps. It is probably more than coincidence that these critical zones are: (*a*) the most common sites of attritional changes in tendinous structures about the shoulder; (*b*) the areas with most functional demands imposed by phylogenetic changes described above; (*c*) the areas subject to impingement beneath the coracoacromial arch and (*d*) common sites of tendon disruption consequent to attritional change. The concept, then, is a unifying one.

The supraspinatus tendon has a radically different vascular pattern than the other rotator cuff tendons. Relative avascularity was noted at, or within, one centimetre of its insertion into the superior facet of the greater tuberosity of the humerus. This finding is not related to age, and was seen in cadavers under twenty years of age. The investigators indicated that this avascular zone was related to the longitudinal orientation of vessels in a flat tendon (as opposed to blood supply from paratenon in round tendons) and the tension created in the tendon because of its anatomical pathway to insertion. The mechanism was conceived as one of the tendon being "wrung out" by compression of the humeral head when the arm was adducted. Coracoacromial impingement in flexion and abduction is another plausible explanation of vascular compression. Once degeneration in the tendon occurs, further vascular change takes place with ingrowth of granulation tissue increasing intratendinous tension and extending the zone of avascularity wider and wider until spontaneous tendon rupture occurs.

Coracoacromial Arch Impingement

The importance of the coracoacromial arch in the pathogenesis of attritional changes in the rotator cuff has been emphasised by Neer [17,18], Hawkins [9] and others. The coracoacromial arch consists of the coracoacromial ligament, the acromioclavicular joint and the anteroinferior aspect of the acromion. Codman stated that the coracoacromial ligament functions largely to restrain the head of the humerus from gaining a fulcrum on the acromioclavicular joint or on the underside of the clavicle [4]. Evidently the coracoacromial ligament has an important duty and should not be thoughtlessly divided at any operation.

Anterior acromioplasty with excision of the coracoacromial ligament, as well as excision of the outer end of clavicle or any inferior acromioclavicular spurs causing impingement on the underlying supraspinatus tendon is a major contribution of Neer. The "critical area" of tendinous structures (supraspinatus, long head of biceps, and occasionally anterior edge of infraspinatus tendon) lies anterolateral to the coracoacromial arch, as defined. Vertical acromionectomy, either partial or total, has been carried out in the past with many disappointing results because of deltoid weakening, joint or bursal sinuses, scar retraction, and persistent symptoms.

What is the evidence supporting impingement by the coracoacromial arch? The "critical area" of tendinous structures lies below and in front of this arch with the arm at the side, but as the humerus is flexed forward and internally rotated, these structures are impinged by the overlying arch. The posterior two-thirds of the acromion do not contribute to this impingement, and this fact is the basis for Neer's surgical approach to the problem. Furthermore, observations made of full-thickness cuff tears at surgery invariably reveal the greatest thinning and attritional changes in the supraspinatus and/or anterior edge of infraspinatus tendons. Once the cuff is torn, similar changes occur in the exposed long head of biceps. Observations of small tears demonstrate that they almost always start in the "critical area" and propagate from there. Sometimes (but certainly not usually), a small spur is present at the anteroinferior acromial margin and may be accompanied by similar spurring at the acromioclavicular joint and the superior margins of the biceps groove. These spurs should be removed as they contribute to the impingement. The anterior acromial spur may represent an exostosis caused by traction from either anterior deltoid or coracoacromial ligament.

Three stages of impingement have been described. Stage I is that in younger individuals, characterised by oedema and haemorrhage. This is reversible and may not progress to Stages II and III. Not infrequently it is seen in throwing sports.

Management of patients in this group is often non-operative, consisting of rest, analgesics, and avoidance of precipitating arm positions for varying periods of time. Occasionally, excision of the coracoacromial ligament without anterior acromioplasty may be indicated. Calcium deposits may also result in impingement in this age group.

Stage II is characterised by thickening and fibrosis of the bursal structures overlying the tendon and occurs often in the third and fourth decades, precipitated again by overhead use of the arm. If non-operative measures do not relieve the complaint, anterior acromioplasty, coraco-acromial ligament excision, and excision of thickened subdeltoid bursa are indicated. Steroids should be used, if at all, very infrequently in non-operative management because evidence suggests that tendon rupture may be precipitated by such an injection and may interfere with the natural process of healing of such lesions.

Stage III is seen in individuals usually over the age of 40 and is the end stage of impingement. The bony spurs mentioned above may be seen, and rotator cuff tears are present. If symptoms and function fail to improve with non-operative management after six weeks, anterior acromioplasty, excision of coracoacromial or biceps groove spurs, and repair of the rotator cuff may be indicated.

The criteria for cuff repair are: (1) a patient physiologically younger than 65 years of age with clinically or arthrographically demonstrable full-thickness cuff tear; (2) failure to improve under non-operative management for a period of not less than six weeks; (3) the patient's need to use the involved shoulder in overhead elevation in his vocation or avocation; (4) full passive range of motion of the shoulder; (5) willingness on the part of the patient to exchange decreased pain and increased external rotator strength for some possible loss of active abduction of the shoulder, and (6) ability and willingness of the patient to co-operate in rehabilitation.

Not all cuffs are capable of being repaired. Some have undergone such severe attritional change that attempted repair is like sewing the ends of a brush together. It is useful to decompress such shoulders by anterior acromioplasty, even when the cuff cannot be repaired. The patient will appreciate the diminution of pain.

Clinical signs and symptoms of impingement include: (1) reproduction of pain on forced forward flexion of the shoulder; (2) reproduction of pain on forced forward flexion of the shoulder to 90°, followed by forced internal rotation in that position; (3) reproduction of pain in active unassisted shoulder elevation between 70 and 130°; (4) temporary relief of the above three findings by subacromial injection of 10 cc 1% xylocaine; (5) soft-tissue crepitus, most marked in Stage III; (6) weakness of external rotation and abduction, most marked in Stage III; (7) selective supraspinatus and/or infraspinatus atrophy in Stage III, and (8) "fluid sign", or palpable bursal swelling, noted in Stage III.

Radiological findings are usually nil in Stages I and II. In Stage III an anteroinferior acromial spur may be present and is best seen on an anteroposterior view with the tube tilted in a 15° caudal direction. On occasion, the spur may be seen with the tube tilted 25° cephalad. The routine anteroposterior view of the shoulder will usually fail to show the spur. Acromioclavicular joint spurring may be seen on films of this joint. Exostosis at the superior margin of the biceps groove is best seen on bicipital groove views. Prominence of the greater tuberosity with spurring at the facet for supraspinatus insertion can be seen on routine shoulder views. If the cuff is torn, the humerus is displaced upwards; on occasion it may descend downwards (especially in the presence of axillary nerve palsy). Subchondral cysts are sometimes seen at the greater tuberosity. An arthrogram will reveal a full-thickness cuff tear and may demonstrate a "geyser sign" with contrast material entering the acromioclavicular joint. The latter confirms the contribution of inferior acromioclavicular impingement to the resultant cuff tear.

Surgical Technique for Relief of Impingement

The technique for rotator cuff repair is described elsewhere (p. 000).

With the patient in a semi-Fowler (semi-sitting) position, with a folded towel beneath the scapula and the arm draped free, an incision is made along the acromion margin anteriorly to just above the coracoid process. The deltoid is split in the direction of its fibres, a distance of 4-5 cm. The deltoid is detached with a cautery knife, from the front of the acromion and outer clavicle. The coracoacromial ligament is identified, and downward traction is placed on the freely draped arm. In Stage I or Stage II impingement, simple excision of the coracoacromial ligament after identifying its acromial and coracoid insertions is sufficient. In Stage III, after identifying the coracoacromial ligament, the underside of the acromion and acromioclavicular joint are palpated for the presence of spurs. If spurs are present at the acromioclavicular joint, the outer end of the clavicle is removed. An osteotome is directed backwards and downwards from the anterior acromial margin, removing a wedge based inferiorly. This wedge, with coracoacromial ligament attached (detaching the ligamentous insertion into the coracoid), will contain any existent acromial spurs. Bicipital groove spurs, if present, are removed. Meticulous deltoid repair is carried out to the acromion, and the subcutaneous tissue and skin are closed. The wound is dressed and the shoulder is immobilised.

Postoperative management plays an essential part in the quality of the final result. Early assisted shoulder motion is the key to success, but active unassisted forward flexion is prohibited for about ten to fourteen days, to preserve the deltoid repair. Assisted forward flexion and external rotation are performed with the guidance of a knowledgeable physical therapist on the fourth postoperative day. Exercise is performed with the patient supine, minimising the effects of gravity. Once full range of motion is achieved, resisted exercises to increase power and endurance may commence.

I.3. Decompression of the Subacromial Space: An Anatomical Study

U. Laumann

The subacromial space is limited above by the fornix humeri, the common arched roof formed by the coracoid process, coracoacromial ligament and acromion; the inferior limitation is the head of the humerus. On average, this space has a width of 1-1.5 cm and enlarges from before backwards (Fig. 1a and b). In this narrow space a series of soft tissues are included. The osteofibrous covering does not allow any space for increase of volume of the soft tissue; consequently, if the internal pressure increases, a typical compartment syndrome develops with painful restriction of movement. In such cases operative enlargement of the subacromial space is indicated in order to decompress the enclosed soft-tissue structures. Various procedures of decompression were tried on anatomical specimens and investigated from two points of view:

(ii) The extent of the enlargement achieved;
(ii) The biomechanical alteration of function of the shoulder joint.

Anatomy of the Subacromial Space

The soft-tissue structures within the subacromial space may be divided into three segments with the arm in its normal position:

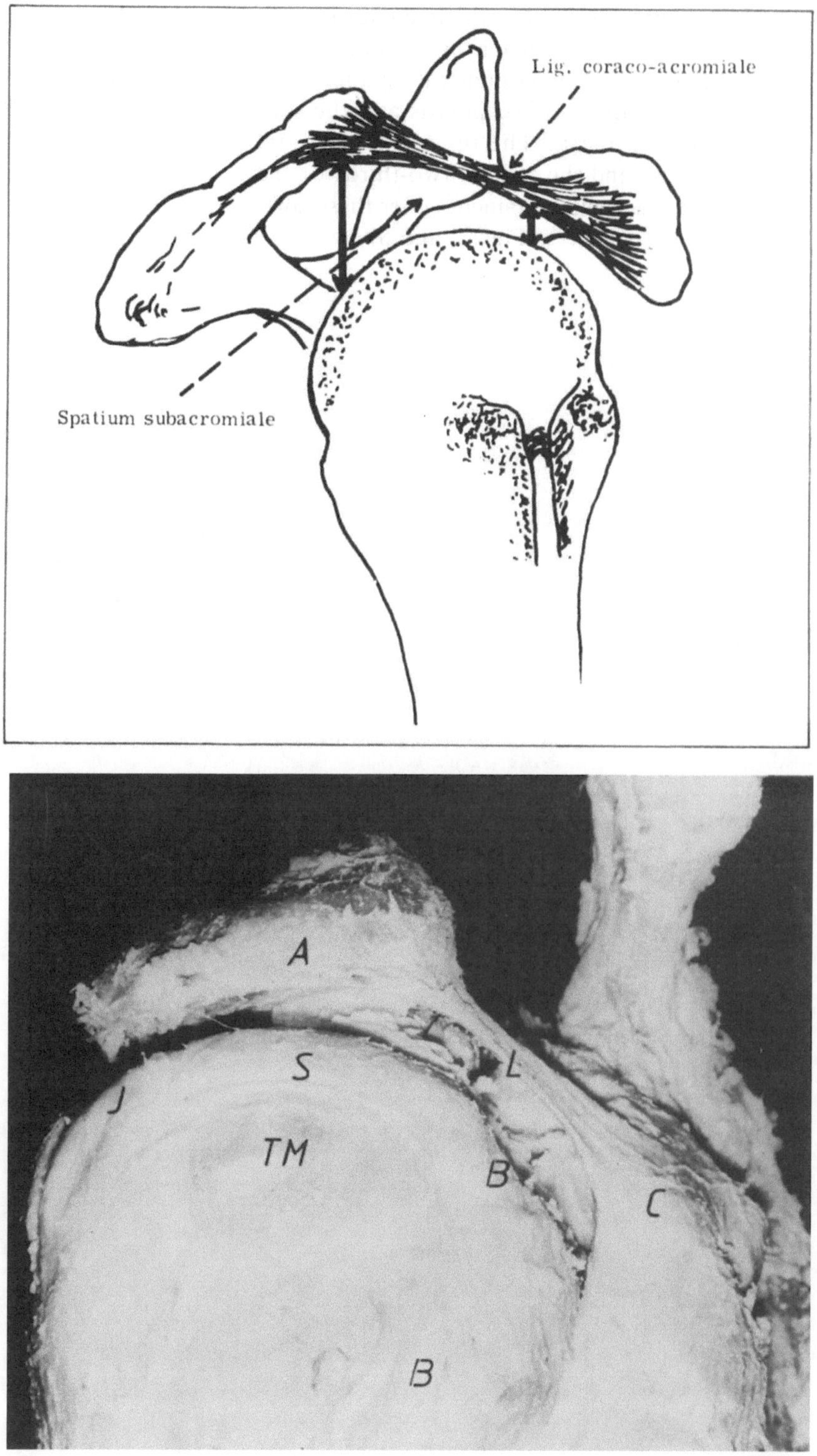

Fig. 1a and b. Subacromial space, lateral view

A = Acromion
L = Coracoacromial ligament
C = Coracoid process
I = Infraspinatus
S = Supraspinatus
B = Biceps, long head
TM = Greater ituberosity

I. A ventral segment which comprises the intra-articular portion of the long biceps tendon, the coracohumeral ligament, the upper part of subscapularis and the subcoracoid bursa. The tip of the coracoid process and the ventral two-thirds of the coracoacromial ligament cover these soft-tissue structures (Figs. 2 and 3).

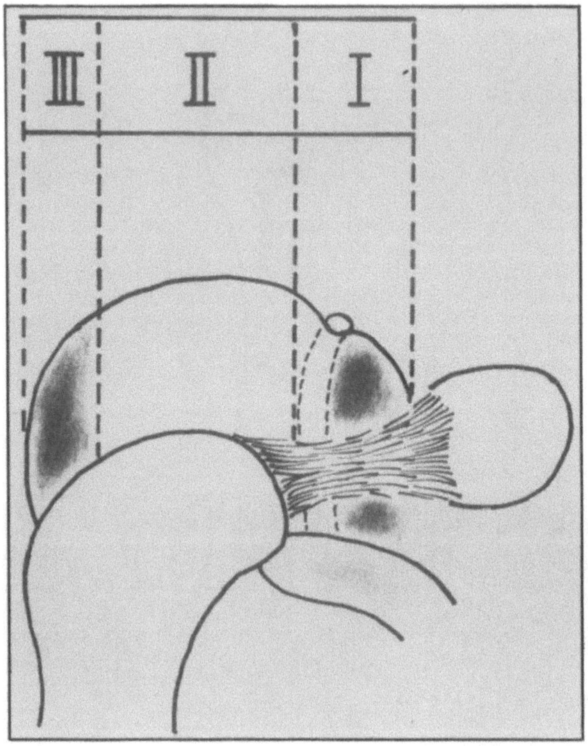

Fig. 2. Fornix humeri, upper superficial aspect, division into 3 segments

II. A median segment comprising the whole of the insertion of supraspinatus tendon and parts of the subacromial bursa; this segment is ventrally covered by the coracoacromial ligament too, the acromioclavicular (AC) joint and the anterior half of the acromion (Fig. 4).

III. A dorsal segment which includes the upper portion of infraspinatus and parts of the subacromial bursa and which is covered only by the dorsal part of the acromion (Fig. 5).

The most narrow part of the subacromial space is in segments I and II. Therefore, an adequate decompression can only be achieved if decompression has been performed within the region of the coracoacromial ligament, the ventral half of the acromion and, when indicated, in the region of the AC joint.

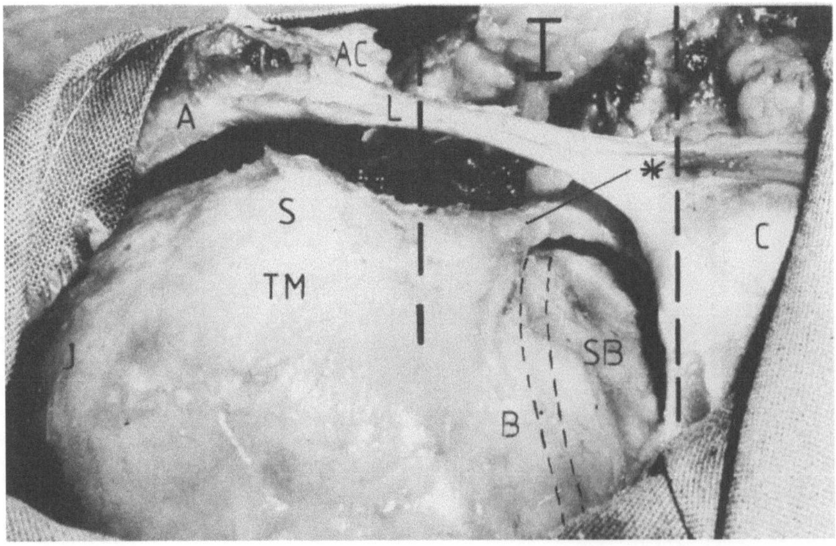

Fig. 3. Subacromial space, segment I, lateral view

AC = Acromioclavicular joint—clavicle resected
A = Acromion
L = Coracoacromial ligament
C = Coracoid process
S = Supraspinatus muscle
I = Infraspinatus muscle
TM = Greater tuberosity
B = Biceps long head
SB = Subscapularis muscle
* = Coracohumeral ligament

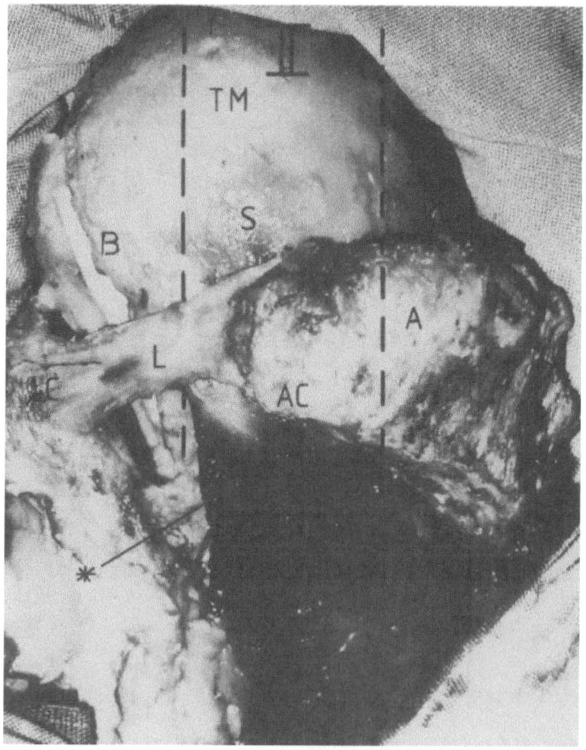

Fig. 4. Subacromial space — segment II, cranial view

TM = Greater tuberosity
B = Biceps long head
C = Coracoid process
L = Coracoacromial ligament
AC = Acromioclavicular joint — clavicle resected
A = Acromion
* = Supraspinatus tendon
S = Supraspinatus muscle

Decompression of the Subacromial Space

In principle, the subacromial space can be increased in two directions (Fig. 6).

A. By superior decompression:
  (i) acromionectomy;
  (ii) lateral acromioplasty;
  (iii) partial anterior acromioplasty (Neer);
  (iv) incision and/or excision of the coracoacromial ligament.

B. By inferior decompression:
  (v) reduction of soft tissue within the subacromial space; (i.e. bursectomy, removal of the intra-articular portion of the long biceps tendon);
  (vi) inferior displacement of the glenohumeral joint by paraglenoid osteotomy (Stamm).

(i) Acromionectomy

In the method described by Smith-Petersen and Armstrong, the acromion is completely resected, the AC joint is thereby destroyed and the coraco-acromial ligament is removed simultaneously. The whole acromial attachment of deltoid and the

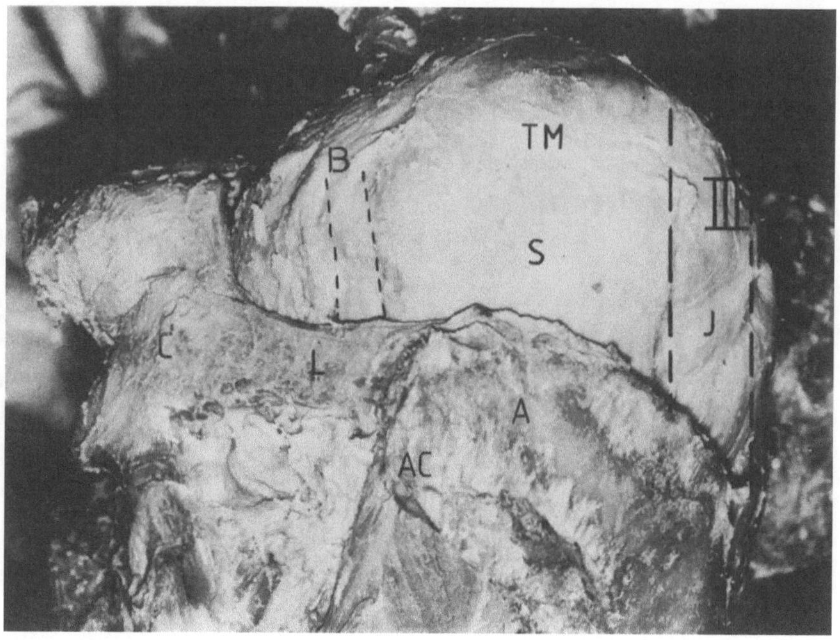

Fig. 5. Subacromial space—segment III, cranial view.

TM = Greater Tuberosity
B = Biceps long head
S = Supraspinatus muscle
I = Infraspinatus muscle
C = Coracoid process
L = Coracoacromial ligament
AC = Acromioclavicular joint—clavicle resected
A = Acromion

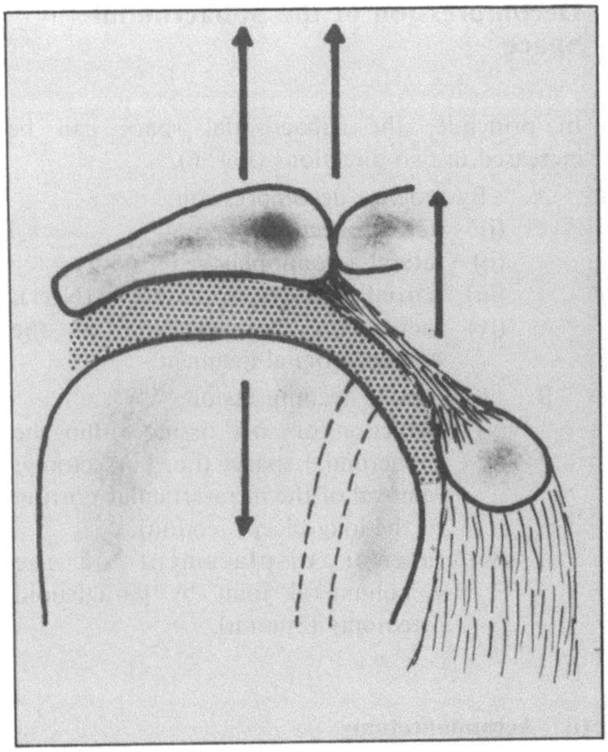

Fig. 6. Methods available to decompress the subacromial space

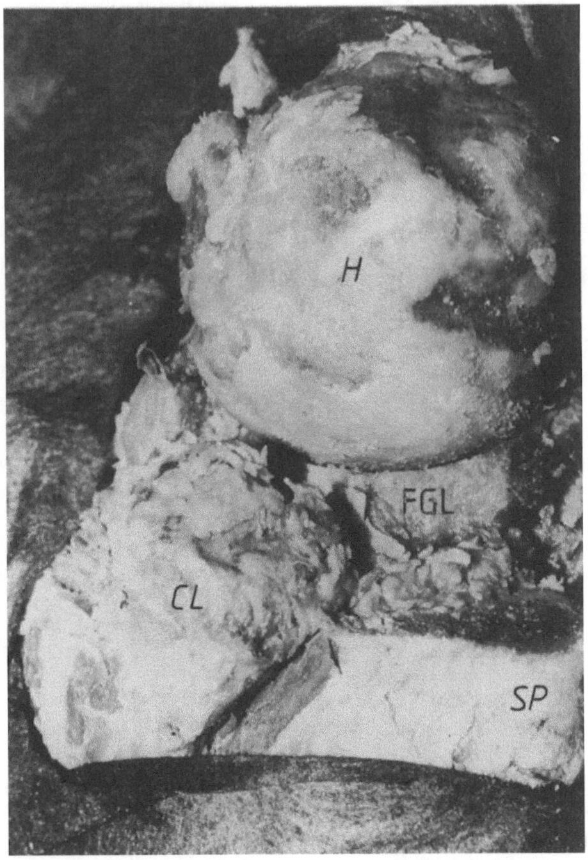

Fig. 7b. Acromionectomy—wide decompression of humeral head

H = Head of humerus
CL = Clavicle
FGL = Glenoid fossa
SP = Spine of scapula

greater part of the oblique fibres of trapezius are detached from their bony attachments (Fig. 7a). As a result there is complete decompression in all the three segments (Fig. 7b).

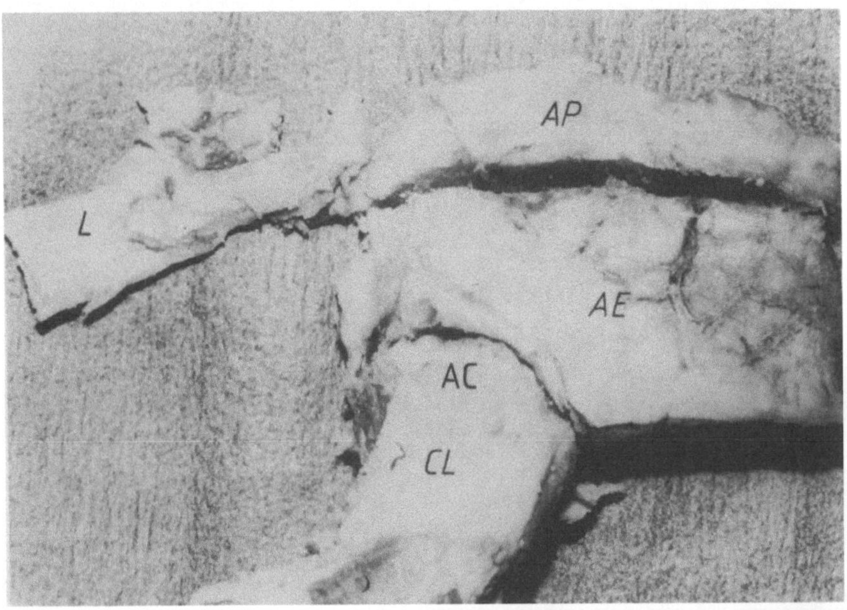

Fig. 7a. Resection levels in lateral acromioplasty (AP) and acromionectomy (AP+AE)

L = Coracoacromial ligament
CL = Clavicle
AC = Acromioclavicular joint

(ii) Lateral Acromioplasty

In lateral acromioplasty, the AC joint is preserved because the acromion is only partially removed; the coracoacromial ligament is partially or completely resected (Fig. 8). If only the lateral third of the acromion and only parts of the coracoacromial ligament are resected, the decompression is not sufficient in segment I nor in segment II, and the fornix humeri is only increased in a sagittal direction. After the removal of two-thirds of the acromion and the whole coracoacromial ligament, there is a complete decompression in segment I. In segment II the decompression is only sufficient when the remaining bony parts of the anterior half of the acromion as well as those of the AC joint have been inferiorally remodelled (Fig. 9).

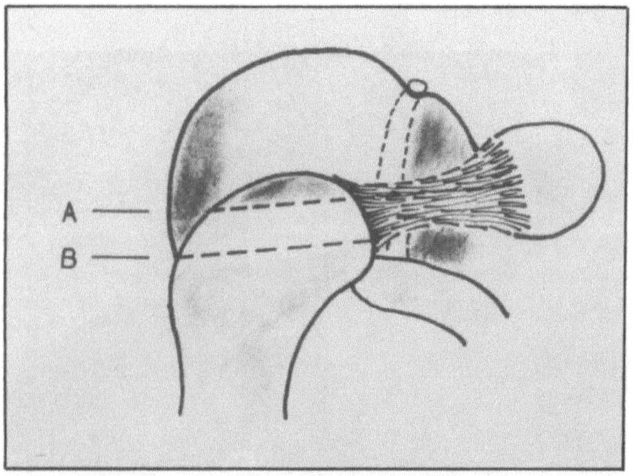

Fig. 8. Resection levels in lateral acromioplasty

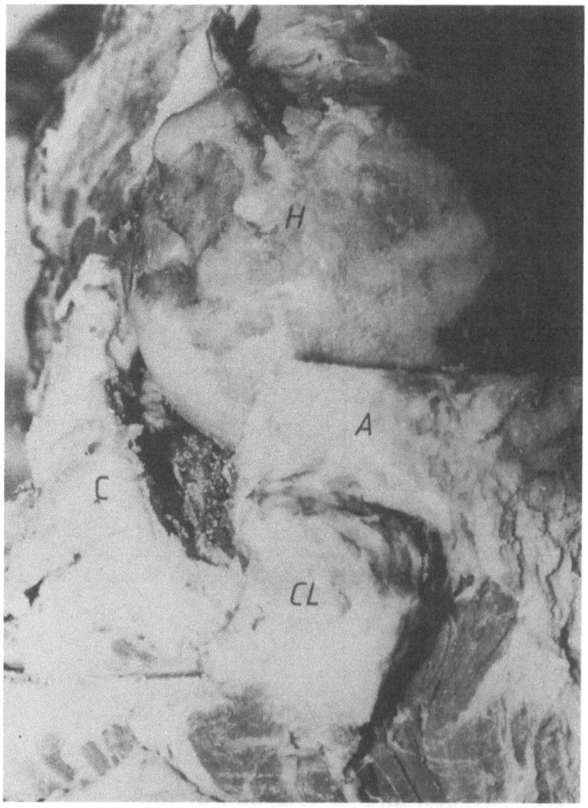

Fig. 9. Lateral acromioplasty with resection of coracoacromial ligament

H = Head of humerus
C = Coracoid process
A = Acromion
CL = Clavicle

(iii) Partial Anterior Acromioplasty (Neer)

In this method, the coracoacromial ligament is entirely removed, and the ventral half of the acromion below is remodelled. The AC joint may also be partially resected, if necessary, whereas the acromioclavicular superior ligament is retained (Fig. 10). Thus segment I is completely decompressed and in segment II, an increase of 0.5 to 0.8 cm can be achieved, which means 50% increase of the original distance (Fig. 11). Deltoid and trapezius remain largely untouched, the function of the clavicle is maintained, and the acromion as the buttress of the humeral head is partially preserved.

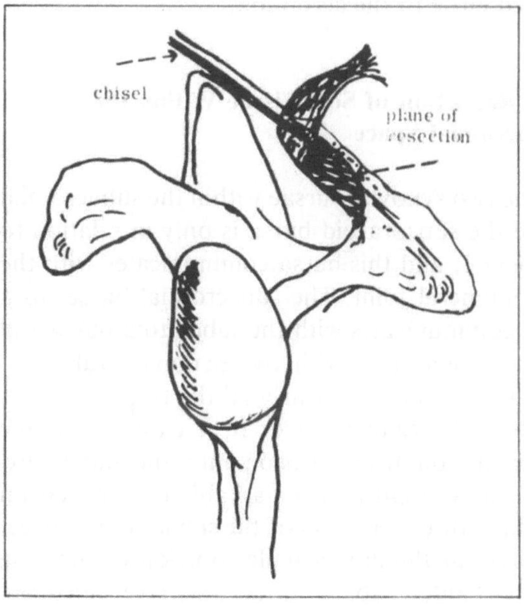

Fig. 10. Neer's partial anterior acromioplasty.

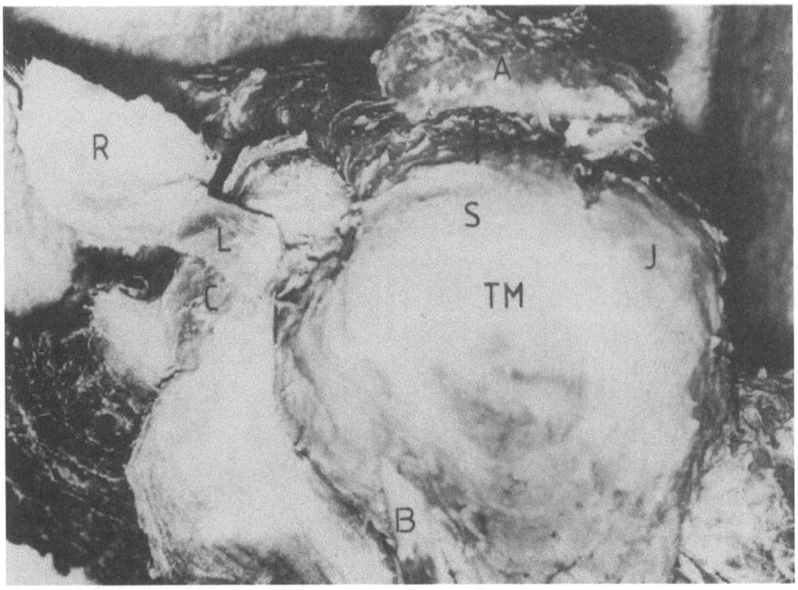

Fig. 11. Condition following Neer's partial anterior acromioplasty: Resection of anterior half of acromion (R) with attached coracoacromial ligament (L)

A = Acromion
C = Coracoid process
S = Supraspinatus muscle
I = Infraspinatus muscle
TM = Greater Tuberosity
B = Biceps long head

(iv) Incision and/or Excision of the Coracoacromial Ligament

If only the coracoacromial ligament is incised or excised, it will lead to a decompression in segment I, while in segment II only the anterior third will be decompressed (Fig. 12). In general, the decompression seems to be better if the ligament is incised close to the acromion.

(v) Reduction of Soft Tissue Within the Subacromial Space

Of the two synovial bursae within the subacromial space the subcoracoid bursa is only in relation to segment I, and this bursa communicates with the glenohumeral joint. The subacromial bursa, as a rule, communicates with the subdeltoid bursa and has no connection with the glenohumeral joint. Usually, it embraces nearly all the three segments of the subacromial space. In a case of chronic inflammation with effusion into the bursa, excision may result in a remarkable decompression in all the three segments of the subacromial space. Excision of the intraarticular portion of the long biceps tendon above does not give adequate decompression in any case.

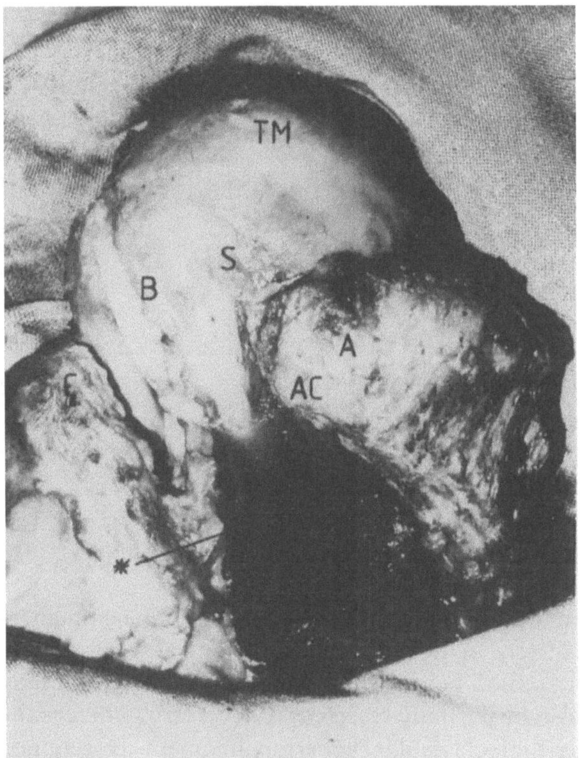

Fig. 12. Resection of coracoacromial ligament: insufficient enlargement of segment II

TM = Greater Tuberosity
B = Biceps long head
C = Coracoid process
A = Acromion
AC = Acromioclavicular joint
S = Supraspinatus muscle and tendon

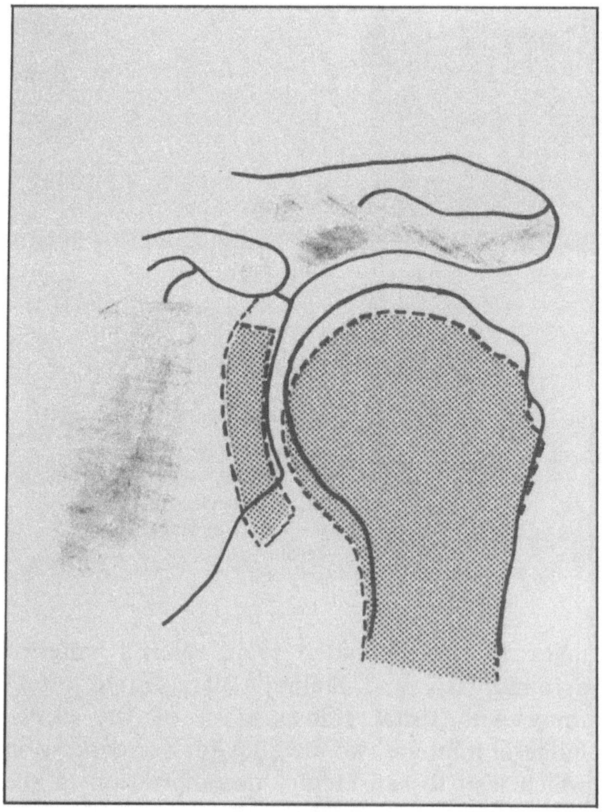

Fig. 13. Stamm's paraglenoid osteotomy

(vi) Paraglenoid Osteotomy (Stamm)

By this method widening of the subacromial space is achieved by distal transposition of the glenohumeral joint through a paraglenoid osteotomy provided that any adhesions to the fornix humeri have previously been completely divided (Fig. 13).

Discussion

Any operative procedure for decompression of the subacromial space which damages essential anatomical structures for the function of the shoulder joint must be abandoned.

Although total acromionectomy leads to the best possible decompression of the subacromial space, it involves considerable functional disadvantages. Deltoid and trapezius, two muscles of essential importance for the function of the shoulder joint, are remarkably weakened through the loss of their bony insertion (Fig. 14). The destruction of the AC joint results in instability of the shoulder girdle which can be compensated only partially by the damaged trapezius. After the loss of the whole upper arch the head of the humerus is without any superior bony buttress, and if there is loss of support due to an inefficient rotator cuff, the consequence is an upward subluxation of the humeral head.

Our investigations indicate that lateral acromioplasty gives satisfactory decompression only if the coracoacromial ligament is completely divided or excised and if the remaining part of the underspace of the acromion is remodelled. This procedure is basically like Neer's partial anterior acromioplasty, which in our opinion is preferable because deltoid and trapezius are only minimally disturbed from their bony insertion; the bony fornix humeri is almost completely retained and the gain of distance is almost the same. Both procedures must be followed by early postoperative physiotherapy in order to avoid subacromial adhesions. The incision and/or excision of the coracoacromial ligament alone in most cases does not result in satisfactory decompression. To be successful this method has to be combined with other procedures of superior decompression.

Bursectomy, as sole therapy for decompression of the subacromial space is only indicated in the exceptional case of an isolated bursitis without any accompanying periarticular alterations. Paraglenoid osteotomy leads to a decompression similar to that attainable by acromionectomy without its disadvantages as the whole fornix humeri remains intact.

The anatomical investigations indicate that for decompression of the subacromial space, Neer's anterior partial acromioplasty and Stamm's paraglenoid osteotomy are the best procedures. Which of the two should be preferred in any particular case depends on the accompanying lesions. In principle, decompression of the subacromial space only results in relief of pain; any functional improvement cannot be expected from these procedures.

Summary

By means of anatomical specimens the utility of various methods for decompression of the subacromial space have been investigated. It has been

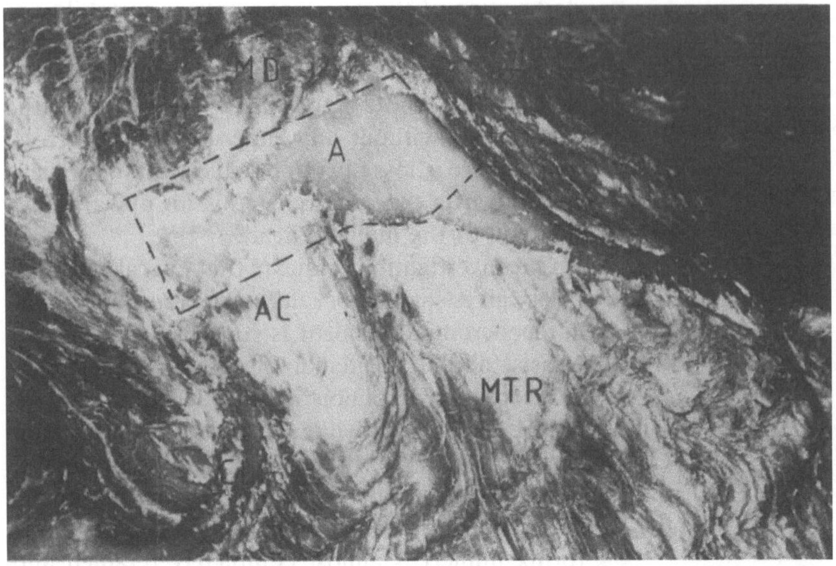

Fig. 14. Oblique fibres of trapezius (MTR) and of the acromial origin of deltoid (MD)

A = Acromion
AC = Acromioclavicular joint
CL = Clavicle
—Resection level in acromionectomy

ascertained that adequate decompression can only be achieved if the subacromial space is widened in the regions of the coracoacromial ligament, the anterior half of the acromion and, at choice, also of the AC joint. Acromionectomy provides the best possible decompression but at the same time involves considerable biomechanical disadvantages to the shoulder joint. Neer's anterior acromioplasty and Stamm's paraglenoid osteotomy with distal transposition of the glenohumeral joint are two methods for decompression which lead to satisfactory decompression of the subacromial space without the disadvantages of acromionectomy.

I.4. The Surgical Treatment of Rotator Cuff Impingement

A. Apoil, P. Dautry, Ph. Koechlin and J. Hardy

The surgical repair of rotator cuff tears appears to be both simple and logical. However, since 1953, we have chosen an alternative technique because we believe that the disability occurs as a result of a conflict between what is left of a torn cuff and the coracoacromial arch: our procedure consists of a superior arthrolysis of the shoulder. This chapter is based on a review of the last 100 patients.

Material

There is a male predominance: 78 men to 22 women. The age ranged from 21 to 78 years, with a mean of 55 years; 5 patients were under 40 years, 4 patients over 70 years. The dominant side was involved in 77 patients.

It was rather difficult to establish the precise onset of the syndrome, but we could classify our patients into three groups of approximately equal numbers.

onset following a significant traumatic episode;
onset following moderate trauma, such as a violent effort or movement;
an apparently spontaneous onset.

The average delay between the onset of symptoms and operation was about 28 months. All the patients who eventually underwent surgery were failures of a strict medical and physiotherapeutic regime of at least 6 months. The average follow-up period is 45 months.

Method

Surgical Technique

i) Position:

The patient is placed supine with his shoulder off the table to allow full mobilisation.

ii) Approach:

We use the deltopectoral approach, curved lateral to the coracoid process. The deeper part of the deltoid muscle is mobilised. The arm is then externally rotated and pushed backwards.

Operative Findings

Sometimes an obvious tear in the cuff reveals the superior part of the humeral head. Most often the enlarged subacromial bursa hides the cuff and has to be excised to show the lesion. Great care must be taken not to mistake this bursa for an intact cuff.

By movement of the arm into abduction, one can substantiate any impingement between the coracoacromial ligament on the one hand, and on the other hand either the edges of the torn cuff or an enlarged capsule.

Management of the Impingement

First, excision of the coracoacromial ligament. Secondly, excision of the lesion consisting of the distal part of the torn cuff inserted on the humeral head and the proximal part of the edge of the tear, which is caught between the head and the glenoid fossa. Firm traction on the arm allows one to see the supraspinatus pathway and the proximal part of the cuff. Finally, excision of the intra-articular part of the biceps tendon, either by direct exposure through a torn capsule or by opening the bicipital groove. Rarely the bicipital tendon is either dislocated in the glenohumeral angle or has completely disappeared. The tendon is divided close to the glenoid fossa and inserted into the bicipital groove or into the pectoralis major with the elbow flexed.

The wound is closed with drainage and the front of a thoracobrachial cast is applied anteriorly to maintain abduction and flexion of the shoulder, the elbow flexed at 90°. The anterior half of the cast is easily applied on a sleeping patient in the supine position and can be completed on the following day.

Postoperative routine

Postoperative routine must be strictly adhered to. From the fourth postoperative day physical therapy is begun by bivalving the brachial part of the plaster which, being opened, allows abduction. The cast must be carefully maintained and corrected daily if necessary. Physical therapy consists of gentle functional movements such as hand to mouth, to head and to neck. Its aim is not to increase muscle power. After the 45th postoperative day, the cast is removed. The patient is then able to put his hand on his head and place his arm in a vertical position. Abduction is maintained thereafter, decreasing regularly over 15 days. A too rapid return to the low vertical posi-

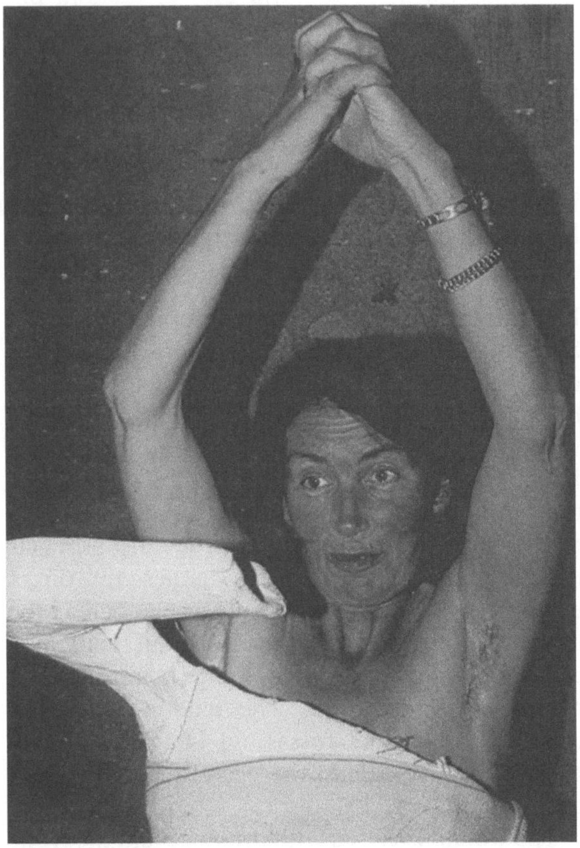

Fig. 1. Postoperative cast and physical therapy

tion might result in an immediate loss of active abduction, which is very hard to regain. When the plaster is finally removed, there is generally a loss of the last few degrees of abduction which is corrected by physical therapy.

The real difficulty during the postoperative period is in gaining abduction between 60° and 90°, which is the preoperative painful arc. Exercise in the supine position and in a swimming pool is of great help.

In cases of residual pain, one to three infiltrations into the painful area with local anaesthetic and steroid might be indicated.

Results

In 100 operations, there was no infection. The results were evaluated according to three criteria: pain, motion, and muscular strength.

Table 1. Pre- and postoperative pain

Grade of pain	Number of patients	
	Preoperative	Postoperative
I	51	1
II	25	4
III	19	45
IV	5	50

Pain

I. Permanent pain by day and night
II. Pain causing marked disability
III. Mild, or inconstant pain resulting in little or no disability
IV. No pain

Table 1 shows that pain was extremely frequent before surgery; 76 patients were graded I or II. Following operation 95 patients were graded III or IV. None of the patients became worse following operation.

Active Motion (Table 2)

We graded elevation of the arm neither in the strict plane of abduction nor in the plane of flexion, but in the plane of the scapula with abduction of the arm in 30° to 40° of flexion. We measured the global abduction which combines movement in the scapulothoracic and the scapulohumeral articulations. Among the 10 patients with abduction reaching 90° to 120°, there was an improvement compared to the preoperative motion. In 55 patients external rotation was decreased compared to the other side. But this loss did not result in disability except in 3 patients who had an external rotation less than 10°.

Table 2. Pre- and postoperative motion

Degree of mobility	Number of patients	
	Preoperative	Postoperative
0-60	61	4
60-90	24	5
90-120	6	10
120-180	5	26
180	4	55

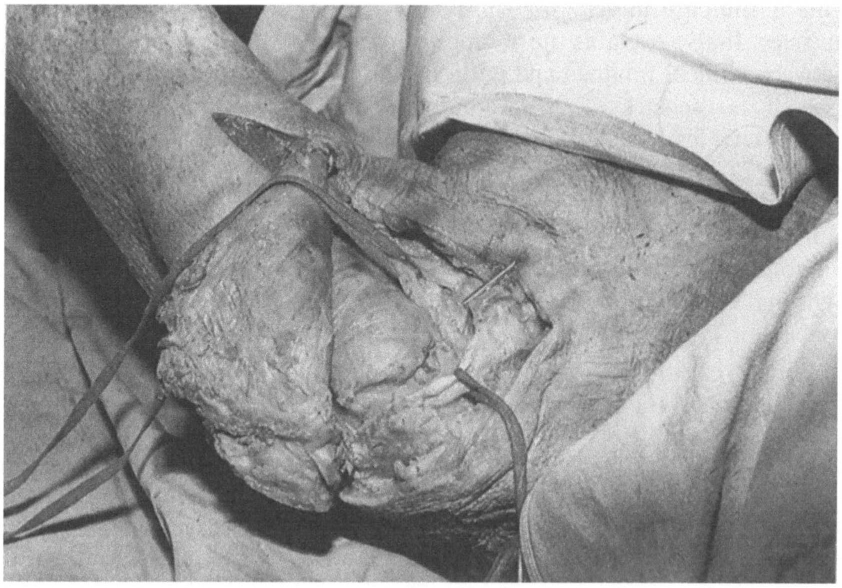

Fig. 2. Cadaveric view of the biceps tendon and the coracoacromial arch in the functional position (abduction, flexion, internal rotation)

Muscle Power

In view of the deliberate sacrifice of the rotator cuff or at least the supraspinatus, we looked for a decrease of muscular power in abduction and external rotation compared to the other side. Of 100 patients, 18 had significant decrease of strength, and 40 had a moderate decrease. However, there was no relation between this decrease of strength and the existence of a lesion of infraspinatus or teres minor. The decrease of power caused only moderate functional disability. Almost all of the 100 patients noted early tiring on repeated effort in the flexed position as well as difficulty in maintaining this position. This is of particular importance in some occupations such as painters. The final result is reached after 3 to 9 months following operation. The average delay before resuming work is 15 weeks.

Overall Results

Fifty-seven patients had normal painless function of the affected shoulder (grade IV), and 180° of elevation; some of the patients complained of early tiredness when working in flexion; 24 patients had mild pain and elevation between 120° and 180°, which is a good result (grade III); 19 patients had a poor result, occasionally due to pain graded I or II, more often because of elevation less than 120°. As judged subjectively by the patients' own evaluation of the operation, 3 were not satisfied.

Discussion

In contrast to anatomical descriptions, in the functional position the shoulder is internally rotated and flexed, bringing the supraspinatus muscle directly under the coracoacromial ligament. In this position the space between the acromial process and the rotator cuff is wide, and the biceps tendon is located under the fibrous arch, behind the tip of the coracoid process where the coracoacromial ligament and the coracobrachialis exchange some fibres.

The muscles of the rotator cuff are tensors of the superior part of the capsule, and the supraspinatus tendon merges with the capsule. The muscles of the rotator cuff stabilise the head and prevent it from ascending during abduction and flexion. It is an important zone of compression, protected by the subacromial ligament where the constant strain on the rotator cuff might result in conflict. For this reason we support a mechanical theory of cuff lesions without, of course, denying a role to degeneration due to disease.

If a tear of the rotator cuff occurs in this critical zone without resulting impingement between the edges of the tear or the biceps and the coracoacromial ligament, painless abduction is possible.

This is the case in very lax shoulders with weak muscles. It also explains the absence of parallelism between clinical findings and pathological lesions, as well as the lack of symptomatology in most rotator cuff lesions. Although one can say that the muscles of the rotator cuff play a role in elevation of the arm, one can also say that they are not indispensible.

From these anatomical and physiological formulations we can draw the following therapeutic conclusions:

Repair of the edges of a tear by suture is difficult and the results are inconstant when the tendon is diseased.

The logical procedure is to correct the elements of the impingement consisting of the coraco-acromial ligament and the edges of the torn cuff.

The shoulder can regain normal active motion by excision which results in a superior fibrous scar. This scar must fit so that movements occur without creating conflict. For this reason it is necessary to maintain abduction for 45 days in order to obtain a smooth sliding scar, and the return to the neutral position must be slow to allow adaptation. We have had an opportunity to substantiate these findings in a patient who required surgical revision when he fell and damaged his shoulder four years after a successful operation.

The role of the biceps tendon must be emphasised; it is partly responsible for pain, and it was found diseased in most of our cases. Its excision and distal reinsertion were a routine part of the operation.

Conclusions

Most rotator cuff tears are well tolerated, and operation is only indicated after failure of other forms of treatment for a period of six months. Very often the symptoms disappear with physical and anti-inflammatory treatment.

We found arthrography of the shoulder to be of no use in the diagnosis of impingement syndromes.

The aim ot the operation is to suppress the mechanical process, which is why it is better to wait for the inflammatory aspects to resolve. It should be noticed that the pain is not always relieved immediately after operation. If excision of inflammatory tissues, especially a diseased subacromial bursa, has been performed, the natural resolution of the inflammatory process, helped if necessary by steroid infiltrations, will give good results. The postoperative management, though very exhausting, is absolutely necessary, and one has to be certain of full co-operation by the patient. Several failures are due to poor physical therapy. Those patients who have been warned in advance of the difficulties in maintaining a flexed position, are generally satisfied. The lack of stability of the head in the glenoid due to the absence of the musculotendinous cuff and the biceps tendon is responsible for this disability, and many patients had to change their occupation.

No parallel between the pathology and the clinical signs, neither pre- nor postoperatively, could be established. It seems, however, that the best results are obtained in anterosuperior tears.

Although good results can be claimed, there were some failures, especially in flexion, due to lesions of infraspinatus, teres minor and subscapularis.

To summarise, the indication for surgical repair of a rotator cuff rupture is very rare except for typically traumatic lesions in young active patients.

I.5. Acromioplasty in the Treatment of Rotator Cuff Impingement: A Preliminary Report

Jan Thorling and Lennart Hovelius

The painful arc syndrome of the shoulder is a clinical entity with night pain and painful abduction and elevation of the arm. The pathogenesis is diverse but impingement of the structures in the subacromial space against the coracoacromial arch has been emphasised as one important cause during recent years [12,13,17]. In about 10%-20% of the patients the symptoms become refractory to conservative treatment (rest from heavy work, physiotherapy, local injections of steroids) and surgical treatment has to be considered [13]. Our results of acromionectomy, lateral as well as total, have often been more or less disappointing. There has, therefore, in our Departments for many years, been considerable hesitation to operate on patients with a painful arc syndrome. The purpose of this paper is to give a preliminary report of the results obtained after acromioplasty [17] and simple excision of the coracoacromial ligament [20] in patients with chronic disability of the shoulder recognised as rotator cuff impingement.

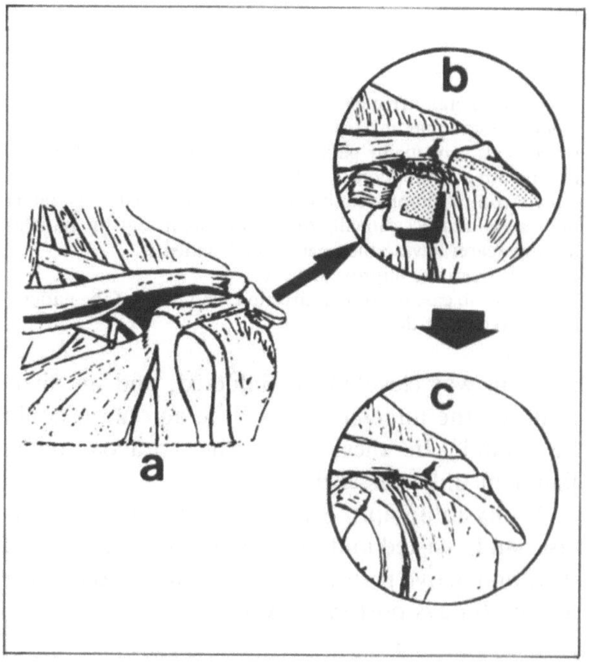

Fig. 1. a The anatomy of the coracoacromial arch **b** The anterior process and lateral portion of the undersurface of the acromion have been osteotomised. **c** The ligament has been cut across at the coracoid process and removed with its bony attachment at the acromion

Patients and Methods

To judge the value of surgical treatment a small amount of local anaesthetic infiltrated in the subacromial space should give temporary alleviation of the symptoms – especially pain. Since 1977, 20 patients have been operated on. The duration of symptoms averaged 46 months, with a range from 12 months to 10 years. All had previous conservative treatment. Radiological examination including arthrography was performed preoperatively. Total rupture of the rotator cuff was diagnosed in two patients, but in all the others no pathological changes of the shoulder girdle were detected.

The subacromial space was exposed through a curved incision from the coracoid process to the lateral margin of the acromion. Beginning at the acromioclavicular joint deltoid was split in the direction of its fibres about 5 cm distally and detached from the anterior edge of the acromion and the acromioclavicular joint capsule.

In 14 patients anterior acromioplasty according to Neer [17] was performed. In this procedure the anterior edge of the acromion and the lateral portion of its undersurface was removed with an osteotome giving a wedge-shaped piece of bone including the entire attachment of the coracoacromial ligament. The ligament was then cut across the coracoid process (Fig. 1).

In 6 patients there was evidence of impingement against the coracoacromial ligament only when

Table 1. Results at follow-up for 14 patients operated upon by acromioplasty and 6 patients by excision of the coracoacromial ligament alone.

	Acromioplasty		Excision of the coracoacromial ligament	
	No.	%	No.	%
Excellent	7	64	3	67
Good	2		1	
Fair	5	36	2	33
Poor	–		–	
Total	14		6	

Excellent. Totally free of symptoms: 10 patients
Good. Occasional mild pain but no limitation of shoulder movement; no night pain and the patient was back to preoperative occupation: 3 patients
Fair. Definitely improved, but some pain persisted on shoulder movement and occasionally during the night, but the patients did not regret having the operation: 7 patients
Poor. No definite improvement: 0
There was no case of wound infection, and none of the patients had weakness of deltoid

the arm was elevated or abducted, and no alteration of the undersurface of the acromion could be found. In these cases the coracoacromial ligament only was excised.

A physiotherapist encouraged pendulum exercises and assisted motion from the second or third day, and active forward elevation was avoided for about 10 days postoperatively.

Results

The operative findings in the 20 patients were:

total rupture of the rotator cuff in 2 patients

partial rupture in 7 patients;

tendinitis or chronic subacromial bursitis in 11 patients.

The patients have been followed-up for an average period of 15 months after operation with a range of 6 to 42 months. The period of follow-up for the "excellent" and "good" groups averaged 18 ± 8.5 months (range 6-42 months); and for the "fair" group, 11 ± 4.6 months (range 6-12 months). At the follow-up the result of the operation was assigned to one of four groups.

Discussion

There was no difference in the results obtained in the 14 patients following anterior acromionectomy and the 6 patients following simple excision of the coracoacromial ligament, with about 65% "excellent" or "good" and 35% "fair" results. However, when studying these patients it is our impression that improvement was more rapid in those who had undergone acromioplasty compared to those who had an excision of the coracoacromial ligament alone. We therefore now recommend acromioplasty as advocated by Neer for all patients with a chronic painful arc syndrome that can be recognized as being due to rotator cuff impingement. It is also interesting to notice the longer period of follow-up for the patients with "excellent" or "good" results in comparison with the patients with "fair" results, which suggests that it probably takes some time to get full recovery from the underlying disorder which causes rotator cuff impingement.

I.6. Re-alignment of the Acromion in the Treatment of Chronic Rotator Cuff Ruptures

P. Grammont and G. Lelaurin

In order to ease the passage of the greater tuberosity under the acromion during abduction, we have devised an operation for combined translocation, rotation and elevation of the acromion (TRE).

Clinically a large number of painful and inefficient shoulders are due to progressive wear and inflammation of the rotator cuff, of the acromion and the acromioclavicular joint. The incidence of these chronic disorders in clinical practice has its correspondence in cadaveric shoulders. We have observed a significant lesion in more than half of the subjects over 50 years old, and we believe that these syndromes have a mechanical origin which causes loss of freedom of functional elements of the shoulder.

We can distinguish (i) glenohumeral movement between the head of the humerus and the corresponding glenoid cavity, which is characterised by a centre of rotation as fixed as possible and where the ligaments are predominant; and (ii) shoulder girdle movement generally between the acromioclavicular arch and deltoid above and the whole upper end of humerus below. This movement is mechanically characterised by a moment of force due to muscular action, which depends on the synergistic coupling actions of deltoid and rotator cuff muscle groups. In this analysis we have set aside the question of scapulothoracic movement.

If the shoulder is not stable at the glenohumeral joint at the commencement of abduction, the vertical component of deltoid will cause an upward subluxation of the humeral head and increase friction between the acromion and underlying tuberosity. The rotator cuff and long head of biceps reinforce the shoulder ligaments to maintain a stable centre of rotation. In so doing they prevent the ascending movement of the head of the humerus and protect themselves against wear.

In the act of lifting, deltoid acts in such a way that acromial-tuberosity friction is unavoidable and therefore leads to cuff degradation.

Methods

We have developed a technique of acromial displacement in three spatial planes in order to re-establish the equilibrium between glenohumeral and subacromial movements. The technique was developed on the lines of the following hypothesis:

Elevation of the acromion creates a passage for the supraspinatus muscle, depresses the greater tuberosity which impinges at 60° of abduction, increases the distance between the centre of shoulder and the acromial head of deltoid, and increases the mechanical independence of these two elements of shoulder movement.

Lateral transfer of the acromion modifies the action of deltoid at the commencement of abduction. The undesirable elevating force of deltoid is diminished and the pure abduction force is favoured. This is confirmed by Strasser's pulley model where an increase in either arm of deltoid at the beginning of abduction requires a decrease of the applied force to obtain the same degree of movement.

Rotation around the coracoclavicular ligaments of the acromioclavicular arch has the following effects:

It decreases the distance between the acromion and the coracoid process and therefore unloads and elevates the coracoacromial ligament. This important ligament is a cause of tuberosity impingement and operative displacement makes it unnecessary to divide the ligament.

The second effect is a forward displacement of the anterior part of deltoid which increases its mechanical power.

The third effect is to transfer the posterior part of deltoid from an adductor to an abductor position which increases the abductor muscle power.

Since anterior rotation of the acromion corresponds to posterior rotation of the glenoid, a relative retroversion is created which provides a more stable position of the humeral head during active movement.

Clinical Experience

Indications for operation

The patient has a painful shoulder; he cannot sleep on it; he has restricted movement so that he can neither comb his hair, shave himself, nor take a book off the shelf. This is particularly important if the predominant arm is involved. There is weakness in the shoulder, particularly when it is loaded during movement. There may be pain arising from the tendon of long head of biceps which limits such action as carrying an object with the arm to the side of the body. This type of shoulder frequently is the site of recurrent small haemorrhage, mainly in elderly patients. During operations we have noted synovial haemorrhagic tears due to acromioclavicular erosion.

Clinical examination of such a shoulder often reveals almost normal passive mobility and little pain. Crepitus is noted at about 45°-60° of abduction, corresponding to acromial impingement.

It is important to exclude a disorder arising from the cervical spine or other forms of neuropathy.

Radiographic examination provides important evidence: there is loss of parallelism between glenoid and humeral head, and the humeral head is often subluxated backwards with consequent impingement under the acromion. Such impingement is amplified by isometric abduction effort. In our practice, two radiological views are taken: the first is the standard anteroposterior view angled slightly downwards, the second is a scapular profile, called the "tangential view" by McLaughlin. Both views show loss of space between humeral head and acromion.

Although we performed arthrography in many cases, we do not use it as a routine, because the clinical signs are more dependable in judging the degree of contact between humeral head and acromion than are any attempt to measure the dimensions of a rotator cuff tear. Often arthrography has previously been performed elsewhere and reveals a large tear.

Surgical Technique

The patient is placed in the lateral position, the leg underneath being extended and the leg above flexed. The head of the table is raised and supports are placed under knee and foot to avoid slip. Further supports are necessary fore and aft on the patient's body. This provides a 45° head-up tilt with lateral inclination. The blood pressure must be monitored; it is found to be more stable when using venous compression elastic stockings.

A posterior skin incision is performed along the lateral two-thirds of the spine of the scapula. Trapezius and deltoid attachments are split in continuity with the periosteum of spine and proximal acromion. This bone is exposed subperiostally and care is taken to preserve the integrity of the suprascapular nerve. This part of the spine of the scapula looks like a strong vertical shaft, large enough to receive a 3.5 to 4.5 mm screw.

The spine is then divided with a saw in the plane of the inferior face of the acromion; it requires some experience to define this plane, and it is helpful to remember that the saw has to be parallel to the upper triangular facet of the acromion which is located between the posterolateral angle and the pillar of the spine of the scapula.

After section of the bone the distal part of the acromion is mobilised upwards to display the underlying supraspinatus and any tear of the rotator cuff; the acromion is mobilised and sometimes the posterior aspect of the acromioclavicular joint requires to be freed in order to permit displacement of the acromion by translocation, rotation and elevation. This manoeuvre provides excellent separation between the acromion and clavicle and removes any impingement. Some 15-20 mm of displacement of the acromion and spine is readily obtained.

The osteotomy is fixed in the new position by a vertical compression screw and circumferential steel wire. If this is judged to be inadequate a bone plate is used. Occasionally, the displacement is so marked that a bone graft should be inserted at the osteotomy. Trapezius and deltoid are re-attached after suction drainage has been instituted. A second subcutaneous drain is used. At the end of the operation the arm is placed in a light abduction brace for 45 days which permits daily passive outward rotation of the arm and isometric contraction of the deltoid. Active mobilisation is then initiated, especially in abduction and outward rotation to the arm.

Results

All 16 patients were reviewed from one to three years following operation. There was diminution of pain in every case; after the second year most of them were quite painless, especially during the night; 4 patients had intermittent pain on occasions only.

The passive range of motion was fully maintained but took as long as one year to achieve. On occasions we found it necessary at the third month following operation to mobilise the shoulder under analgesia. The active range of movements was better in every case than the preoperative range. Half the patients recovered full movements by the end of two years.

Loss of power remains an unsolved problem; all patients were unable to do long and hard work following operation.

Complications

In two women whose acromions were frail, a pseudarthrosis developed, and a second operation was required with bone grafting in order to achieve fusion. Generally in women and small persons the frailty of the bone is such that the osteotomy should be plated.

Discussion

Best results were obtained in men aged 50 years who had suffered a chronic rupture of the rotator cuff giving rise to pain. The best results were in those patients who had had pain for very many years and had exhausted all medical, physical and other forms of conservative therapy. Better active movements were observed in those patients in whom the cuff had not been fully exposed during operation and when no attempt had been made at any repair. This procedure is not planned to treat the lesion itself but rather the painful effects of it.

References

1 Armstrong JR (1949) Excision of the acromion in treatment of the supraspinatus syndrome. J Bone Jt Surg 31-B: 436

2 Bateman JE (1972) The shoulder and neck. Philadelphia/London/Toronto. W Saunders

3 Brewer BJ (1979) Ageing of the rotator cuff. Orth Transactions Vol.3, No.1

4 Codman EA (1934) The shoulder. Thomas Todd Co. Boston

5 Depalma AF Surgery of the shoulder. Philadelphia/Toronto, Lippincott 1973

6 Eulert J, Gekeler J (1976) Le ligament acromio-coracoidien et ses rapports avec le tendon du muscle susépineux. Rev Chir Orthop 62: 60

7 Gschwend N (1968) Die operative Behandlung der progressiv chronischen Polyarthritis. Stuttgart, Thieme

8 Hammond G (1962) Complete acromionectomy in the treatment of chronic tendinitis of the shoulder. J Bone Jt Surg 44-A: 494

9 Hawkins R, Kennedy JC (1980) Impingement syndrome in athletes. Am J Sports Med 8, No 3: 151-158

10 Ippolito E, Natali PG, Postacchini F, Accinni L, DeMartino C (1980) Morphological, immunochemical and biochemical study of rabbit achilles tendon at various ages. J Bone Jt Surg 62-A: No 4, 583-598

11 Kennedy JC, Willis RB (1976) The effects of local steroid injections on tendons: A biomechanical and microscopic correlative study. Am J Sports Med 4: 11-21

12 Kessel L, Watson M (1977) The painful arc syndrome. Clinical classification as a guide to management. J Bone Jt Surg 59-B: 166

13 Laumann U (1980) The so-called "periarthritis humero-scapularis" — possibilities of an operative treatment. Arch Orthop Traumat Surg 97: 27-37

14 Laumann U, Hertel E (1978) Biomechanische Probleme bei der Acromion-Plastik am Schultergelenk. Arch Orthop Traumat Surg 93: 49

15 Lindblom K (1939) On pathogenesis of ruptures of the tendon aponeurosis of the shoulder joint. Acta Radiologica 20: 563

16 Moseley HF, Goldie I (1963) The arterial pattern of the rotator cuff of the shoulder. J Bone Jt Surg 48-B: 780

17 Neer CS (1972). Anterior acromioplasty for the chronic impingement syndrome in the shoulder. J Bone Jt Surg 54-A: 41

18 Neer CS (1976) Anterior acromioplasty for the chronic impingement syndrome in the shoulder — a preliminary report. J Bone Jt Surg 54A: *1* 41-50

19 Neer CS (1979) Instructional Course Lectures. American Academy of Orthopaedic Surgeons

20 Pujudas (1970) ?????????

21 Rathbun JB, Macnab I (1970) The microvascular pattern of the rotator cuff. J Bone Jt Surg 52-B: 540-553

22 Rothman RH, Parke WW (1965) The vascular anatomy of the rotator cuff. Clin Orth 41: 176

23 Samilson RL, Binder WF (1975) Symptomatic full thickness tears of the rotator cuff — an analysis of 292 shoulders in 276 patients. Orth Clin of NA Vol 6 2: 449-466

20 Samilson RL, Raphael RL, Post L, Noonan C, Siris E, Raney FL (1961) Arthrography of the shoulder joint. Clin Orth 20: 21-32

25 Samilson RL, Raphael RL, Post L, Noonan C, Siris E, Raney FL (1961) Shoulder arthrography. JAMA 175: 773-778

26 Smith-Petersen MN, Aufranc OE, Larson CB (1943) Useful surgical procedures for rheumatoid arthritis involving joints of the upper extremity. Arch Surg 46: 764
27 Stamm TT, Crabbe WA (1972) Paraglenoid osteotomy of the scapula. Clin Orthop 88: 39
28 Weigert M (1976) Acromionplastik – Technik und Ergebnisse. Orthop Praxis 12: 898

Section II. Rotator Cuff Rupture

Moderator—Dr. James E. Bateman

II.1. The Correlation of Clinical Evaluation with Operative Findings and Prognosis in Rotator Cuff Rupture

Bo J. Lundberg

The significance of degenerative changes due to ageing in the aetiology of ruptures of the rotator cuff tendon is generally accepted [11, 38, 55]. The average age of these patients is therefore high; after the age of 60 ruptures even occur spontaneously. Fortunately, in most cases adaptive mechanisms allow the defective tendon apparatus to function with only slight or temporary discomfort. About one out of ten patients may require operation on account of persisting functional disturbance and pain [19, 4]. The difficulty is in predicting the cases which need to be repaired. Early intervention should give better results when severe symptoms are present [29]; however, expectant treatment for 1-6 months is accepted [15]. Arthrography reveals only the presence but seldom the size of a tear, which could be of value as regards selection for surgery and planning the operation.

The present study of the relation between clinical evaluation and operative findings throws new light on these matters. Correlation with the results of surgery also gives an idea of what the patient and doctor may expect of the treatment.

Material

In a series of 67 operatively verified cases in 52 men and 14 women, average age 57 and 58 years, 26 showed a rupture of the rotator cuff greater than 3 cm in width; 30 a medium-sized complete tear within the range of 1-3 cm; 11 were classified as small, less than 1 cm at the greatest width, 2 of which were incomplete. They all suffered from pain preoperatively. 24 were unable to raise the arm, 25 showed reduced strength but 18 had intact function in this respect (see Table II.1). The average preoperative disability was 6 months, ranging between 1 month and 2 years. The majority, 53 cases, were related to trauma, 8 of which were minor injuries. The remaining 14 (2 large, 7 medium-sized, and 5 small tears) had no such incident. Of the 45 following severe trauma, 10 were caused by dislocation of the shoulder. The diagnosis was confirmed by arthrography in 55 out of 59 cases. Four negative and 3 with doubtful radiographs showed concealed tears at operation [5].

A conventional surgical method was practised according to the principles of McLaughlin [38], Neer [45], and Wolfgang [66]. A wider exposure of the operative field was achieved by dividing the outer portion of the acromion in 30 cases. The biceps tendon was resected in 17 cases because of degenerative changes associated with large ruptures of the cuff in 12, with medium ruptures in 4, and with a small rupture in 1 case. The distal portion of the biceps tendon was fixed into the bicipital groove. In only 1 case was the intra-articular portion used to cover the cuff defect. Complete restoration by suture was possible in all small and medium ruptures, except one. In the majority of

Table 1. The relationship between clinical evaluation and the size of rupture

Size of rupture	Preoperative function			Total
	Unreduced	Reduced	Highly reduced	
Small	7	3	1	11
Medium	11	13	6	30
Large	0	9	17	26
Total	18	25	24	67

the large ruptures complete closure could not be achieved; in 4 cases defects wider than 1 cm had to be left open. In 10, however, restoration to normal by tight suture was possible.

The arm was immobilised in abduction for six weeks, gradually reduced after three weeks when active exercises were commenced. The results were evaluated when no further improvement could be expected, on average six months after operation. At that time follow-up arthrography was performed in 21 cases. The cases were rated as follows:

Good: No complaints; capable of doing their previous work, with extent and power of elevation normal or insignificantly reduced.

Fair: Subjectively and objectively improved; at least capable of active elevation with a straight arm.

Poor: Unimproved or not capable of full elevation with a straight arm.

Results

On the basis of the above criteria the results of treatment were available in 66 cases, of which 34 rated "good", 23 "fair" and 9 "poor".

The main symptom of the smaller ruptures (i.e. pain) was alleviated successfully, but the lifting power remained reduced in the same proportion as preoperatively (Table 1 and 2). The 30 medium-sized ruptures improved greatly following operation, and twice as many were able to elevate with full strength. The large ruptures also derived benefit from the operation. Two-thirds of the cases with highly reduced function improved after operation. On the whole, operational repairs considerably reduced the number of cases with significantly poor function (24 of 67 preoperatively as against 9 of 66 postoperatively – Table 3). Statistical calculation showed highly reduced function to be significantly more common with large ruptures ($P<0.01$) Table 1. (The method of Chi-square with Yates correction was used throughout.) The size of rupture and results of operation were significant only to the level of $0.2>P>0.1$, i.e. larger ruptures have a tendency to less successful results, but this is not statistically significant. An analysis between pre- and postoperative function showed probability but not significance ($0.05<P<0.1$) that cases with highly reduced function had less good prospects of surgery.

Table 2. The relationship between size of rupture and results

Size of rupture	Postoperative results			Total
	Good	Fair	Poor	
Small	8	3	0	11
Medium	21	6	3	30
Large	5	14	6	25
Total	34	23	9	66

Table 3. The relationship between clinical evaluation and results

Preoperative function	Postoperative results			Total
	Good	Fair	Poor	
Unreduced	15	3	0	18
Reduced	11	11	3	25
Highly reduced	8	9	6	23
Total	34	23	9	66

A frequent but passing complication in 20 cases was reduced passive mobility, but in 7 cases this was present before operation. One case, complicated by infection, improved after revision. Following the repair of a large rupture one case of "shoulder-hand" syndrome developed.

Of the 21 arthrographies at follow-up, 2 large, 8 medium, 4 small ruptures had normal radiological anatomy. Seven showed persisting leakage through the repaired cuff, 4 large and 3 medium-sized, in 2 of which small defects had been left at operation. Of these 7 patients, 2 were rated "good", 4 "fair" and 1 "poor" functional results.

In considering the quality of the repair, we found that the majority (12) of the 16 successfully repaired by suture, had normal arthrographs and in 4 the repair had regressed with leakage of the contrast material. Of the 5 patients with incomplete repair, 2 had normal arthrographs at the follow-up examination.

Discussion

Experience of symptomatology, pathology and treatment of 67 patients with ruptured rotator cuff has enabled a more critical appraisal of the indications and timing of operation. Since the recognition of the lesion by Codman in 1934 [10], the work of McLoughlin [39, 41], DePalma [19], Rowe [60], Neviaser [46] and Debeyre [15] amongst others, has evolved the principles of today. After his further experience Codman reviewed his classical series of 100 consecutive early cuff repairs and stated certain requisites for successful results, and drew attention to the cogent contra-indications to early operation in the majority of cuff ruptures, mainly for the reasons mentioned in this introduction.

Comparative random studies to establish the significance of Codman's views are desirable, but have not been carried out. There does, however, seem to be great unanimity that early repair is mandatory when a large rupture is suspected in the 50- to 60-year-old patient who has sustained an injury [4, 11, 15, 29, 41, 60]. Our figures (Table 1) suggest that such a rupture can be expected in more than two-thirds of those unable to achieve abduction.

However, those large ruptures in this study who obtained "good" and "fair" results were operated upon after an average time of 5 months, those with "poor" results even earlier, after an average of 4 months. These results do not support the views for early surgery. Wolfgang's study [66] indicated the same. Treatment must of course be tailored to the individual, but generally, delay *seems* to be more helpful rather than damaging. The configuration of the rupture in relation to how reparable it is, is probably of greater importance. In our present series, large tears were recognised as easy to repair in six cases, when the cuff had been disinserted without any substantial loss of tissue. Most of the others were technically difficult to handle due to the lack of tendon tissue. The side-to-side repair combined with the end-to-bone repair was practised, and some tension at the suture was accepted instead of shortening the insertion too much by a proximal siting of the bone trough. Insufficient closure had to be accepted as an unavoidable disadvantage, but as it mimics nature it should function as long as the repaired tendon is able to retain the head of the humerus, thus allowing normal action of the deltoid. Nevertheless, the results of repair of large ruptures were better in the 10 patients with complete closure (3 "good", 7 "fair") compared with the 15 patients with inadequate closure (2 "good", 7 "fair" and 6 "poor").

The transacromial approach was not used, nor was the advancement of the supraspinatus muscle according to Debeyre [15] or grafts for closure [29, 46]. However, with reservation for differences in assessment, compared to the series of McLaughlin and Asherman [39], Wolfgang [66] and Heikel [29], our experience of small and medium-sized ruptures showed similar figures of 80% "good" and "fair" results despite deficiencies in repair. Debeyre's [15] isolated ruptures treated with simple suture are on the same level.

The advantage of Debeyre's method of advancing the supraspinatus muscle, however, becomes obvious when comparing the outcome of our 25 large ruptures and his 11. Not only was he able to complete suture in all of them, but half of his cases also showed very satisfactory results compared to 1 out of 5 in our series. Even if the difference between the unimproved 6 of 25 and 1 of 11 respectively is not significant, and even if Wolfgang [66] was so successful in using the conventional method practised here that he obtained as good results in the large tears as in the smaller ones, Debeyre's method [15] seems superior because it overcomes the problem of lack of tendon tissue. Unfortunately the advancement of the supraspinatus does not give the best functional improvement and cases of denervation have been described by Mallet and Patte [36]. Instead of advancement, Mallet, using a modified Debeyre technique, prefers to suture with tension into a bone trough.

Our data indicates less good prospects of surgery in the larger tears. This is close to McLaughlin's opinion [41] that the person disabled by a massive cuff rupture should not usually expect anything more than a reasonably comfortable and useful shoulder following repair. It should be remembered that when operation for one reason or another is not advisable the condition may be tolerable due to the development of compensatory use [60]. The long-term effect of an untreated rupture is not yet known. Operation may well be mostly a measure of symptomatic relief. Postoperative management is also rather frustrating when, as in this series, most cases need an abduction device for at least six weeks to release tension both at the suture line of the tendon and the reinserted deltoid. Despite active exercises a common complication was a secondary "frozen shoulder" [35] which is, however a reversible condition, which is not always the case with the most serious shoulder-hand syndrome following trauma and forced immobilisation which carries great risk of permanent disability.

Considering these negative factors, frequent with large tears, the patient totally disabled after trauma should have time to consider and be fully informed before operative repair is attempted. With restricted passive mobility even longer delay is indicated until full passive movements have been achieved and the residual consequences of the cuff lesion alone can be considered. Arthrography is indicated to confirm the diagnosis.

Arthroscopy should make it possible to determine the size and type of lesion. The proficiency of the surgeon is an important factor in deciding upon operation. The transacromial postero-superior approach gives an excellent view, but a lateral incision also gives good access when combined with resection of the outer border of the acromion and has the twofold benefit of exposure and avoiding impingement and secondary wear.

This study confirms early observations [12, 45, 61, 64] of the association of cuff rupture with lesions of the biceps tendon. A cuff tear may predispose to lesions of the biceps tendon, as suggested by Samilson *et al* [61]

Postoperative arthrography provided interesting information on the results of repair. One-third showed cuff defects, the majority of which had occurred after satisfactory closure, but the results were still acceptable. Furthermore, some kind of secondary healing probably occurs since some incompletely sutured tendons showed no evidence of a leak in the postoperative arthrograph. Arthrography, however, is of limited value because of false negative findings and the inability to reveal concealed, partial, or incomplete tears as well as degenerative, inflammatory or other qualitative changes. The relief of pain generally and the functional improvement of the medium-sized tears provide the best indication for surgical treatment. Too aggressive an attitude is not good strategy; much encouragement over a long period of time is of the greatest value.

Summary

Based on an analysis of the relation between clinical evaluation and operative findings at 67 rotator cuff ruptures, highly impaired function was significantly more common in large ruptures. Good results are generally achieved in small and medium-sized tears. Those who had a later repair did better than the rest, and there was therefore no disadvantage in delay of operation. The results of repair were generally less successful in larger than in small or medium-sized ruptures, but not at a statistically significant level. Cases with pre-operative severely reduced function had less good prospects of surgery, excellent results being achieved in only 1 out of 5 patients.

Postoperative arthrography indicates that most completely sutured tendons remain intact, one fourth had arthrographic recurrence without any obvious clinical deterioration. Two incompletely repaired tendons had normal arthrographs at follow-up.

II.2. The Transacromial Approach for Rotator Cuff Rupture

Lipmann Kessel

Indications

The transacromial approach is the most benign surgical procedure for the full exposure of lesions in the subacromial region. The principal indication is for inspecting and treating ruptures of the rotator cuff:

(i) Fracture with displacement of the greater tuberosity (this is effectively a total disinsertion of the rotator cuff).

(ii) Rotator cuff rupture in which a repair is indicated either for pain or for loss of function.

(iii) Persistent subacromial painful arc syndrome which may be due to a healed attrition rupture of the cuff with secondary bursitis.

Merits of the Approach

Almost every technique for exposing the subacromial region carries with it the risk of some morbidity due to dehiscence of the origin of deltoid. The subacromial approach carries no such risk and therefore considerably extends the scope of operations in this area. It is aesthetically satisfying because it does not alter the contour of the shoulder and leaves a neat posterior scar.

History of the Transacromial Approach

The development of the approach arose from a number of disparate sources. Some 50 years ago Fowler [24] mentioned, but did not describe in detail, a coronal acromion-splitting incision to the torn rotator cuff; Diamond [22] in his elegant monograph *The Obstructing Acromion* showed how the trapezius and deltoid form a continuous sheet by way of the periosteum over the acromion; Debeyre et al. [15] recommended division of the acromion and detachment of the trapezius from the spine of the scapula in their operation to advance the supraspinatus muscle laterally in order to enable a cuff defect to be sutured without tension. Lorden Trickey (personal communication) has for many years used a similar direct approach for the fixation of fractures of the greater tuberosity. In 1954 McFarland and Osborne [42] described how the hip joint could be approached without impairing the integrity of the important lateral musculature by detaching the insertion of gluteus medius in continuity with the origin of vastus lateralis in a single continuous sheet with the underlying periosteum.

If one combines all these surgical and anatomical concepts, one arrives at the present operation [31, 32].

Development of the Transacromial Approach

All previous procedures recommended simple division of the acromion and its subsequent reconstitution with wire or other forms of suture in order to stabilise the orogin of deltoid. In this operation, two thick osteoperiosteal flaps are raised from the superior surface of the acromion before the acromion itself is divided. The ultimate suture of these thick osteoperiosteal flaps is sufficient to stabilise both trapezius and deltoid without formal repair of the acromion, because the pull of the two muscles tends to approximate rather than to distract the suture line.

The subacromial space can conveniently be decompressed either at the beginning of the operation or at the end by filleting out the anterior part of the acromion underneath the osteoperiosteal

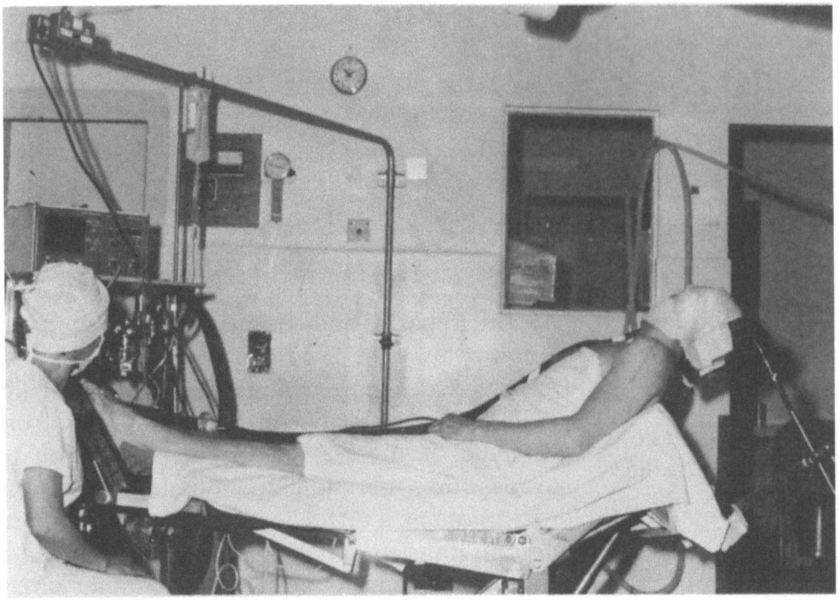

Fig. 1.

flap. That part of the acromion which lies beneath its surgical section and the acromioclavicular joint can be entirely removed.

The Operative Procedure

The patient is placed in a semi-sitting position with a sandbag tucked well under the scapula; a head-rest is used; the whole arm is fully draped (Fig. 1). The shoulder region is thus completely exposed and available, whilst the arm can be moved into any position in the course of the operation. A slight lateral tilt of the table away from the side of operation facilitates the ease of approach.

The surface-marking of the incision is conveniently defined by pressing an index finger into the supraspinous fossa: on one side the finger palpates the back of the clavicle; on the other it is in contact with the spine of the scapula (Fig. 2).

The skin incision extends 3 cm proximal and 5 cm distal from the acromion process (Figs. 3, 4, and 5). Trapezius and deltoid are split in the line of their fibres up to the acromion. Deep to the trapezius is a constant pad of yellow fat overlying supraspinatus, and beneath the deltoid lies the large subdeltoid bursa. Both these structures conveniently define the depth of the muscles. The axillary nerve hugs the humerus beneath the deltoid, and provided one does not go more than

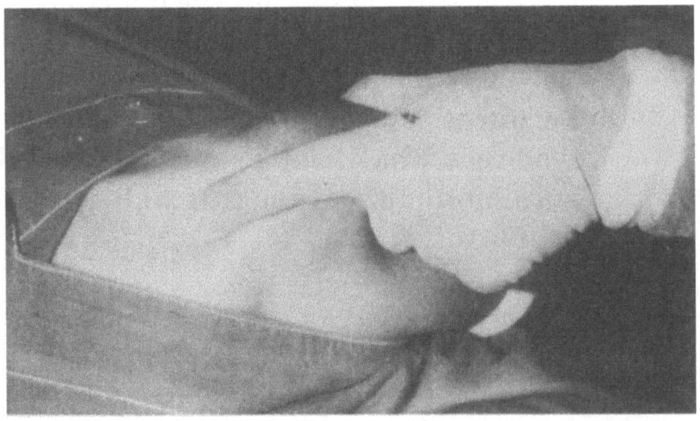

Fig. 2.

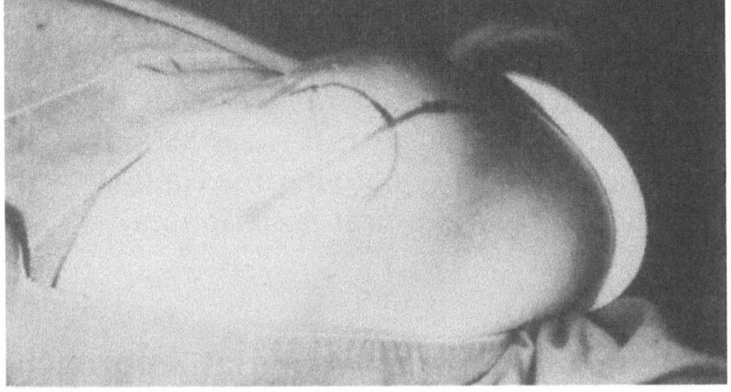

Fig. 3.

5 cm (3 finger-breadths) distal to the lateral edge of the acromion and is careful not to retract downwards with violence, it should not be in any danger. The line of the incision across the acromion is coagulated, and flaps of conjoint aponeurosis, periosteum and bone are raised with an osteotome from the superior surface of the acromion (Figs. 6a, 6b). These flaps are continuous proximally with the insertion of the trapezius and distally with the origin of deltoid. The acromion is divided with an oscillating saw. Retraction of the two halves of the acromion with a self-retaining retractor exposes the subdeltoid bursa. The roof of

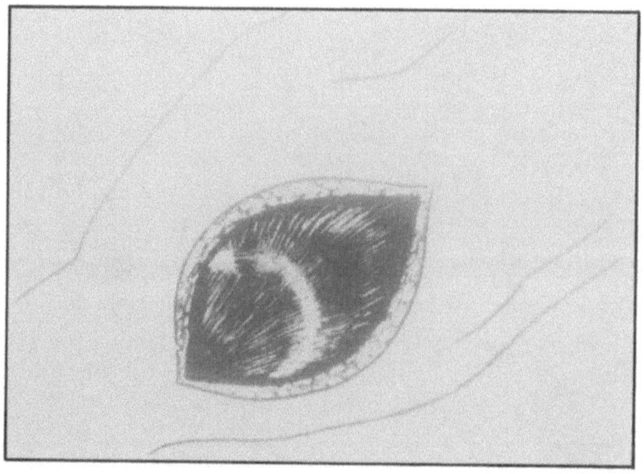

Fig. 4.

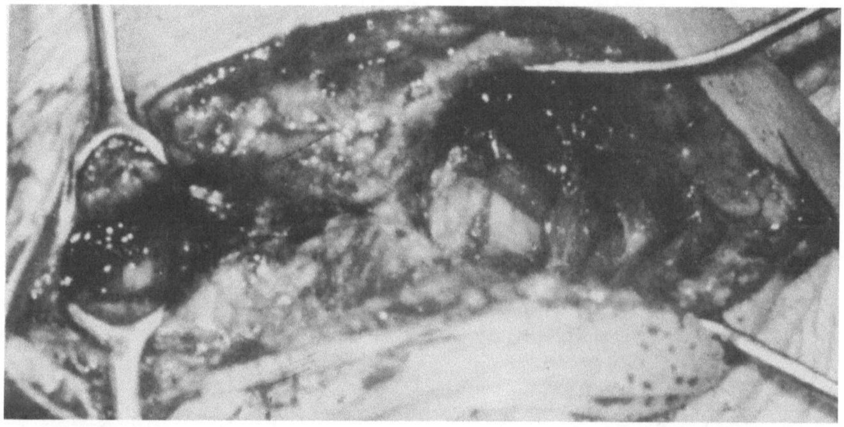

Fig. 5.

a

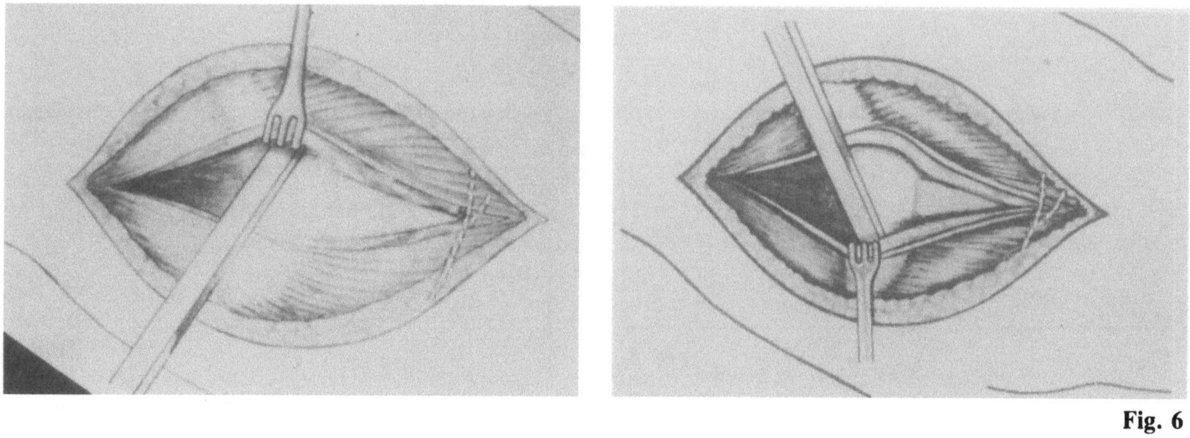

b

Fig. 6

the bursa is formally opened. By medial and lateral rotation of the arm the whole of the insertion of the rotator cuff may then be paraded into view. When the appropriate surgical procedure has been completed, the retractor is released and the fragments of acromion fall together and are held with a towel-clip for simple interrupted suture of the osteo-aponeurotic flap, deltoid and trapezius. Vacuum drainage is employed (Figs. 7-10).

There are two variations in closing the wound which are occasionally useful (Figs. 11 and 12): in order to obtain adequate decompression of the sub-

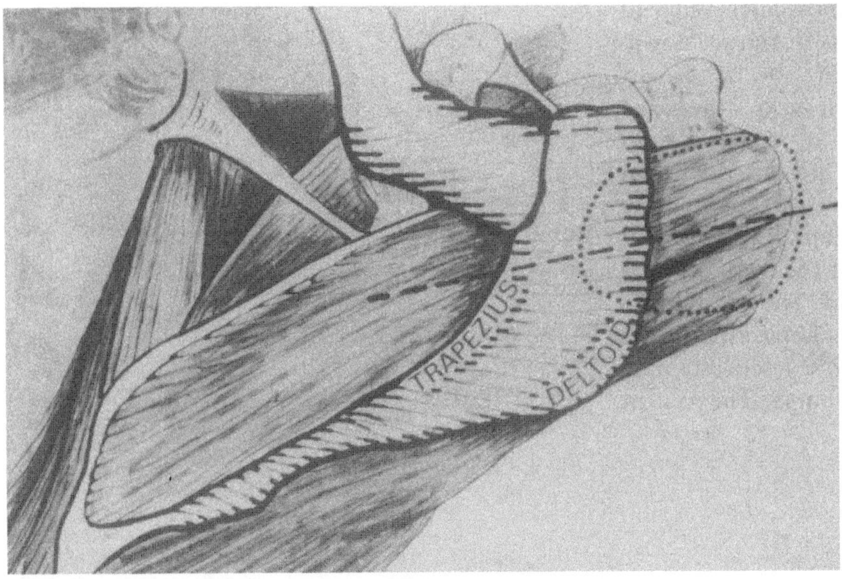

Fig. 7.

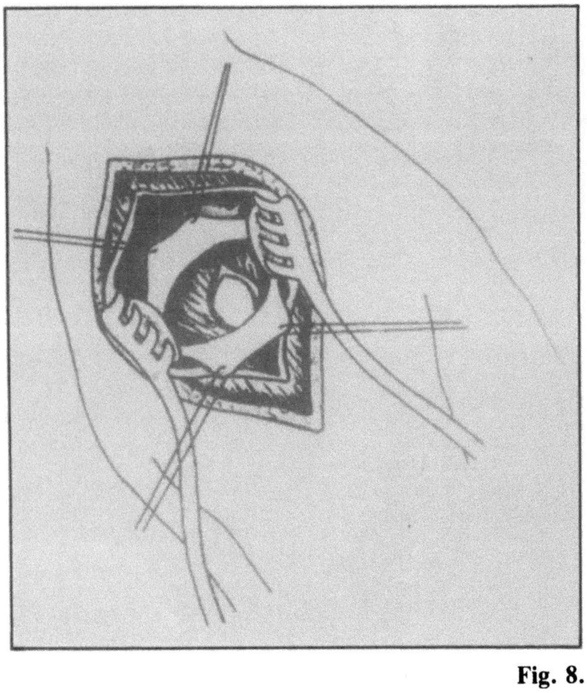

Fig. 8.

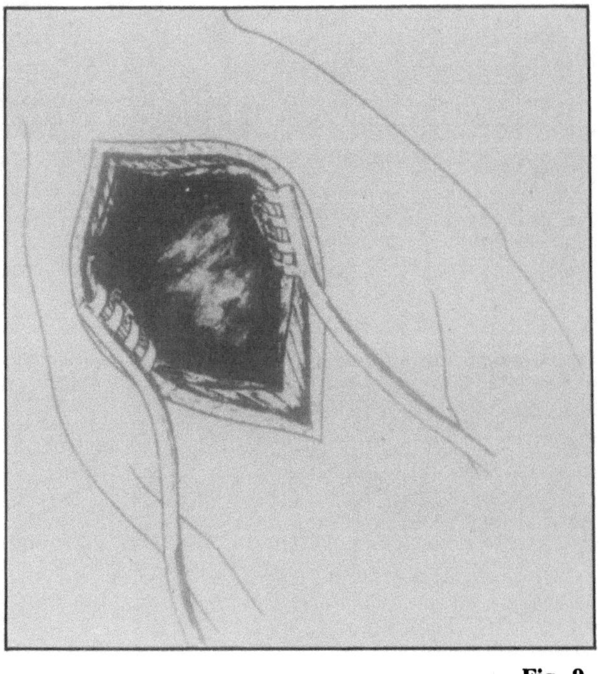

Fig. 9.

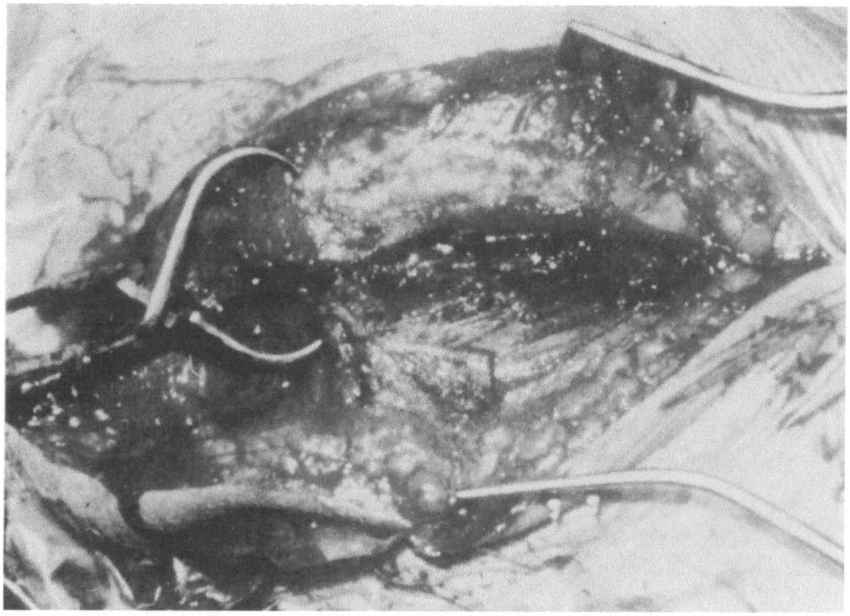

Fig. 10.

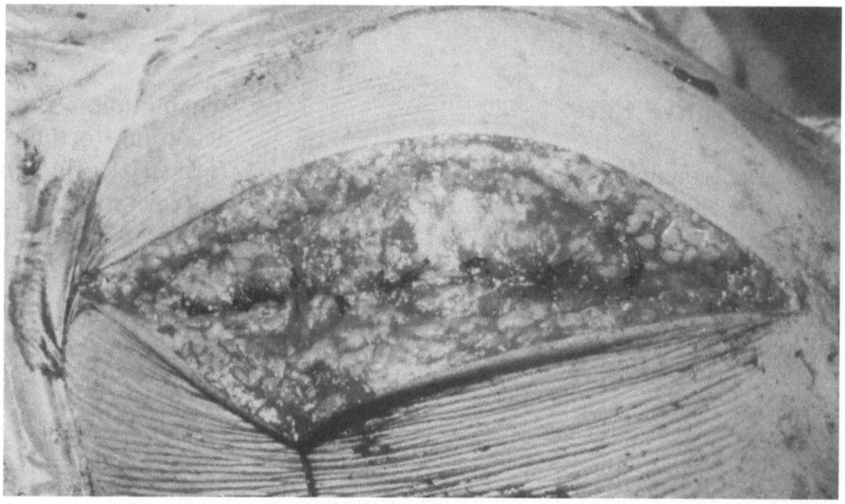

Fig. 11.

acromial space following repair of a rupture of the rotator cuff, it may be considered desirable to allow the split acromion to spring apart and remain un-united by sealing its cut edges with bone wax. Alternatively, the anterior fragment of the acromion may be completely resected: that part of the acromion between the surgical division and the acromioclavicular joint is shelled out subperiosteally, and inevitably carries with it the attachment of the coracoacromial ligament. With or without these minor variations of closure, effective functional and cosmetic repair is obtained by suture of the anterior and posterior aponeurotic flaps in continuity with trapezius and deltoid.

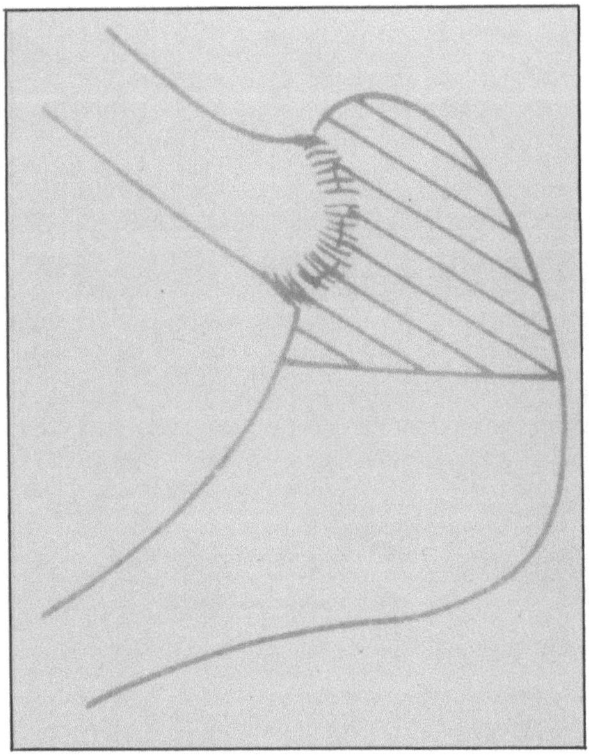

Fig. 12.

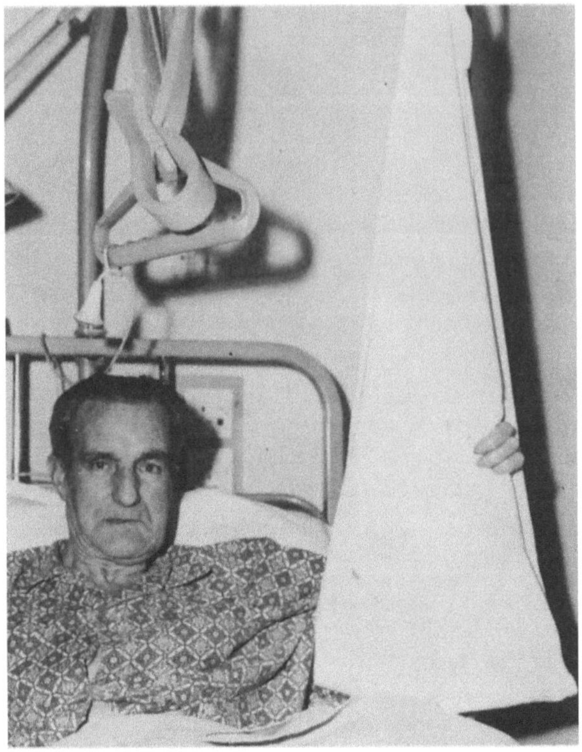

Fig. 13.

Postoperative Care

The arm is maintained in abduction in a simple roller-towel hammock (Fig. 13). Passive mobilisation may be commenced forthwith. Active muscle rehabilitation is delayed for a length of time according to the procedure which has been performed. During the first three weeks following any operation on the subacromial joint it is essential to maintain full passive movements.

II.3. A Method for Reconstruction of the Rotator Cuff After Rupture

Kauko A. Solonen

In ruptures of the rotator cuff of the shoulder the most important component is the supraspinatus tendon. Since the fundamental work of Inman and his co-workers in 1944 [30], we know that this muscle acts simultaneously with the deltoid throughout the entire range of abduction of the shoulder. The supraspinatus is also a forward flexor and outward rotator. Glenohumeral movements are possible, however, without its active contribution, its role being purely quantitative. In the varying positions of the humerus, supraspinatus serves to maintain the fulcrum of the humeral head in the glenoid fossa.

In many cases the inconvenience of rotator cuff injury can be relieved conservatively. Simple surgical procedures are available for the relief of pain. In many cases, however, it is desirable not only to relieve pain and achieve free motion but also to restore the power of glenohumeral abduction and outward rotation. The treatment of a patient with a torn rotator cuff must be individually determined. Repair or reconstruction will be required when the patient has significant disability or pain, if conservative treatment has failed, if the diagnosis of a complete tear has been confirmed, if passive mobility is complete or nearly so, and if the patient is in general able to undergo a major operation as well as the demanding after-treatment. There is no particular age limit.

Several operative methods of repair have been published lately, but the one most widely used is

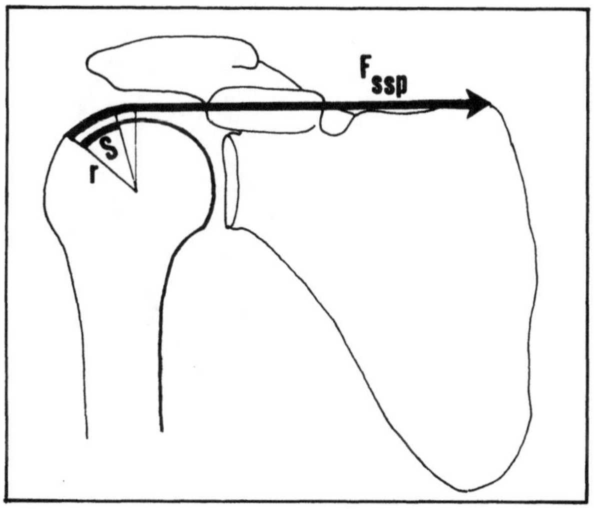

Fig. 1. If the insertion of supraspinatus tendon is transferred proximally by the distance S, the following results can be predicted: the excursion amplitude of the supraspinatus will be reduced by: $S/r \cdot 360°/2\pi$. If r = 25 mm, S = 15 mm, the reduction is 34°, i.e. more than ⅓ of the original supraspinatus amplitude. ($_{ssp}$ = the supraspinatus force)

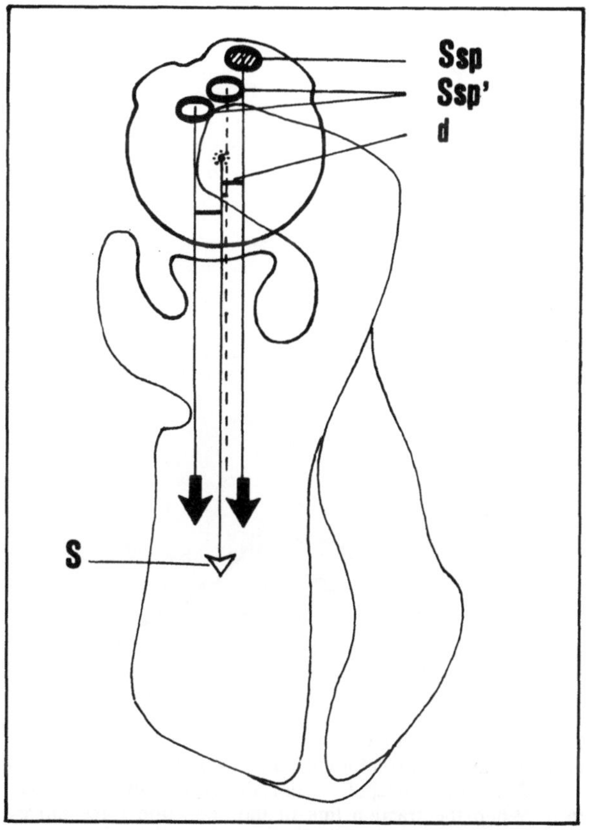

Fig. 2. The effect of displacement of supraspinatus insertion on outward rotation. Ssp' = the original attachment. Ssp = new attachment. Black arrows = the supraspinatus force. If the lever (d) shortens, the outward rotation momentum decreases. If the momentum line lies anterior to the support line (S), the supraspinatus force causes inward rotation

still that of McLaughlin [38], in which the insertion of the supraspinatus tendon has to be moved proximally, so that the effect of the muscle as well as the rhythm of the glenohumeral motion will be altered (Figs. 1 and 2).

A massive tear of the rotator cuff causes upward subluxation of the humeral head. The deformity is roughly analagous to the buttonhole deformity in a finger: the humeral head has lost its stability because of the large defect in its tendinous roof, the pull of the deltoid muscle moves the head upwards and the tension of subscapularis and infraspinatus muscles cause their superior fibres to glide even beyond the "equator" of the humeral head. As a result these muscles come to act more or less as adductors, actively preventing the abduction effect of the deltoid. In these cases it will be impossible to achieve active abduction without reconstruction of the rotator cuff (Fig. 3). The principle underlying the technique to be described is that normal joint function depends on restoration of the anatomy. The laws of mechanics have to be respected as well as those of biology.

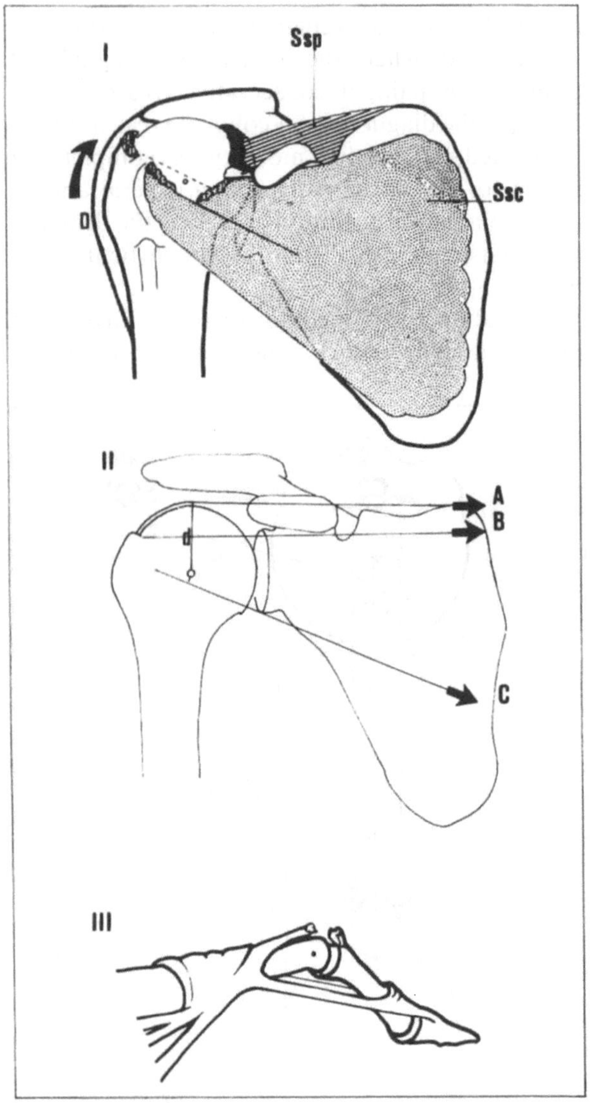

Fig. 3. Upward subluxation of the humeral head after massive tear of the rotator cuff. Ssp = torn supraspinatus, Ssc = partially torn subscapularis, dorsally the infraspinatus is also torn. When the traction line of the abduction force moves closer to the rotational axis (from A to B in Fig.3.II), the momentum decreases because the lever shortens. If the traction line goes below the rotational axis, the abductor is converted into an abductor (C). The deltoid pulls along a line close to the longitudinal axis of the humerus. (Take care not to do acromionectomy!) Compare with a buttonhole deformity of a digit (III)

Method

The approach is started as a short longitudinal or sabre-cut incision (Fig. 4). The rotator cuff is exposed between the deltoid fibres. If there is a large defect, the incision is lengthened along the scapular spine. Deltoid is usually not detached from the margin of the acromion. It is often help-

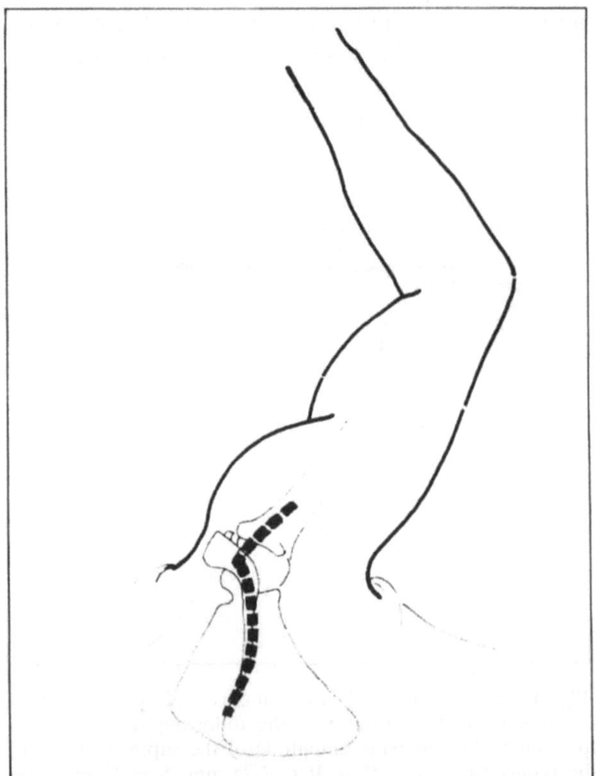

Fig. 4. The routine skin incision

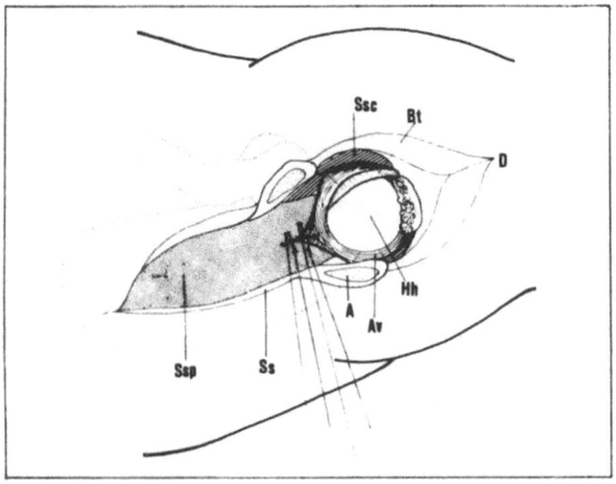

Fig. 5. After excision of the avascular margin (Av), the defect in the rotator cuff may be reduced with a few transverse proximal sutures Ssp = supraspinatus muscle, Ss = spine of scapula, A = base of acromion after severance, Hh = humeral head, D = split deltoid muscle, Bt = biceps tendon, Ssc = subscapularis

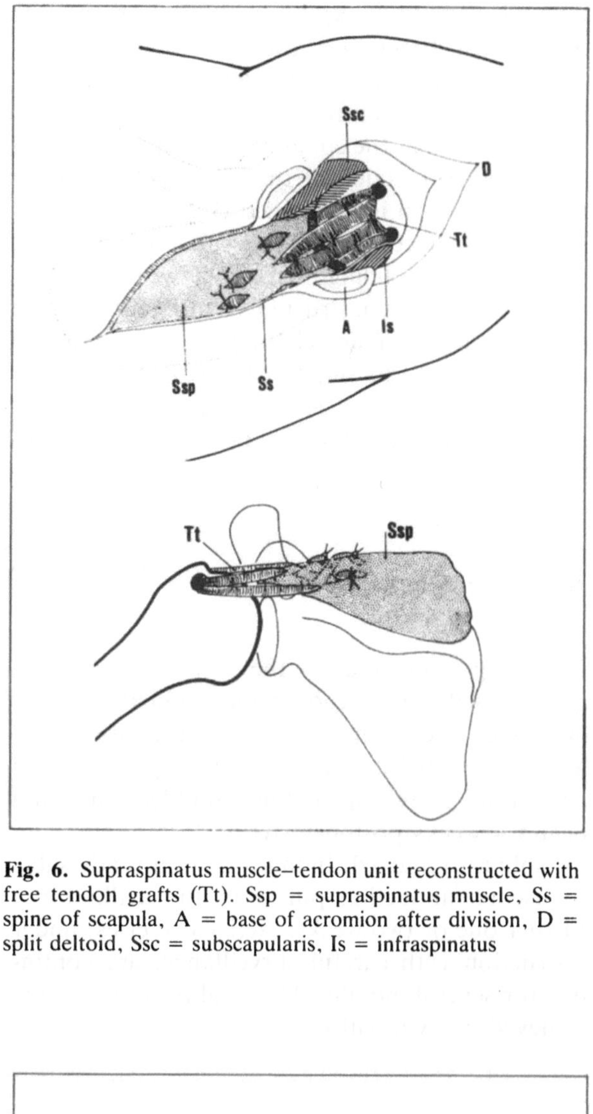

Fig. 6. Supraspinatus muscle–tendon unit reconstructed with free tendon grafts (Tt). Ssp = supraspinatus muscle, Ss = spine of scapula, A = base of acromion after division, D = split deltoid, Ssc = subscapularis, Is = infraspinatus

ful to sever the acromion in line with the scapular spine. Trapezius insertion is elevated subperiosteally from the lateral part of the scapular spine. The subacromial bursa, if not severely inflamed, is dissected free and turned aside, but left. The adhesions are removed, and the degenerated avascular margins of the rent are excised. If anatomical repair is not possible without undue tension, reconstruction is resorted to. The arm is held in abduction. The rupture, usually in the supraspinatus tendon only, may be diminished with a few transverse sutures (Fig. 5). The remaining defect is bridged with free tendon grafts from e.g. plantaris longus, or 2 or 3 long toe extensors (Fig. 6). Fascia lata may be suitable. The transplants are tunnelled through the greater tuberosity, flattened out and sutured under reasonable tension to the pulled-down proximal end of the ruptured muscle and side by side to each other. If the acromion has been left in place, the grafts are carefully brought underneath the process, avoiding the suprascapular nerve and vessels, and fixed into the proximal end of the ruptured muscle-tendon unit. If infraspinatus and subscapularis tendons are ruptured, they are repaired or reconstructed in the same way as the supraspinatus tendon. The reconstruction is completed by side-to-side approximating suture of the new supraspinatus tendon to the subscapularis and infraspinatus tendons. Extensive defects of the rotator cuff may have to be closed with grafts laced through all damaged tendons (Fig. 7). This

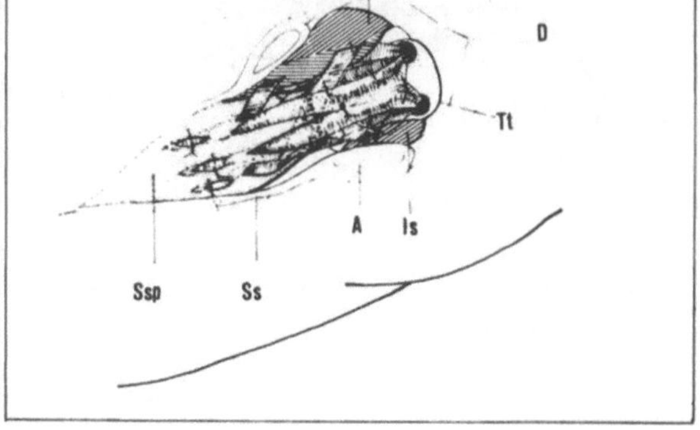

Fig. 7. Large rupture extending to the subscapularis and the infraspinatus tendons closed with grafts laced through all three tendons (See legend of Fig. 6)

method, however, leads to limitation of the independent function of the muscles concerned.

After reconstruction, the detached trapezius is re-attached with sutures passed subperiosteally or through holes in the spine of the scapula. If need be, a wedge resection of the inferolateral margin of the acromion is performed (Fig. 8). Acromionectomy is never done. The subacromial bursa may be used as gliding material between the acromion and the reconstructed rotator cuff. If the acromion has been detached, it is sutured back so that it comes to lie slightly elevated (Fig. 9). The coracoacromial ligament is resected if deemed advisable. Throughout the operation an atraumatic technique is essential.

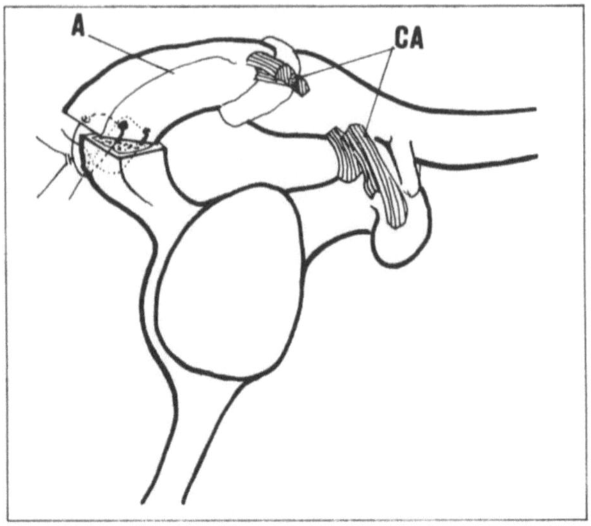

Fig. 9. The detached acromion is sutured back slightly elevated, CA = resected coracoacromial ligament

After-treatment

Following operation, the upper limb is immobilised on a ready-made abduction splint (airplane). Active movements of the elbow and hand are started 2-3 days after the operation and abduction exercises of the shoulder joint are begun 4 weeks postoperatively. Two weeks later the splint is removed. In many cases it is advisable to use an abduction pillow in the axilla for a further one or two weeks. Active exercises, under instruction with careful surveillance, are continued for several months. The final result is usually achieved in six months.

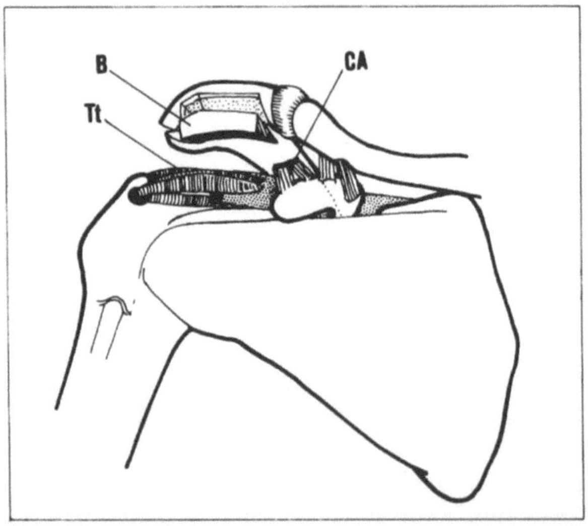

Fig. 8. A wedge (B) resected from the inferolateral margin of the acromion. CA = resected coracoacromial ligament, Tt = tendon grafts to the supraspinatus muscle

Discussion and Conclusions

In massive tears or defects of the rotator cuff of long duration it is not possible to reconstruct the tendons anatomically or to restore the normal function of the muscles involved by the methods generally adopted. If the anatomy is altered, we cannot expect to restore physiological function. Anatomical reconstruction of the muscle-tendon units gives the glenohumeral joint a better chance to regain normal or near normal activity. The supraspinatus muscle, although only a secondary mover, plays an important role in glenohumeral function.

The results in a series of over 80 patients, using the technique described, are favourable. I personally have used the technique with slight variation for 11 years in more than 50 cases. The results are gratifying (to be published).

Summary

Based on considerations of the mechanics of shoulder movements, a method was planned to restore the anatomy and undisturbed function of the rotator cuff using free tendon transplantation. The method appears useful and the results in a series of over 80 patients are gratifying.

II.4. Rotator Cuff Repair by Muscle Advancement

D. Patte, J. Debeyre and D. Goutallier

Rotator cuff rupture surgery cannot claim to relieve pain. It must, therefore aim only at repairing the anatomical lesions causing the functional disability. Despite the wealth of plastic surgical procedures described since Codman's first setbacks, reconstructive surgery may still be impossible or unreliable due to the extensive loss of tendinous material and widespread necrosis of the edges. To overcome the technical difficulties which have led these operations into disrepute, J. Debeyre [14] came upon the idea of performing a disinsertion-advancement of the entire supraspinatus muscle, and sometimes of the infraspinatus as well. We have steadily improved the accuracy of the technique over the past twenty years [15, 16, 17, 18] and have refined the indications for operation with improved results. We consider our technique to be reliable since we have a record of 250 operative procedures to support our judgement.

General Principles

1. The Need to Excise Necrotic Tendon Tissue

We believe that the term ''rotator cuff rupture'' is a misnomer because it suggests a traumatic discontinuity amenable to suture. It is in fact a degenerative trophic perforation which causes a loss of substance through necrotic tendon (Fig. 1).

The distal insertion area of the tendon vanishes and prevents any suture so that re-insertion into bone is required.

The proximal part, subject to the diverging pull from the constituent muscles, becomes concave when it retracts and rounds off the perforation.

Active inward rotation of the arm causes infraspinatus to slide over the posterosuperior aspect of the head which thereby becomes further ''uncuffed''

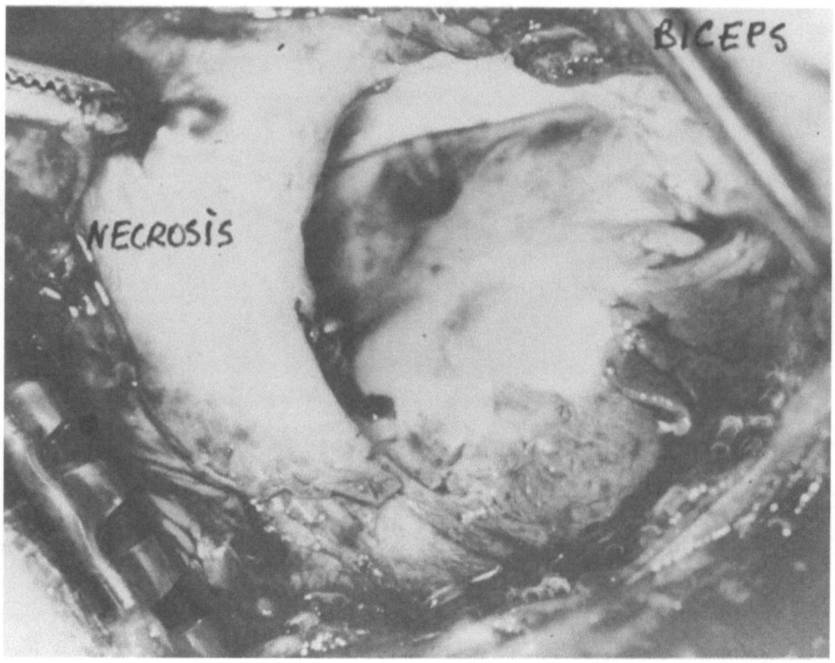

Fig. 1. Preoperative photograph of the lesion taken from above shows that it looks more like a "trophic perforation" than a "rupture"

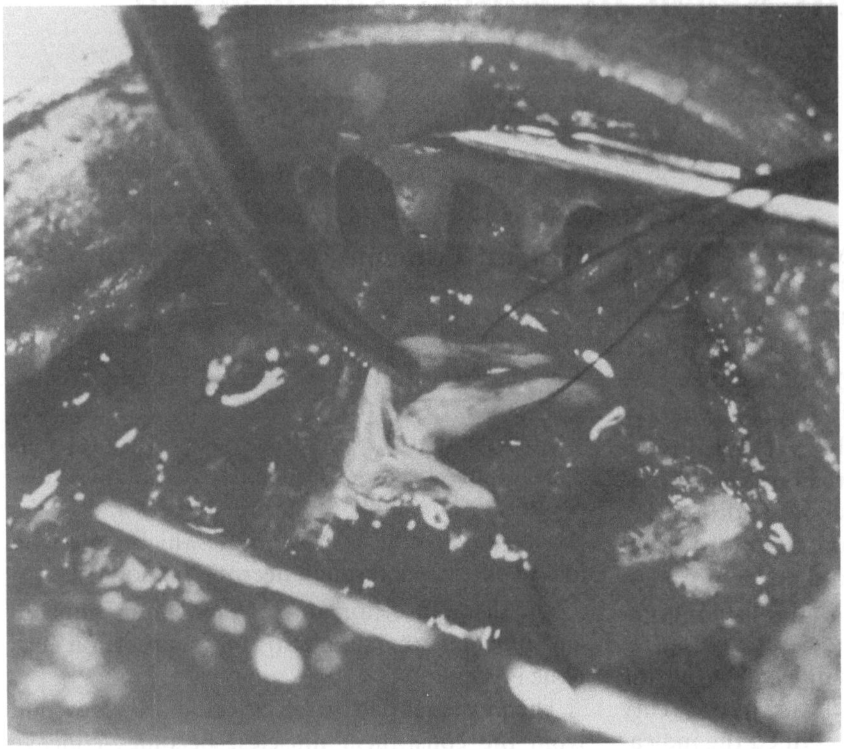

Fig. 2. Tendon splitting induced by necrosis

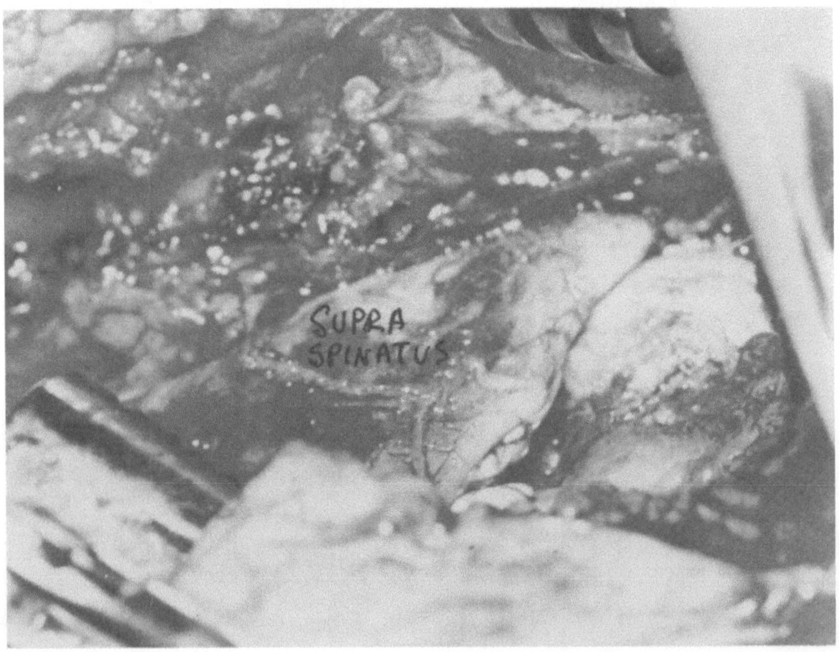

Figs. 3 and 4. The lower articular side of the tendon is necrotic, making it unfit for reconstructive surgery

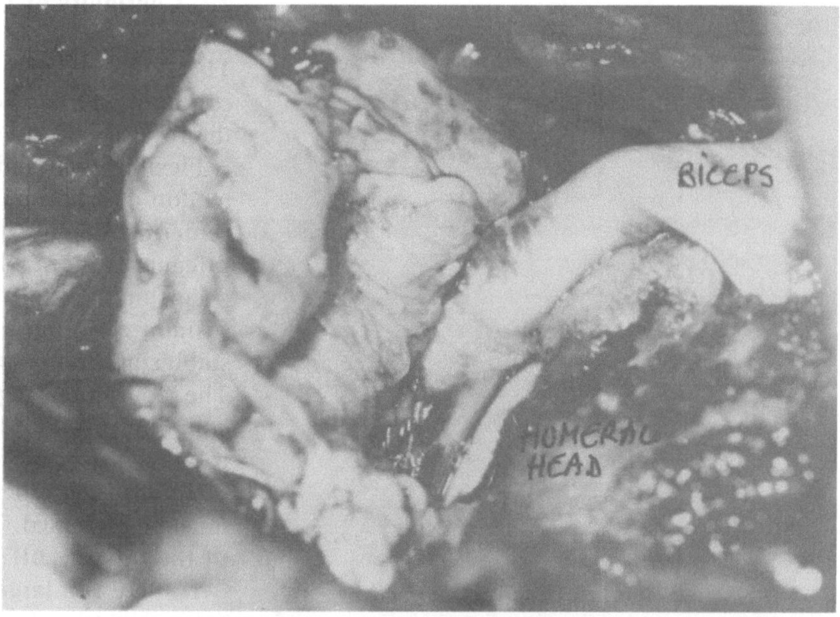

Fig. 4. Interior surface of supraspinatus

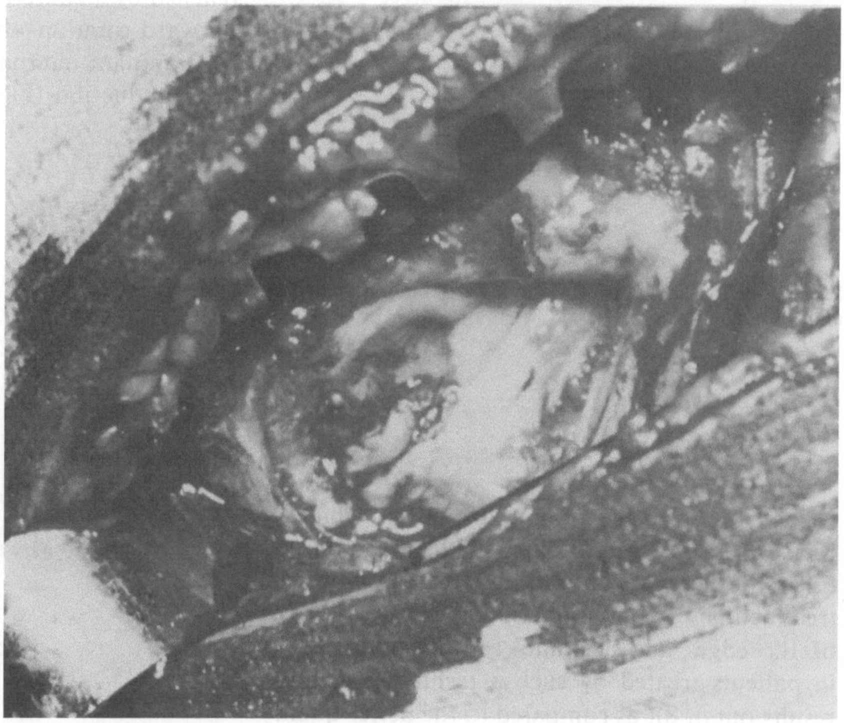

Fig. 5. Recent anterosuperior triangular rupture

and the head is subjected to the released upward force of deltoid (fig. 2).

Necrosis of tendon may spread farther and undermine the thickness of the tendon (Fig. 3), particularly on its inferior articular aspect (Figs. 4 and 5), making it unfit for repair. The excision of the necrosed tissue which is essential, further increases the loss of substance.

There is a wide spectrum between a large avulsion causing the "bald" head of an old rupture, which gives rise to subacromial rather than general shoulder arthritis, and the limited triangular-

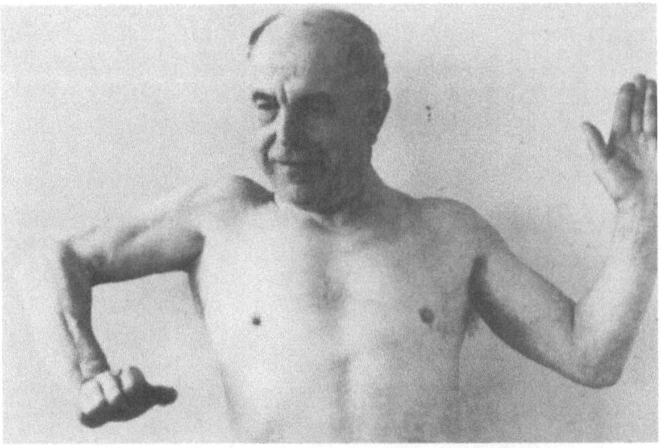

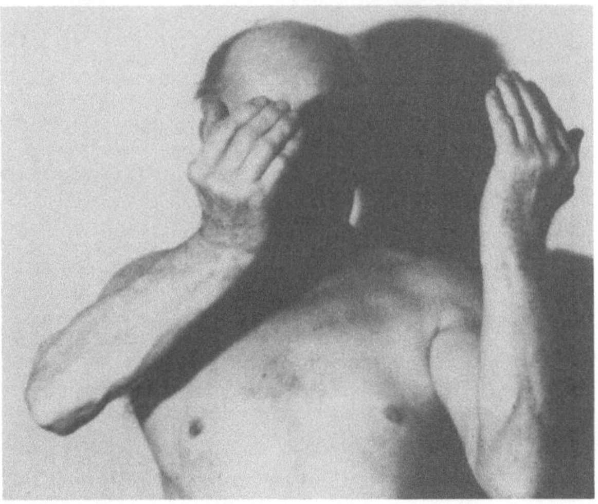

Figs. 6 and 7. Automatic return of inward rotation hindering abduction and flexion

shaped and somewhat anterior lesion which is focused on the intra-articular path of the biceps. Even in these apparently easy cases, however, treatment by longitudinal suture causes necrosis of the edges and accounts for the poor results in patients treated by such a technique (4 good results out of 8), as compared to the better quality of results following transosseus reinsertion after excision of necrotic tissue (6 good results out of 7).

When appreciable loss of substance has occurred, and when the edges are poorly vascularised, i.e. in most surgical cases, the basic tenets of tendon surgery of secure and tension-free reinsertion across bone of a live tendon, is not possible unless one uses a device like muscle advancement.

2. Continuity of Cuff Reconstruction

This is the second mandatory rule. The anatomical conditions to ensure the dual mechanical role of the rotator cuff must be restored.

Flexible ball-and-socket interlocking at the tendon insertion must be achieved to allow active centering of the head into the glenoid, which safeguards the stability required for movement to occur and curtails the constraints required to sustain elevation without fatigue. This is the stabilising component of rotator cuff function. The continuous equilibrium of the mechanical coupling, produced by the varying action of the rotator cuff muscles on the one hand and by the deltoid on the other during elevation of the arm, must be preserved. This is the dynamic component of the rotator cuff muscle function.

If there is a large lesion, the separate repair of supraspinatus alone (which is all that can be reached by an anterior approach), does not restore outward rotation–abduction coupling, so that the predominant internal rotators continue to impede both abduction (Fig. 6) and flexion (Fig. 7). On

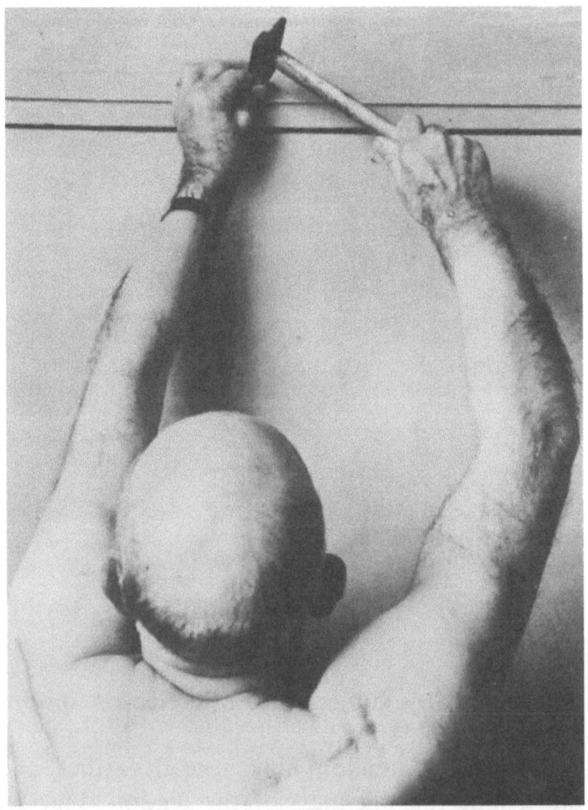

Fig. 8. Infraspinatus repair is needed to recover active outward rotation and powerful elevation

the other hand, repair of infraspinatus, which is the only genuine external rotator muscle of the shoulder, is vital to restore the balance and to guarantee enough muscular force in the elevated position (Fig. 8). It is striking to observe the difference in results when the supraspinatus has been repaired, and when it has not (Table 1).

Table 1. Postero-superior ruptures and extensive avulsions: 40 results (average 13 years)

	Favourable results
Fully repaired cuff	21/29 (72%)
Non-repaired infraspinatus	6/11 (50%)

3. Restoration of Subacromial Gliding

When the cuff has been repaired, a free gliding space must be restored under the inextensible coracoacromial vault (the so-called second articulation of the shoulder – De Seze [20]).

The bursal giding space usually recovers spontaneously, so that no additional operative step is required. However, there are "tight" shoulders inducing more pain than loss of function, causing a painful anterior arc during flexion in the position of inward rotation, which indicates an anterior impingement between head and vault.

Many authors advocate anterior decompression procedures to an extent that they entirely forget the glenohumeral mechanism. We do not support them, but like Neer [45] and others, we are not opposed to supplementary surgery of this kind.

Resecting the coracoacromial ligament is not enough, and we add a resection of the protruding and sometimes osteophytic anterior acromial beak, and often a resection of the acromioclavicular joint (Fig. 9). The quality and speed of pain relief achieved in 8 out of 10 recent cases have convinced us to continue.

In the shoulder, even more than in other joints, one must refrain from too mechanical a concept of pain. Like Macnab [43], we believe that the inflammatory reaction secondary to necrosis of

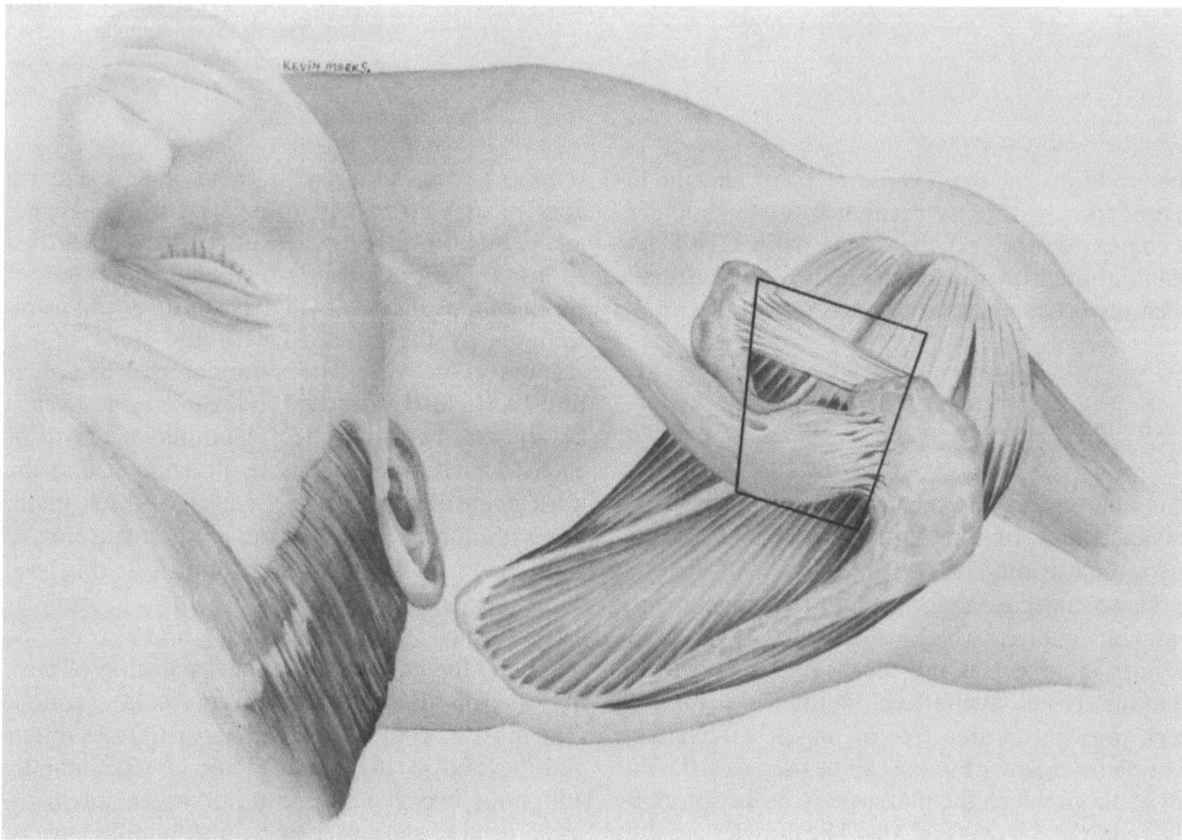

Fig. 9. Coracoacromioclavicular vault resection

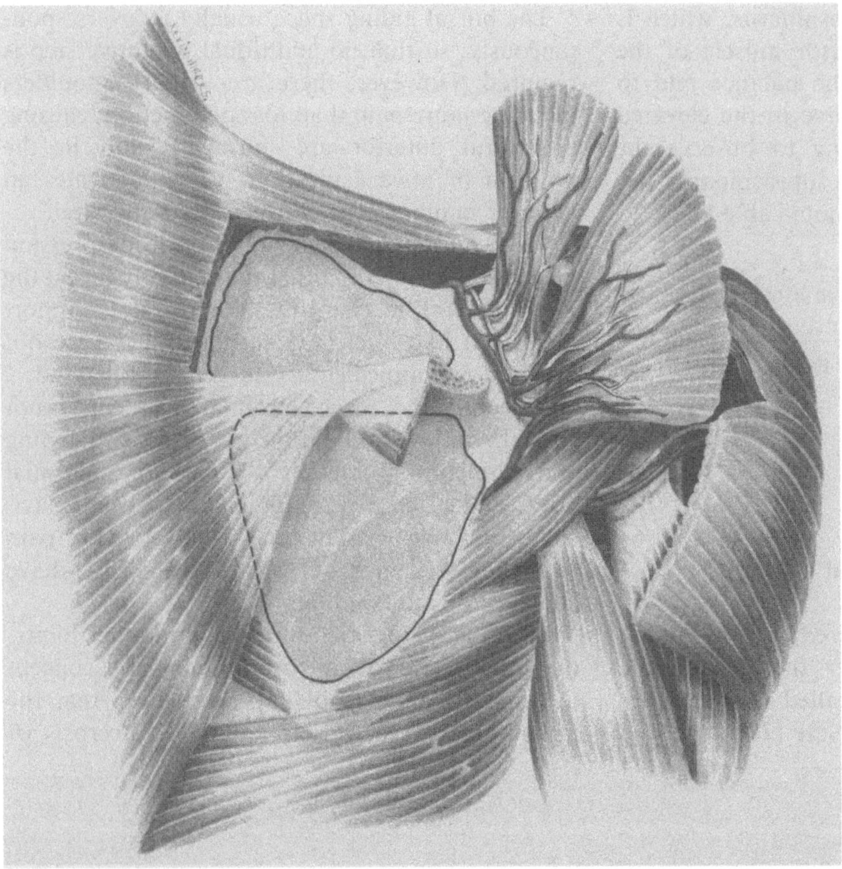

Fig. 10. Suprascapular neurovascular hinge

the tendon is the main cause of pain, and the inflammatory sensitivity peculiar to some shoulders accounts for the fact that some patients still feel pain although correct mechanical conditions have been restored.

Technique

The anatomical arrangement allows disinsertion-advancement of the entire supraspinatus and infraspinatus muscles.

These muscles share a suprascapular neurovascular pedicle which is unique. It is easily defined as it enters the supraspinous and infraspinous fossae, at the level of the distal third of each muscle, an area free of muscle attachment. The neurovascular bundle can be used as a flexible pivot about which the muscle may be advanced by the required 3-4 cm (Fig. 10). The muscles are thus disinserted from the medial two-thirds of their fossae, taking along with them their enclosing aponeuroses up to where the neurovascular pedicle enters the fossae and can be easily identified – for the supraspinatus by the thick iridescent supraspinous ligament (Fig. 11) and for the infraspinatus by the outer edge of the spine of the scapula (Fig. 12). The terminal neurovascular branches, closely attached to the deep side of each muscle are therefore safe. The outer one-third of each fossa is free of muscle attachment and the muscles easily move up to the neck of the scapula. Teres minor is dissected out with infraspinatus after ligaturing the only anastomosis at this level with the posterior branch of the subscapular artery which hugs the axillary margin of the scapula. One has to ensure the separation of teres major from its conjoint intermuscular septum. One must of course heed the nerve to teres minor and beyond it the axillary nerve. Occasionally adhesions between the posterior aspect of infraspinatus and the posterior deltoid bundle have to be freed to achieve full release of the muscle.

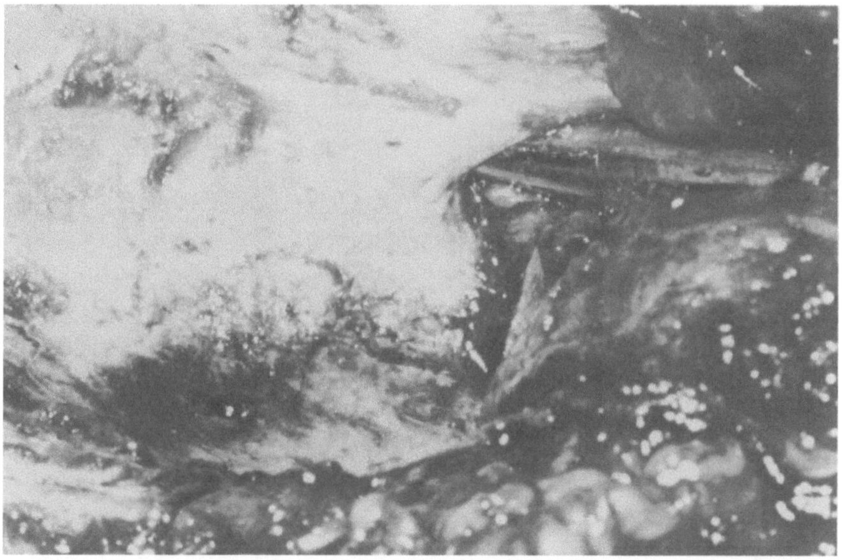

Fig. 11. The supraspinous ligament is the landmark showing where neurovascular bundle enters supraspinous fossa

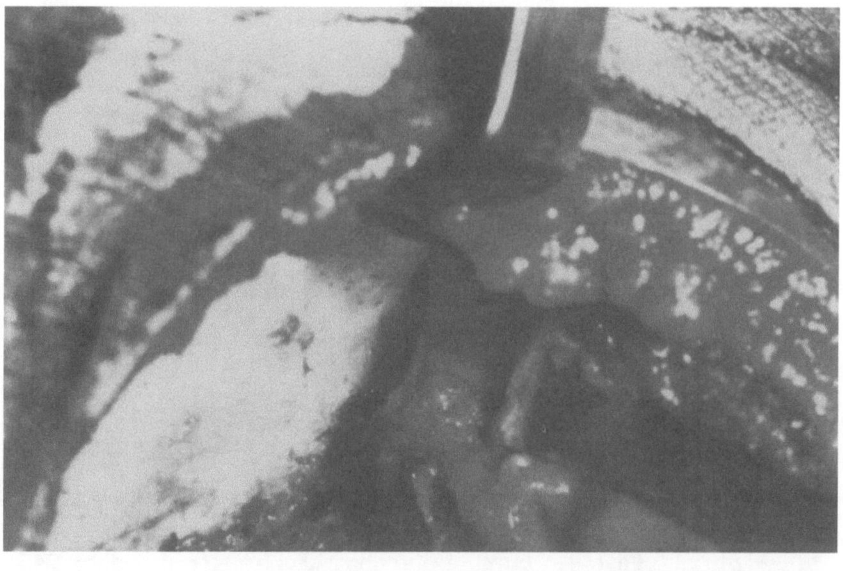

Fig. 12. The outer edge of the spine is the landmark for the infraspinous fossa

Posture and Surgical Approach

This varies with the site and size of the lesion.

The posterosuperior, supraspinous and trans-acromiodeltoid approach (1 in Fig. 13) with the patient lying prone remains the most widely used method. It leads straight on to the upper aspect of the cuff by dividing the acromion in the coronal plane (Fig. 14), running parallel to the fibres of the trapeziodeltoid mass.

The anterolateral coracoacromial approach in a semi-sitting posture may be preferred when the lesion is thought to be anterosuperior and when it is planned to combine cuff repair with coracoacromioclavicular vault resection (2 in Fig. 13). The incision is shaped like a shoulder tab and subtotal T-shaped disinsertion and separation of anterior deltoid fibres is performed.

A separate infraspinous approach with the patient lying prone or in lateral decubitus is used if muscle slide of infraspinatus is planned (4 in Fig. 13). The lower fibres of trapezius are displaced inwards, latissimus dorsi downwards and the posterior bundle of deltoid upwards. This gives wide

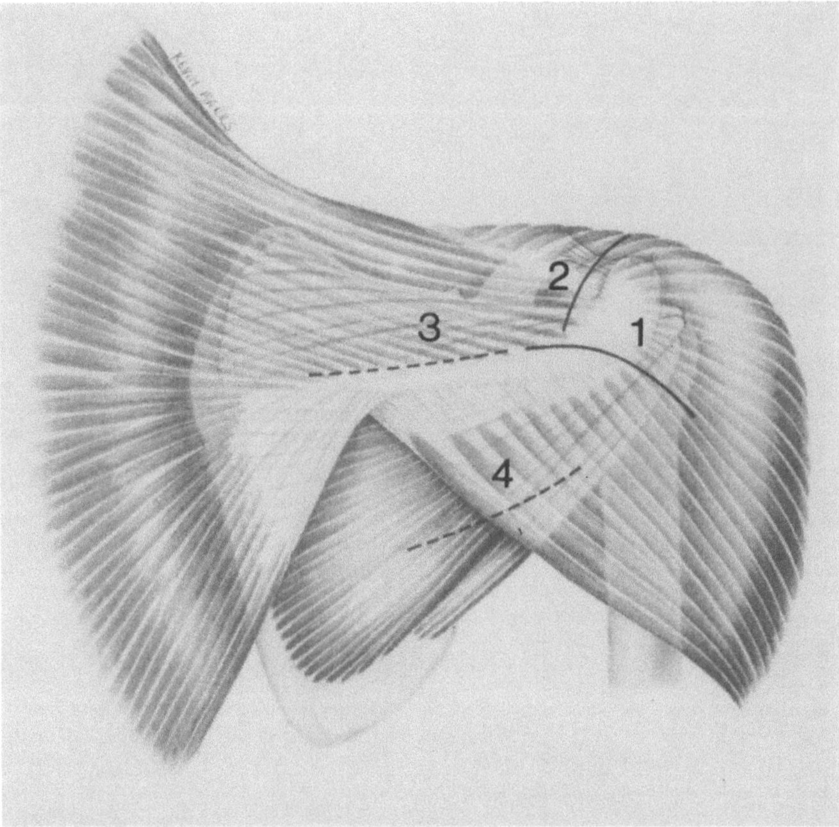

Fig. 13. Surgical approaches (1) Posterosuperior supraspinous and transacromiodeltoid approach, and prolongation into the supraspinous fossa (3). (2) Anteroexternal coracoacromial approach. (4) Subspinous approach.

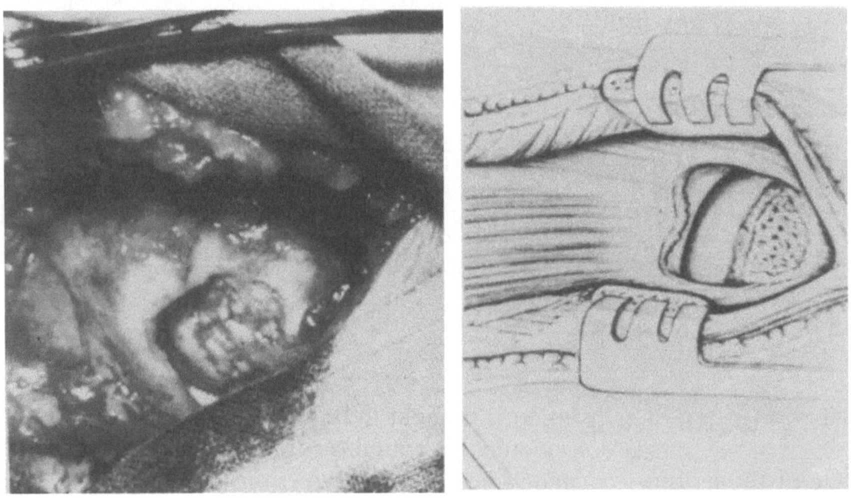

Fig. 14. Direct approach to the upper side of the cuff

access to the subspinous fossa up to and beyond the outer edge of the spine of the scapula.

The patient's posture and the surgical approach must be carefully selected on the basis of the clinical signs and symptoms with particular reference to outward rotation and the precise definition of the lesion provided by antero-posterior and lateral arthropneumotomography as devised by Bernageau[6]. It is a useful examination, and its reliability was confirmed by comparing findings at operation in 50 patients (Figs. 15, 16, 17). It is, however, a difficult technique and as yet not very widely used.

The choice between direct re-insertion and re-

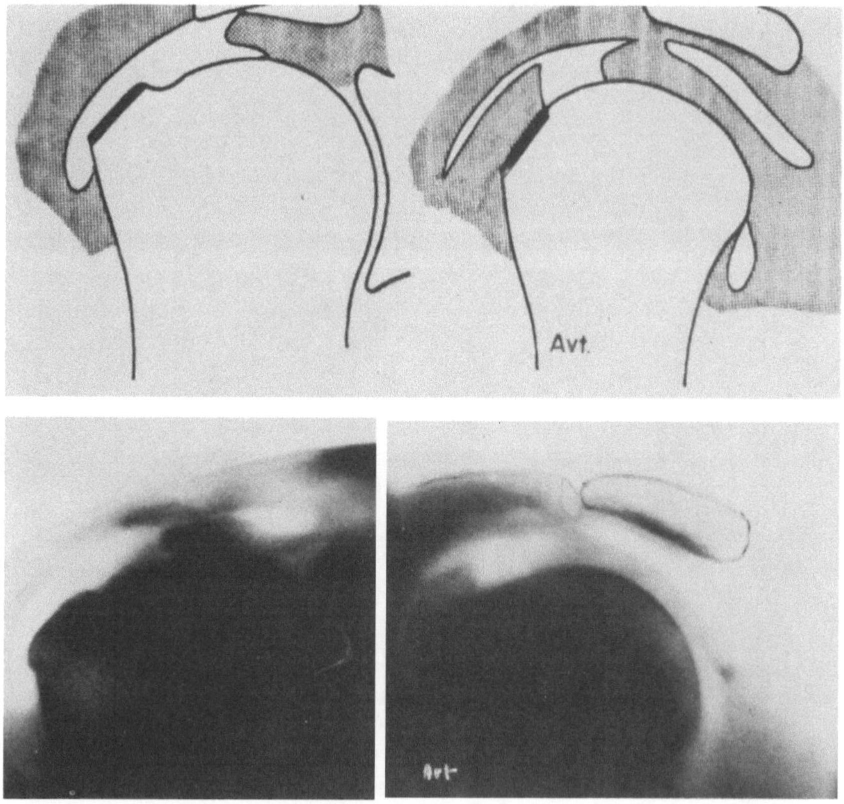

Fig. 15. Anteroposterior and arthropneumotomography— Small superior rupture (Stage I)

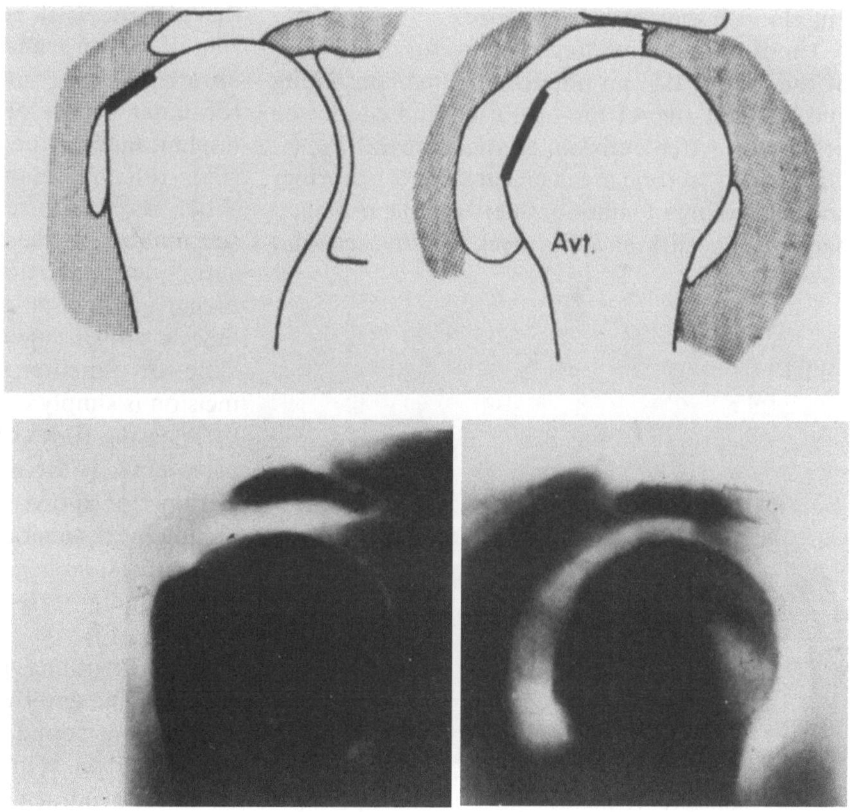

Fig. 16. Anteroposterior and lateral arthropneumotomography—Average antersosuperior rupture (Stage II)

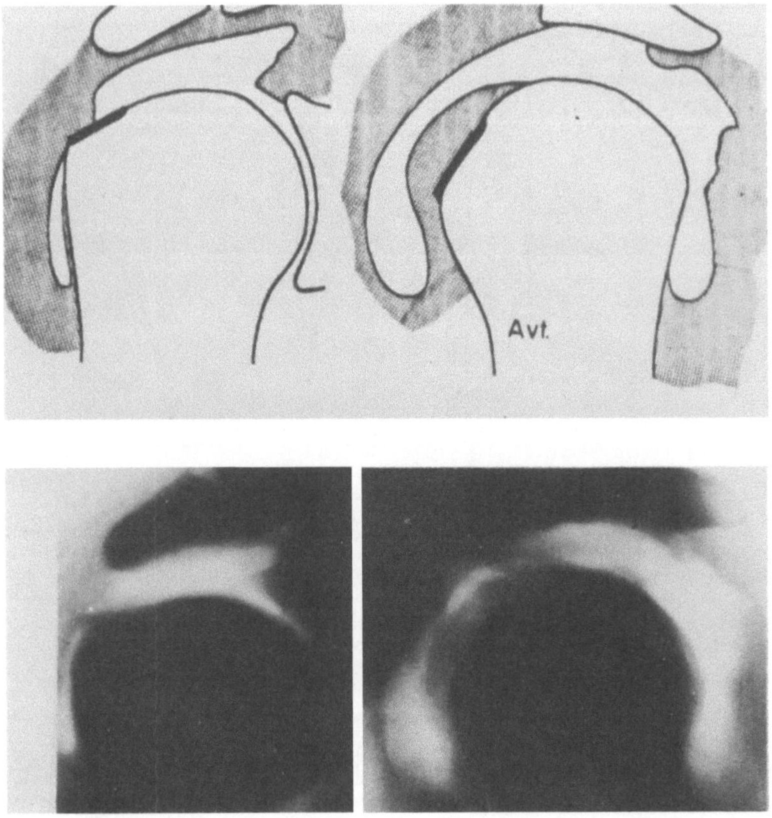

Fig. 17. Anteroposterior and lateral arthropneumotomography —Large posterosuperior rupture (Stage III)

insertion after advancement, of one or both muscles is a matter of experience.

The first operative step is a careful assessment of the lesion. It is an important, time-consuming and difficult step of the operation and cannot be neglected. After excision of the synovial bursa, scar tissue, necrotic areas unsuitable for suturing, and the freeing of adhesions between the proximal part of the cuff and the neck of the scapula, muscle quality and elasticity are tested to assess the prospects of repair. If suitable tissues are found, secure transosseus re-insertion with non-absorbable wire sutures secured in a U-shape to the outer aspect of the tuberosity ensures good implantation of the tendinous flap into its groove (Fig. 18) and retains the head of the humerus. When direct suture is not possible, rather than succumbing to the temptation of performing an acrobatic re-insertion by a strongly abducted and precarious tendon suture, we prefer to perform muscle advancement despite the subsequent decline in function. For the infraspinatus, the incision is simply extended to 1 cm from the spine by releasing fibres of the trapezius in line with the osteotomy of the acromion, if the original posterosuperior approach has been used; or, after resecting the acromioclavicular joint and opening up the supraspinous fossa, if the more recently devised anteroexternal approach has been used (3 in Fig. 13).

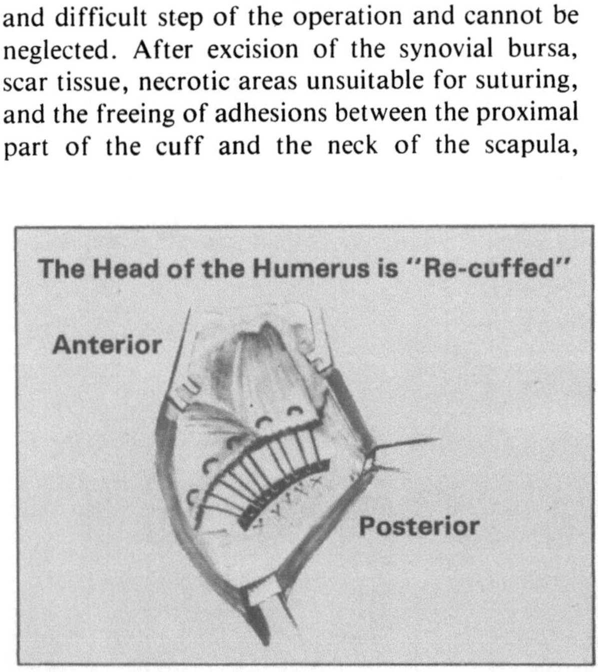

Fig. 18. Transosseus re-insertion

The cuff still has to be entirely rebuilt to correct tension. The anterior edge of the proximal flap is sutured to sound anterior tissue beyond the tendon or biceps in order to protect it and to stop its entrapment at that level.

Postoperative Management

This is of cardinal importance. The arm is immobilised in a thoracobrachial cast in abduction and outward rotation: the more posterior the lesion, the more outward rotation. The cast is retained from 30 to 45 days. It is replaced by an abduction cushion as soon as active horizontal abduction can be easily sustained. Rehabilitation must be started at once and gently and gradually to suit the individual patient. Manual attention by a physiotherapist who listens to what his patient has to say is the kind of rehabilitation that is required. Intelligent co-operation between patient and experienced physiotherapist largely determines the result, probably more by preventing irreversible damage than by improving the result of the operative procedure, which has in any event already been defined by the size of the lesion and the quality of the reconstructive surgery.

Conclusions

Twenty years' surgical experience involving upwards of 250 operations cannot be assessed in a few sentences. Continuous follow-up leads us to regard muscle advancement as the only currently available technique able to remodel a sturdy, continuous and mobile cuff meeting the three criteria listed above. One should not hesitate to use it when ideal conditions do not exist for direct re-insertion of the cuff.

The percentage of good results has increased steadily over the years (Table 2). It has continued to improve since 1977 and now regularly exceeds 70%, probably because indications are most carefully defined, surgical technique is more precise, and after-care more gentle, thus avoiding the iatrogenic neurological or painful dystrophic complications which were previously encountered when this kind of treatment was started.

Table 2. Trend of results

	Favourable	Improved	Failures
1960-1967 110	57 (52%)	28 (25%)	25 (23%)
1967-1977 40	27 (67.5%)	8 (20%)	5 (12.5%)

Improved surgical approaches and techniques of operation based on a more accurate preoperative diagnosis of the lesion have also contributed in an important way to the improved quality of our results. Supra- and infraspinatus muscle advancement in a single muscle flap substantially improves the pseudoparalytic outward rotation of the shoulder as well as muscular power. Coraco-acromioclavicular vault resection protects the repaired cuff and thereby seems to produce a faster, more complete and lasting result, with less pain.

II.5. Transfer of Subscapularis and Teres Minor for Massive Defects of the Rotator Cuff

Robert J. Neviaser and Thomas J. Neviaser

The repair of an acute, large tear of the rotator cuff is not a difficult surgical problem. However, the failure to diagnose the lesion at an early stage and to understand the importance of its early repair has resulted in considerable difficulty with later reconstruction of the lesion. Until recently, the only useful procedure was the insertion of the tendons into a trough in the humeral head at whatever point they happened to reach [38]. This often relieved pain but left weakness in abduction.

Because of dissatisfaction with the inconsistency of the results by McLaughlin's technique [38, 39, 40, 41], two procedures were developed: the intra-articular portion of the biceps tendon was employed to bridge small residual defects in the cuff, or freeze-dried rotator cuff graft was used to cover large defects [46, 48]. These two methods have consistently produced a high percentage of good results. Unfortunately, freeze-dried cadaver grafts are increasingly difficult to obtain. This scarcity is a result of the stringent criteria placed upon the source of such grafts, i.e. individuals under the age of 45 who have no history of malignancy and whose cause of death was not sepsis.

It therefore became necessary to develop a satisfactory alternative to the freeze-dried cuff graft when the residual tendinous defect was too large to be bridged by a biceps graft and no cadaver graft was available. For the past six years, the tendons of subscapularis and teres minor have been transferred in patients with large, chronic tears of the rotator cuff for which no other satisfactory technique was possible. It is the purpose of this report to describe the technique and discuss its results.

Materials and Methods

Seventeen patients have undergone transfer of subscapularis and teres minor tendons for large tears of the rotator cuff. All of these tears were chronic, i.e., of more than three weeks' duration; the longest was one year. At the time of repair, 16 out of 17 patients could abduct the involved arm 30° or less. The remaining individual had 90° of abduction preoperatively. All patients complained of pain, especially at night, and all underwent arthrography to confirm the diagnosis. In each case contrast medium escaped into the subdeltoid bursa. The amount of contrast medium in the bursa showed no correlation with the size of the defect of the cuff, an observation consistent with past experience. As in any operation to reconstruct the rotator cuff, the primary goal was to relieve pain.

There were 15 males and 2 females; 11 patients had undergone previous attempts to repair the cuff by other surgeons, obviously without success. Their ages ranged from 42 to 70 years (average 58.2 years). Their occupations included farming, watch-repairing, maintenance, housework, and various clerical and desk jobs.

Operative Technique

The operation is performed under general endotracheal anaesthesia with the patient in a sitting position. An anterosuperior approach is used at the level of the acromioclavicular joint. The deltoid fibres are split at the same level and the muscle dissected subperiosteally from the superior margin of the clavicle, acromioclavicular joint and acromion as far laterally and posteriorly as necessary for adequate exposure [48, 49, 51, 52]. The coracoacromial ligament is resected and an anteroinferior oblique acromioplasty [45] as well as an acromioclavicular arthroplasty is carried out. The bursa is divided and tagged for closure later but is dissected free from the cuff and deltoid to improve the exposure. The rupture of

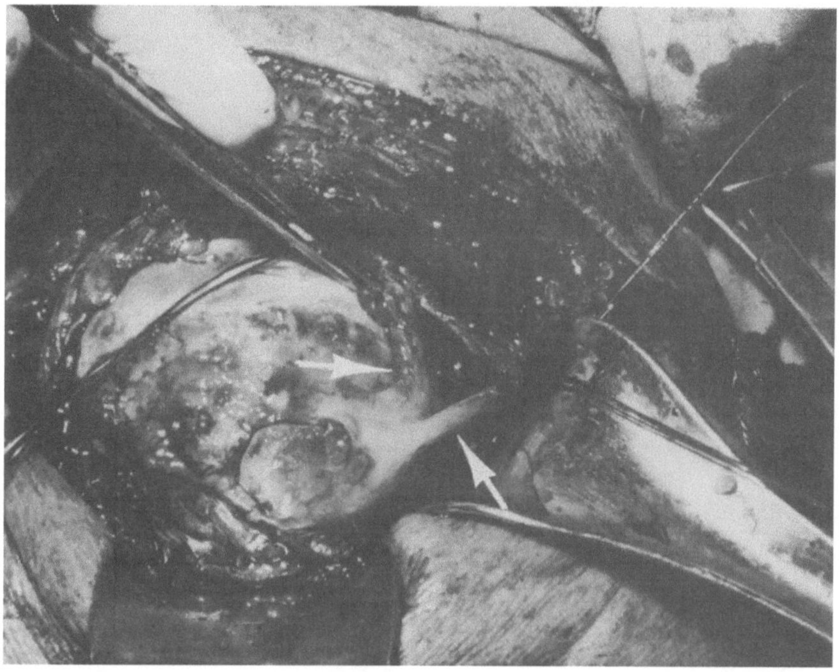

Fig. 1. The interval between the subscapularis (*arrow on right*) and underlying capsule (*arrow on left*) has been developed

the cuff is then clearly seen and every effort made to mobilise the tendons to diminish the size of the defect.

If the residual gap from the torn tendons to the tuberosities is too large for either a direct suture or a biceps graft and no freeze-dried cadaver rotator cuff is available as a graft, the transfer of the tendons is undertaken. The intervals between the subscapularis and the underlying articular capsule anteriorly and the teres minor and the capsule posteriorly are identified. Each tendon is dissected free from the capsule as far as possible up to its insertion and then detached, leaving the capsular attachments intact (Fig. 1). The tendons are mobilised sufficiently to allow each to be shifted upwards. A trough is made with a gouge in the anatomical sulcus between humeral head and tuberosities. The tendons are transferred upwards so that the superior margin of one touches the corresponding border of the other. These edges are sutured together. The lateral ends of the new combined tendon are inserted into the trough and secured through drill holes to the humerus with the knots lying below the tuberosities on the lateral cortex of the upper humerus (Fig. 2). The remaining interval in front between the undisturbed articular capsule and the lower border of subscapularis is sutured (Fig. 3). The interval behind between teres minor and capsules is also closed. If the size of the defect permits, a single tendon—either subscapularis or teres minor—can be used alone.

The bursa is repaired and deltoid replaced over the acromion and clavicle; the split in its fibres being repaired with inverted sutures.

The arm is immobilised at the side in a Velpeau for six weeks. The seventh week is spent by the patient on pendulum exercises. Full rotator cuff rehabilitation is started in the eighth week.

Results

All patients were followed for a minimum of one year; the longest follow-up was six years. The grading of end-results was based on relief of pain and the degree of shoulder abduction. An "excellent" result was one in which there was virtually no pain and abduction greater than 120°. A "good" result was one in which there was occasional pain on use but none at night and abduction from 90-120°. A "fair" result was one with some nocturnal pain and abduction from 60-90°. A "poor" result was one with abduction of less than 60° with or without decrease in pain.

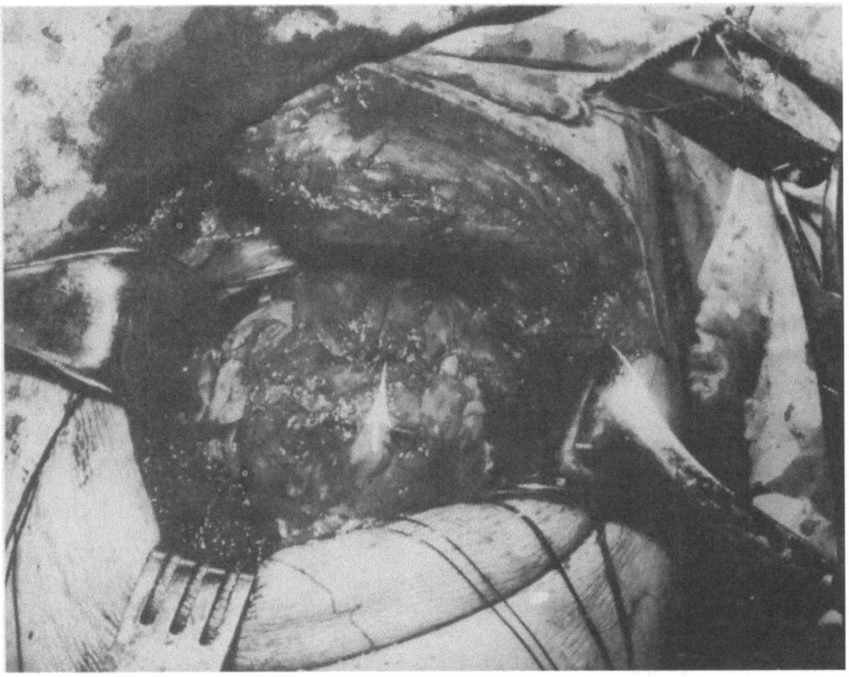

Fig. 2. Tendons of subscapularis and teres minor have been transferred superiorly and fixed to trough (*arrow*) made in sulcus between anatomic neck and the tuberosities

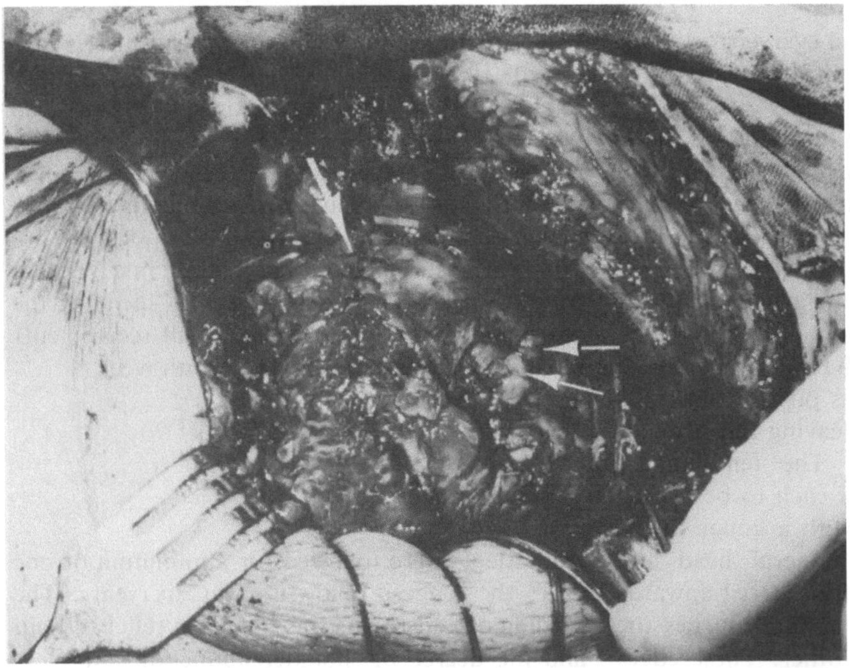

Fig. 3. New common border between transferred subscapularis and teres minor is sutured (*single arrow*). Inferior border of transplanted subscapularis and superior border of remaining anterior articular capsule are sutured together (*double arrow*). Same closure is done posteriorly between inferior margin of the teres minor and superior margin of the posterior articular capsule

Using this classification, there were five excellent and seven good results. There were no fair results, and five were graded as poor.

An analysis of the poor results revealed that in three cases there was relief of pain but no gain in motion. Each of these patients had undergone previous surgery which left them with a deltoid detached from the acromion and retracted distally. Attempts to restore the function of the deltoid were not successful.

The remaining two poor results were true failures of the procedure. One patient had rheumatoid arthritis. Her tissues were of very poor quality, increasing the likelihood of failure to heal. The other patient was immobilised for only four weeks and had recurrence of pain very early in his course of rehabilitation. Improved patient selection and an adequate period of immobilisation should reduce the failure rate.

Discussion

This procedure should be viewed as a salvage operation. It is indicated for chronic, massive tears of the rotator cuff. Ideally, these problems can best be handled by use of freeze-dried cadaver rotator cuff. Transfer of subscapularis and teres minor was developed as an alternative to these grafts because of difficulty in obtaining them.

This combination of transfers has not been previously reported. In his book, Bateman [5] briefly mentions transferring subscapularis tendon for rotator cuff ruptures. He does not provide sufficient detail to determine how closely that transfer resembles the one described here.

The majority of the failures were due to poor deltoid function resulting from previous surgery. This emphasises that proper handling of the deltoid during surgical exposure and closure is critical to satisfactory recovery of shoulder function. The remaining causes of failure in this series should be obviated by careful patient selection and an adequate period of immobilisation.

If there is a choice between tendon transfer and the use of freeze-dried rotator cuff, the graft would be preferred because of a slightly higher rate of excellent and good results as well as a lower rate of failure of the procedure. Nevertheless, transfer of the subscapularis and teres minor tendons has proved to be a satisfactory salvage procedure for relieving pain and improving movement.

Summary

Seventeen cases in which the tendons of subscapularis and teres minor were transferred superiorly for massive, chronic defects of the rotator cuff have been presented. This approach has proved to be satisfactory for relief of pain and improvement of movements, when the deltoid function is unimpaired.

II.6. Long-Term Results of Rotator Cuff Repair

Claes Petersson

Many investigators have reported their results after rotator cuff repair. In most reports the time interval between operation and follow-up examination does not exceed 5 years; only rarely does it exceed 10 years. The purpose of the present study is to evaluate the long-term results of rotator cuff repair after 12 to 19 years and to compare these results with those of an initial evaluation undertaken at the end of the convalescence.

Material and Methods

The original group consisted of 53 men and 13 women with an average age of 57 years operated on between 1961 and 1968 in Malmo General Hospital, all by the same surgeon, who had reported the results of the original follow-up examination on average 6 months following the operation. The second re-examination was undertaken in 1979 and early 1980. The average time interval between operation and re-examination was then 14 years (range 12-19). Of the original 66 patients 19 had died and 5 were lost for follow-up for other reasons; 42 patients with 43 operated shoulders were therefore available for examination, 32 men (average age 70, range 56-85), and 10 women (average age 68, range 30-83).

The operative findings were:

Partial tear	1
Complete tear	
Small (< 1 cm)	5
Medium (1-3 cm)	21
Large (> 4 cm)	16

The surgical procedure consisted in: exploration only in two shoulders; tendon suture end-to-end or with re-insertion of the proximal margin of the tear to the head of humerus in 21 cases; suture combined with resection of the lateral end of the acromion in 20 cases.

The rating of the long-term results was based on interview and physical examination, and the results were classified with respect to patient satisfaction and the total range of active straight arm elevation. The rating of patient satisfaction included pain and function:

Good. Pleased: no pain and no impairment of function.

Fair. Pleased, but with mild or moderate pain and with restriction in some activities.

Poor. Not pleased, with moderate to severe pain and impairment of function.

The range of motion was classified:

Good. Elevation > 150°
Fair. Elevation 90°-150°
Poor. Elevation < 90°

For a total score the mean of the two ratings was used in order to get a scoring value comparable with that of the initial evaluation.

In 35 shoulders radiological examination was performed at the time of re-examination. In 39 patients preoperative arthrograms were available. Unfortunately, because of their extremely unpleasant recollections of this examination, all patients objected to having it repeated.

Results

The initial and the re-examination ratings are compared in Table 1. There was no significant difference between the two evaluations. In the interval between the two evaluations 5 patients had improved equivalent to one grade on the rating scale from fair to good, and 1 from poor to fair; 8 patient ratings dropped— 6 one grade from

Table 1. Rotator cuff repair: ratings 1969 and 1980

	1969		1980		
	Number	%	Number	%	Difference
Good	27	63	25	58	−2
Fair	12	28	12	28	0
Poor	4	9	6	14	+2

Table 2. Relationship between size of rupture and ratings (results from 1969 in brackets)

Size of rupture	Rating		
	Good	Fair	Poor
Small	3 (4)	2 (2)	1 (0)
Medium	16 (19)	4 (1)	1 (1)
Large	6 (4)	6 (9)	4 (3)

good to fair, 1 one grade from fair to poor, and 1 two grades from good to poor.

Table 2 demonstrates the relation between the size of rupture and the long-term results (the results of the first evaluation in brackets). In the interval between the evaluations 1 patient with a small tear had dropped one grade from fair to poor, and 1 from good to fair. One patient with a medium-sized rupture had dropped from good to poor, and he required a further operation of anterior acromioplasty *ad modum* Neer in 1979 because of severe pain arc. Three patients with medium-sized tears dropped from good to fair. In the group of patients with large ruptures, 4 patients had improved from fair to good, whereas 2 dropped from good to fair and 1 from fair to bad. Table 3 shows the relation between some other factors which might influence the result and the long-term ratings.

Table 3. Relationship between factors with a possible influence on results and the long-term results

	Shoulders	Results		
		Good (%)	Fair (%)	Poor (%)
Sex				
Women	10	60	30	10
Men	33	58	27	15
Age (years)				
40–49	8	63	37	
50–59	19	58	26	16
60–69	13	47	30	23
Type of trauma				
No trauma	10	70	20	10
Fall on the level	12	33	33	33
More severe trauma	14	57	36	7
Glenohumeral dislocation	7	72	14	14
Operation				
Suture only	21	67	19	14
Suture and acromion resection	20	60	30	10
Resection of degenerated biceps tendon	11	64	27	9

Radiographic examination of 35 shoulders showed superior migration of the humeral head in 11 shoulders and radio-opaque deposits in the subacromial region in 13 shoulders. Of the 11 shoulders with superior migration 7 were rated good, 3 fair, and 1 poor.

Of the 13 shoulders with radio-opaque deposits 7 were good, 4 were fair and 1 was poor. There was a coincidence between superior head migration and radio-opaque deposits in 7 cases. (Figs. 1a,b, and 2a,b).

Case Report

A man, aged 83, who had an operation in 1966 at the age of 70, for a large cuff rupture and who was rated good both at the primary evaluation and at the re-evaluation, died from a rectal carcinoma some weeks after re-examination. Radiographic examination of his shoulders showed superior migration of both humeral heads, and post-mortem dissection of the shoulders disclosed a large lesion on the operated side with nests of sutures. On the left, non-operated side, there was an equally large lesion (Figs. 3a, and 4).

Discussion

The long-term results of rotator cuff repair in this study were good in 58%, fair in 28%, and poor in 14%. In the interval between the first and the second evaluation there was no significant change in rating. The long-term results were better if the tear was small or medium-sized or if the patient was under 50 at the time of operation; the results tended to be worse if the tear was large or the patient over 50. The patients who had injured their shoulder by falling at ground level had a worse long-term result than those with a more severe injury. The type of operation did not influence the result. Wolfgang in 1974 presented the results of a re-evaluation of 46 shoulders 18 months to 20 years after repair [67]. He found excellent to good results in 74% and fair to poor results in 26%, and stated that the results after

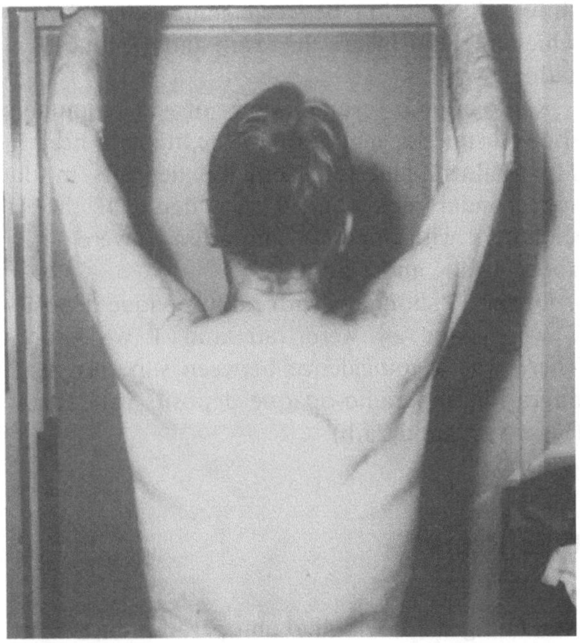

Fig. 1a. Operation in 1965 at the age of 63 for a large rupture of the left rotator cuff. At follow-up in 1979 he was pain-free and was rated "good"

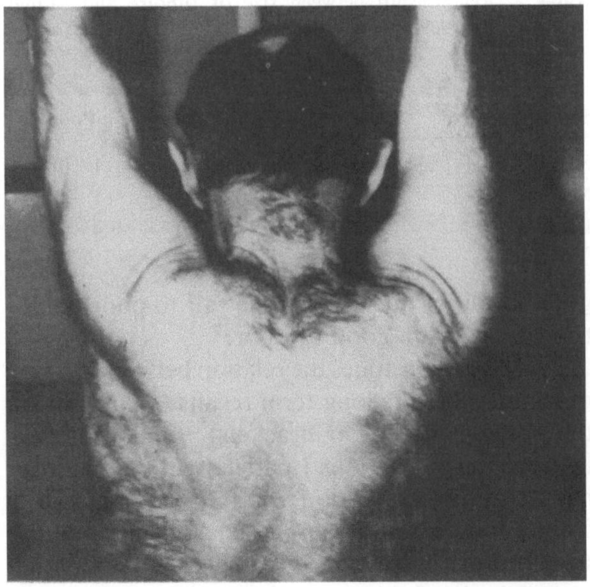

Fig. 2a. Operation in 1964 at the age of 51 for a large cuff rupture of the right shoulder. At follow-up he was pain-free, had good elevation and was rated 'good'

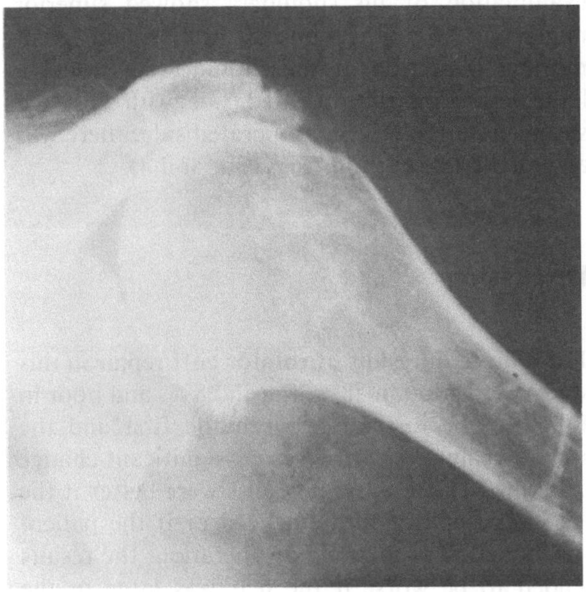

Fig. 1b. Radiograph of the left shoulder in slight abduction. Superior migration of the head of humerus with an acromiohumeral impingement

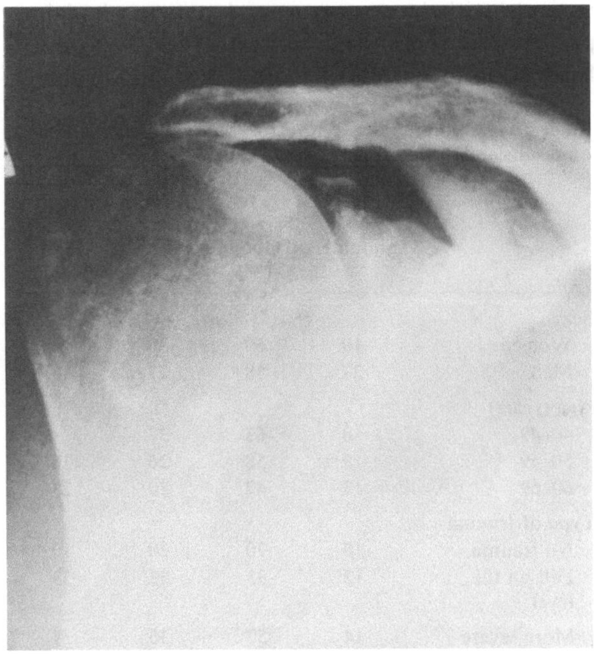

Fig. 2b. Radiograph of the right shoulder. Superior migration of the head of humerus. Multiple radio-opaque deposits

rotator cuff repair are not likely to change after six to nine months. He also pointed out that after repair, recurrence of the tear with or without associated symptoms may be frequent. In our investigation, 11 out of 35 patients, one-third of the radiologically examined shoulders, had signs of superior migration of the head of the humerus. Cotton and Rideout [13], Weiner and Macnab [64], and Kotzen [33], found that superior migration of the head is associated with complete rupture of the cuff. We performed no shoulder arthrographs in this study but in one case a post-

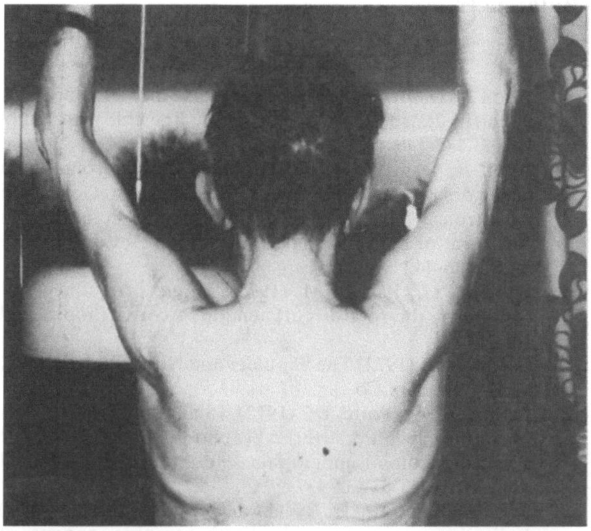

Fig. 3a. **Operation in 1966 at the age of 70 for a large cuff** rupture of the right shoulder. At follow-up he was rated "good"

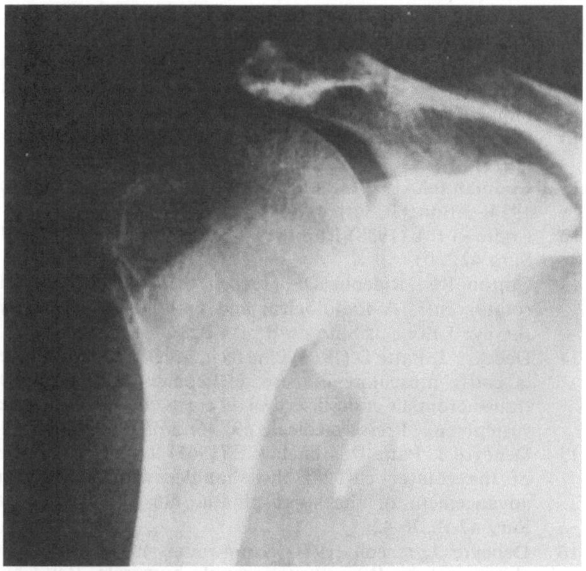

Fig. 3b. Radiograph of the right shoulder. Superior migration of the head of humerus

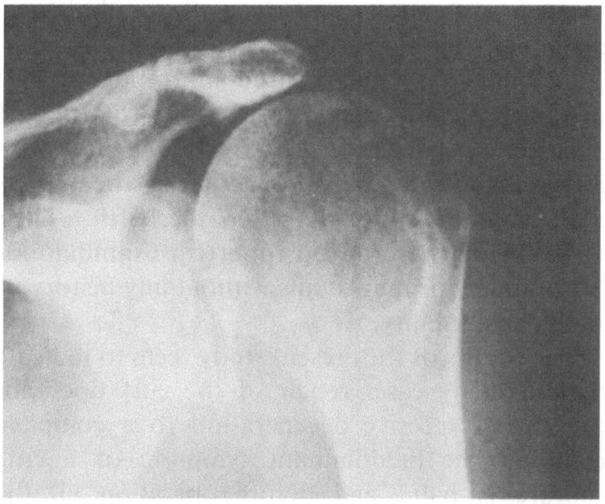

Fig. 3c. Radiograph of the left shoulder. Superior migration of the head of humerus

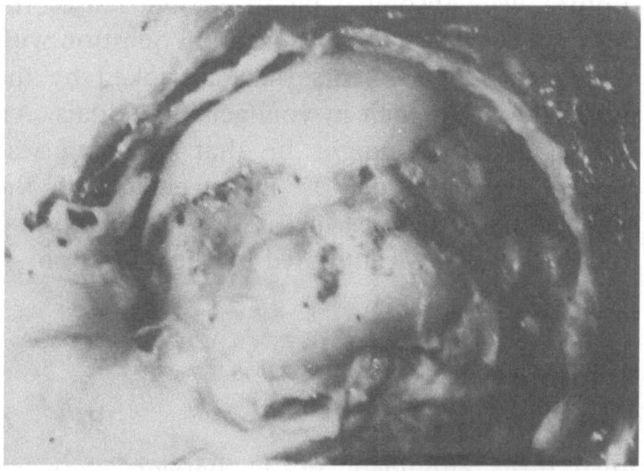

Fig. 3d. **Post-mortem dissection of the right shoulder** disclosed a total rupture of the cuff with the humeral head articulating against the acromion. The trough cut in head and the holes for the sutures can be seen

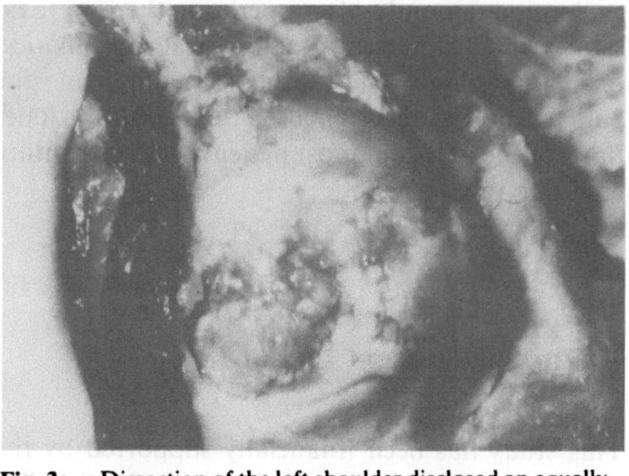

Fig. 3e. Dissection of the left shoulder disclosed an equally large rupture with acromiohumeral new joint formation and with severe destruction of the articular cartilage along the lateral edge

mortem dissection confirmed the radiological diagnosis.

DePalma [19] and Cotton and Rideout [13] described the progressive degenerative rotator cuff alterations that occur past middle life with increasing incidence and severity of the lesions each successive decade after the fifth. Their observations were on post-mortem examinations of shoulders of individuals without any history of shoulder disability.

The results of the present study seem to indicate that in many cases repair of the cuff does not prevent progressive degeneration to a complete rupture. The predominant symptom of a cuff rupture is pain, and before operation all the patients complained of shoulder pain or had a painful arc. At re-examination 25 patients, of whom 7 showed radiological evidence of complete rupture, were absolutely pain-free. One reason for this may be that in the age group in question with a mean age of 70 years the load taken by the shoulders is less than in younger individuals. An additional reason might be that the pain was elicited by irritation or impingement of the subacromial structures such as the bursa and that this irritation was eliminated by the operation.

Summary

Forty-three shoulders in 42 patients with an average age of 70 were evaluated between 12 and 19 years after rotator cuff repair. The long term results were good in 58%, fair in 28%, and poor in 14%. In comparison with the results of an initial evaluation 6 months after operation there were no significant differences. Radiological examination of 35 shoulders and autopsy findings in one patient showed recurrence of the rupture in one-third of the cases but most patients with re-rupture could be rated as good.

Acknowledgement

This study has been financially supported by the Herman Jarnhardt Foundation and the Swedish Medical Research Council.

References

1 Apoil A, Dautry P (1977) Le syndrome dit "de rupture de la coiffe des rotateurs de l'epaule". Rev chir orth Suppl II, 63: 145-149

2 Apoil A, Dautry P (1978) Chirurgie du syndrome de la coiffe des rotateurs de l'epaule. 1 vol. Docum. Geigy. 43p

3 Armstrong AC (1949) Excision of the acromion in treatment of the supraspinatus syndrome. J Bone Jt Surg 31-B: 436-442

4 Bakalim G, Pasila, M (1975) Surgical treatment of rupture of the rotator cuff tendon. Acta Orthop Scand 46: 751

5 Bateman JE (1972) The Shoulder and Neck. Philadelphia, W.B. Saunders Co

6 Bernageau J, Patte D, (1972) Bilan radiologique pré-operatoire de la Periarthrite Scapho-humerale. Interêt de l'arthro-pneumo-tomographie. Journal de Radiol et d'electro. T53,5: 432-437

7 Bernageau J, Patte D, Ryckewaert A, Goutallier D (1975) Indications respectives de l'arthrographie opaque et gazeuse et de l'arthro-pneumo-tomographie de l'épaule. Actualité Rheumatologique. Exp Scientif Paris 234-238

8 Bernageau J, Patte D (1977) Interêt de l'arthro-pneumo-tomographie dans le bilan pré-operatoire des ruptures de la coiffe des rotateurs posant un probleme chirurgical. Rev. du Rhumat. 44, 4: 285-289

9 Buechel FF, Pappas MJ, DePalma AF (1978) Total shoulder prosthesis with floating socket. Journal of biomedical materials research. 12. 89-114

10 Codman EA (1934) The Shoulder. Brooklyn, Miller (1975)

11 Codman EA (1937) Rupture of the supraspinatus, 1834 to 1934. J Bone Jt Surg 19: 643

12 Codman EA (1938) Rupture of the supraspinatus. Am J Surg 42: 603

13 Cotton RE, Rideout DF (1964) Tears of the humeral rotator cuff. A radiological and pathological necropsy survey. J Bone Jt Surg 46-B: 314-328

14 Debeyre J, Patte D (1961) Une technique de reparation de la coiffe musculotendineuse de l'épaule. Voir d'abract trans-acromiale et desinsertion du corps charnu du muscle sus-epineux. Presse medicale 69, 46: 2019

15 Debeyre J, Patte D, Elmelick E (1965) Repair of rupture of the rotator cuff of the shoulder with a note on advancement of the supraspinatus muscle. J Bone Jt Surg 47-B: 36-42

16 Debeyre J, et coll (1971) Symposium sur le traitement chirurgical des Periarthrites scapulo-humerale. Rev Chir orth 57, 8: 602-634

17 Debeyre J, Patte D, Mallet J (1972) Symposium sur la periarthrite scapho-humerale. Hans Huber, Berne: 63-85

18 Debeyre J, Patte D Traitement chirurgical de la pariarthrite scapho-humerale. Encyclopedia Medico-chirurgicale: Techniques chirurgical T.II: 44285

19 DePalma, AF (1950) Surgery of the shoulder. Lippincott, Philadelphia, p 438

20 De Sèze S, Ryckewaert A, Caroit M, Hubault A, Poinsard G, Renier JC, Welfling J (1960) Les ruptures traumatiques de la coiffe des rotateurs. Rev. Rhumatisme. 27 II: 443-453

21 DePalma AF (1963) Surgical anatomy of the rotator cuff and the natural history of degenerative periarthritis. Surg Clin N Amer 43: 1507-1520

22 Diamond B (1964) The obstructing acromion. Charles C. Thomas, Springfield, Ill.

23 Duchenne GB (1945) (quoted in Steindler A 1955)
24 Fowler EB (1932) Rupture of spinati tendons and capsule, repaired by a new operation. Illinois Med J 61: 332-334
25 Godsil RD, Linscheid RL (1970) Intratendinous defects of the rotator cuff. Clin Orthop 69: 181-188
26 Gschwend N, Zippel J, Liechti R, Grass S (1975) Die Therapie der Rotatorenmanschettenruptur an der Schulter. Arch Orthop. Unfall-Chir 83: 129-143
27 Hammond G (1962) Complete acromionectomy in the treatment of chronic tendonitis of the shoulder. J Bone Jt Surg 44-A: 494-503
28 Harrison JH, MacLaughlin HL (1962) Rupture of the rotator cuff. J Bone Jt Surg 44-A: 979-983
29 Heikel HV (1968) Rupture of the rotator cuff of the shoulder. Acta Orthop Scand. 39: 477-492
30 Inman VT, Saunders JB, Abbott LC (1944) Observations on the function of the shoulder joint. J Bone Jt Surg 26: 1-30
31 Kessel L, Watson M (1977) The transacromial approach to the shoulder for rupture of the rotator cuff. Int Ortho 2: 153
32 Kessel L, Watson M (1977) The painful arc syndrome, clinical classification & guide to management. J Bone Jt Surg 59-B, 2: 166
33 Kotzen L M (1971) Roentgen diagnosis of rotator cuff tear. Report of 48 surgically proven cases. Amer J Roentgenol 112: 507-511
34 Linge B, Mulder JD (1963) Function of the supraspinatus muscle and its relation to the supraspinatus syndrome. An experimental study in man. J Bone Jt Surg 45-B: 750-754
35 Lundberg BJ (1969) The frozen shoulder. Acta Orthop Scand (Suppl 119)
36 Mallet J, Patte D (1971) Ruptures de la coiffe des rotateurs. Rev Chir Orthop 57: 620
37 LeLaurin G (1978) L'osteotomie de translation-rotation-elevation de l'acromion dans les periarthrites scapulo-humerale avec conflit trochitero-acromial. These Dijon. p 62
38 McLaughlin HL (1944) Lesions of the musculotendinous cuff of the shoulder. I The exposure and treatment of tears with retraction. J Bone Jt Surg. 26: 31-51
39 McLaughlin HL, Asherman EG (1951) Lesions of the musculotendinous cuff of the shoulder. IV Some observations based upon the results of surgical repair. J Bone Jt Surg 33-A: 76
40 McLaughlin HL (1962) Rupture of the rotator cuff. J Bone Jt Surg (Am) 44: 979-983
41 McLaughlin HL (1963) Repair of major cuff ruptures. Surg Clin North Am. 43: 1535
42 McFarland B, Osborne G (1954) Approach to the hip. A suggested improvement on Kocher's method. J Bone Jt Surg 36-B: 364-367
43 Macnab I (1971) The painful shoulder due to rotator cuff tendonitis. Rhode Island Med J. 54: 367-374
44 Moseley HF (1972) Shoulder lesions, 3rd edn. Churchill Livingstone, Edinburgh, London
45 Neer CS (1972) Anterior acromioplasty for the chronic impingement syndrome in the shoulder. A preliminary report. J Bone Jt Surg 54-A: 41-50
46 Neviaser JS (1971) Ruptures of the rotator cuff of the shoulder. New concepts in the diagnosis and operative treatment of chronic ruptures. Arch Surg 102: 483-485
47 Neviaser JS (1975) Arthrography of the shoulder. The diagnosis and management of the lesions visualized. Charles C Thomas, Springfield, Illinois
48 Neviaser JS, Neviaser RJ, Neviaser TJ (1978) The repair of chronic massive ruptures of the rotator cuff of the shoulder by use of a freeze-dried rotator cuff. J Bone Jt Surg 60-A: 681-684
49 Neviaser RJ (1980) Tears of the rotator cuff. Orthop Clin of N Amer 11: 295-306
50 Neviaser RJ (1980) Lesions of the biceps and tendonitis of the shoulder. Orthop Clin of N Amer 11: 343-348
51 Neviaser RJ, Neviaser TJ (in press) Lesions of the musculo-tendinous cuff and capsule of the shoulder. Part I: Tears of the rotator cuff. Amer Academy of Orth Surgeons' instructional course lectures, vol. XXX. CV Mosby, St. Louis
52 Neviaser TJ, Neviaser RJ (in press) Lesions of the musculo-tendinous cuff and capsule of the shoulder. Part II: Lesions of the long head of the biceps tendon. Amer Academy of Orth Surgeons' instructional course lectures, vol. XXX. CV Mosby, St. Louis
53 Neviaser TJ (1980) Arthrography of the shoulder. Orthop Clin N Amer 11: 205-217
54 Nixon JE, DiStefano V (1975) Ruptures of the rotator cuff. Orthop Clin N Amer 6: 423-447
55 Olsson O (1953) Degenerative changes in the shoulder joint and their connection with shoulder pain. A morphological and clinical investigation with special attention to the cuff and biceps tendon. Acta Chir Scand (Suppl 181.)
56 Patte D (1963) Traitement chirurgical des ruptures de la coiffe des rotateurs de l'épaule (à propos de 66 observations) Thèse. Paris, AGEMP, p 98
57 Patte D (1972) Traitement chirurgical des ruptures musculo-tendineuses de la coiffe (une experience de 10 ans) Actualité rhumatol, Exp Scientif Paris. 181-194
58 Patte D, Briere de l'Isle R, Charlet-Troude F (1972) Indications thérapeutiques actuelles dans les ruptures de la coiffe de l'épaule. Ann de Med Physique. 15, 4: 421-436
59 Rathbun JB, MacNab I (1970) The microvascular pattern of the rotator cuff. J Bone Jt Surg. 52-B: 540-553
60 Rowe CR (1963) Ruptures of the rotator cuff. Selection of cases for conservative treatment. Surg Clin N Amer. 43: 1531-1534
61 Samilson RL, Binder WF (1975) Symptomatic full thickness tears of rotator cuff. An analysis of 292 shoulders in 276 patients. Orthop Clin N Amer 6: 449-466
62 Simunovic V (1974) Die Ruptur der Rotatorenschlinge am Schultergelenk. Helv Chir Acta. 41: 477-491
63 Steindler A (1955) Kinesiology of the human body. CC Thomas, Springfield
64 Weiner DS, Macnab I (1970) Superior migration of the humeral head. A radiological aid in the diagnosis of tears of the rotator cuff. J Bone Jt Surg 52-B: 524-527
65 Weiner DS, Macnab I (1970) Ruptures of the rotator cuff: follow-up evaluation of operative repairs. Canad J Surg 13: 219-227
66 Wolfgang DL (1974) Surgical repair of tears of the rotator cuff of the shoulder. Factors influencing the result. J Bone Jt Surg 56-A: 14-26
67 Wolfgang GL (1978) Rupture of the musculo-tendinous cuff of the shoulder. Clin Orthop 134: 230-243

Section III. Recurrent Instability

Moderator—Professor Anthony F. DePalma

III.1. Incidence and Prognosis of Shoulder Dislocation: A Preliminary Communication

L. Hovelius, K. Eriksson, H. Fredin, G. Hagberg, J. Weckström and J. Thorling

Dislocation of the shoulder is a well-known condition which has been recognised since earliest times. We are all familiar with the Hippocratic method of reducing the acute dislocation and his method of curing recurrent instability by coagulating the tissues of the inferior part of the joint with a hot iron. Hundreds of papers on the subject have been written since then, but disputes continue as to the best management both for recurrent instability and, in particular, for the young patient with a primary dislocation. Nor do we know the incidence of the disorder in the general population.

This paper deals with the incidence of shoulder joint dislocation (SJD) and also reports the preliminary results of a prospective multi-centre study to investigate the prognosis and treatment of primary dislocation in people under forty years of age.

Incidence

The incidence of shoulder dislocation is very little discussed. Most series relate to *recurrent* dislocation and deal with cases coming to surgery. In these the male : female ratio varies from 2:1 to 6:1 [24, 37, 44, 45, 54, 61] depending upon the selection of patients. Series which contain a high proportion of athletes may report a male : female ratio of 10:1 [60], whilst in series containing a preponderance of multi-directional instability there will be a more equal sex ratio [42]

The relationship between sex ratio and *primary* shoulder dislocation is also of interest. Kazar and Belovsky [25] report that it is age related. For example, in their series in the 20-30 years age group there were five males to each female but after the age of 60 years, primary dislocation was more common in females and after the age of 80 years as many as three-quarters of the patients were women.

What then is the incidence of primary shoulder dislocation in the general population? We have been unable to find any reports of this in the literature although a study of Swedish ice-hockey players revealed an incidence of 8% in the top league [21].

To establish its incidence in the general population we carried out a study of 2092 randomly selected citizens drawn from the whole of Sweden. In the age range of 18-70 years we found an incidence of at least 1.7%, with a preponderance of males in the ratio of 3:1 [22]. Table 1 shows the sex ratio by age group of 264 primary dislocations collected in 28 Swedish hospitals from 1978 through 1979 [23]. In this study the injury is nine times more common in the male in the 21-30 year age group but thereafter the difference decreases with age.

Treatment and Prognosis of Primary Dislocation

One well-known and important feature of the prognosis of primary dislocation relates to its association with age at injury. However, here again there is lack of agreement as to the exact incidence of recurrent instability

Rowe and Sakellarides [56] reported the incidence of recurrence to be: 94% for ages 10-20 years; 79% for ages 21-30 years; 50% for ages 31-40 years; and 14% for ages 51-60 years. By contrast, corresponding figures in the Hungarian series [25] were much lower: 50% for ages 10-20 years; 30% for ages 21-30 years; 7% for ages 31-40; and only 3% for ages 51-60 years.

Most of the recurrences (70%) will occur within 2 years of the initial injury [25,26] and in some series as many as 90% of the recurrences developed within this time [35,38].

Should the shoulder be immobilised after the initial dislocation? Standard orthopaedic textbooks favour this treatment and recommend from four

Table 1. Sex ratio of 264 primary dislocations (1978-79) according to age group

Age in years	Males	Females	Ratio
Less than 20	64	18	3.5 to 1
21 to 30	93	10	9 to 1
31 to 40	55	24	2 to 1
Totals	212	52	4 to 1

to eight weeks immobilisation [21,48,65], although existing studies all seem to be retrospective. One of the most extensive, in which 324 cases were reviewed from the Massachusetts General Hospital in Boston, slightly favoured immobilisation [56], and in another statement Rowe (1979) [53] felt that this method of treatment reduced the rate of recurrence by 15%. Kazar and Belovszky (1969) [25] endorsed the efficacy of immobilisation, but McLoughlin and McLellan (1967) [35] could find no evidence to support the view, nor could Ehgartner (1977) [12] in his series of 102 patients of which 66 were immobilised in plaster and the remainder treated by early mobilisation.

Prominent experts on shoulder surgery in the United States of America also hold differing opinions on the subject. Neer (1977) [43] favours immobilisation for 6-7 weeks, whilst Allman (1975) [2] supports early mobilisation. Rowe's opinion has already been mentioned.

Factors other than age which should also be considered in a discussion of the incidence of recurrent dislocation include fracture of the humeral head or glenoid rim and type of trauma, etc. [51,56], but these are beyond the scope of this paper.

The Present Study

To evaluate the significance of immobilisation and prognosis of shoulder dislocation, a prospective multi-centre study was started in January 1978 in Sweden. Primary dislocations in people aged 40 and younger have been collected from 28 hospitals [23]. They have been treated in two ways: (1) early mobilisation with a sling for not more than one week, and (2) immobilisation by bandaging the arm against the body for three to four weeks. Six of the larger hospitals randomised selection of the type of treatment, whereas the smaller hospitals practised one of the alternatives exclusively. All patients in the immobilisation group were checked after 1-3 months to ascertain the completion of the treatment. By the end of 1979, 264 dislocations had been collected. Table 2 shows the distribution of this material according to treatment and divided into three different age groups. Thirty-nine shoulders were classified as undefined because they could not be placed in either the sling or immobilisation groups. The undefined group included patients who abandoned prescribed mobilisation in less than three weeks, cases on which surgery was done acutely, known alcoholics, and patients with dislocations not reduced within 24 hours.

Table 2. Distribution of early mobilisation (sling) and immobilisation treatment by age group (see text)

Age in years	Immobilised for 3–4 weeks	Early mobilisation (sling)	Indefinable
Less than 22	49	41	
23 to 30	29	39	39
31 to 40	39	28	
Totals	117	108	39

Follow-up review started in January 1980. Two years (± 15 days) after the initial dislocation each patient is sent a questionnaire. The main inquiries concern redislocation, feeling of instability in the shoulder, and whether the patient regards the shoulder as cured. Two-thirds of the patients questioned so far answered the first letter, and most of the remainder responded to a second letter. In some cases the information has been obtained by telephone or even by social welfare committees.

Table 3 shows the results at the end of August 1980 when a little more than one-third of the 264 cases had been followed for two years. A rather large number in ages up to thirty are considered as having an uncertain prognosis. These are cases with *one* redislocation or with a feeling of instability subjectively but no actual recurrent dislocation. Cases with three or more dislocations or subluxations have been defined as recurrent.

So far we have not been able to show that immobilisation of a primary dislocation for 3-4 weeks, as compared to early movement in a sling, prevents the development of chronic shoulder instability.

Table 3. Results of two kinds of treatment (see text) in 90 primary dislocations reviewed two years after injury. Figures in brackets denote shoulders in which surgery has been performed or is planned

Age in years	Treatment	"Cured"	"Unsure"	"Recurrence"
Less than 22	Early mobilisation	7	7	5 (1)
	Immobilisation	7	6	5 (2)
23 to 30	Early mobilisation	13	3	2 (1)
	Immobilisation	6	2	2 (1)
31 to 40	Early mobilisation	9	0	0
	Immobilisation	12	2	2
Totals		54	20	16

What can be said of the prognosis of primary shoulder dislocation? Table 4 shows the two-year follow-up of 101 dislocations out of 264. Included are those shoulders in the undefined treatment group which have also completed two years since injury. It will be seen that in patients under the age of 20 years numbers are equally spread between those who regard themselves as cured, those who have developed recurrent instability and those with a doubtful prognosis. In the age group 21-30 years a greater proportion (60%) regard themselves as cured, and in the older groups of 31-40-year-old patients nearly 80% were cured. The incidence of recurrent dislocation in the later groups is similar (20% and 15%), but the pool of shoulders with an unsure prognosis from which further recurrent dislocators might come is larger in the younger of the two groups (20% to 5%).

When discussing the results of this preliminary report it should be remembered that thus far only a little more than one-third of the 264 dislocations have been followed for two years. Earlier papers [25,56] have shown that about 70% of all recurrences develop within two years of injury. Without doubt the group with unsure prognosis will become smaller with time as some shoulders develop recurrent instability and others become secure. It may also be that some cases in the "cured" groups will also redislocate after more than two years.

Table 4. The prognosis of 101 primary dislocations out of 264 as far followed up two years after the initial dislocation.[6]

Age in years	Cured	Prognosis unsure	Recurrent dislocations
≤20	11	11	11
21-30	25	7	8
31-40	22	2	4

III.2. Conservative Treatment of Shoulder Dislocation in Young Males

Bruce Yoneda, Peter Welsh and D.L. Macintosh

Recurrence of anterior dislocation of the shoulder is generally thought to be related to factors of age, sex, and force of injury. Rowe [51] reported 84% recurrence of dislocations occurring initially in the second decade and 72% of those occurring in the third, whereas only 12% recurred after age fifty. Recurrence is definitely more common in men, with ratios varying from 4:1 to 6:1 in series quoted by Mosely [39]. Bankart [5] believed recurrences were more common in injuries resulting from direct violence, whereas Rowe [51] reported more recurrences in twisting or forced abduction injuries and also believed that recurrences were less common in more violent initial injuries.

Immobilisation following reduction is generally thought to have little bearing on the rate of recurrence. White [67] recommended no immobilisation. McLaughlin and Cavallaro [34] concluded the length of immobilisation had little bearing on recurrence rate. Rowe [51] reported a lower incidence of recurrence in patients treated by four weeks in a sling or three weeks in a sling and swathe, with more prolonged immobilisation not significantly decreasing recurrence. In particular, the high recurrence rate of patients in the second and third decade seemed unaffected by the duration of immobilisation. Opposing this concept of recurrence rate unrelated to immobilisation, Watson-Jones [64] strongly felt that strict immobilisation for at least three weeks resulted in no recurrence.

Clinical Material

In accord with the feelings of Watson-Jones, we think that the recurrence rate of primary trau-

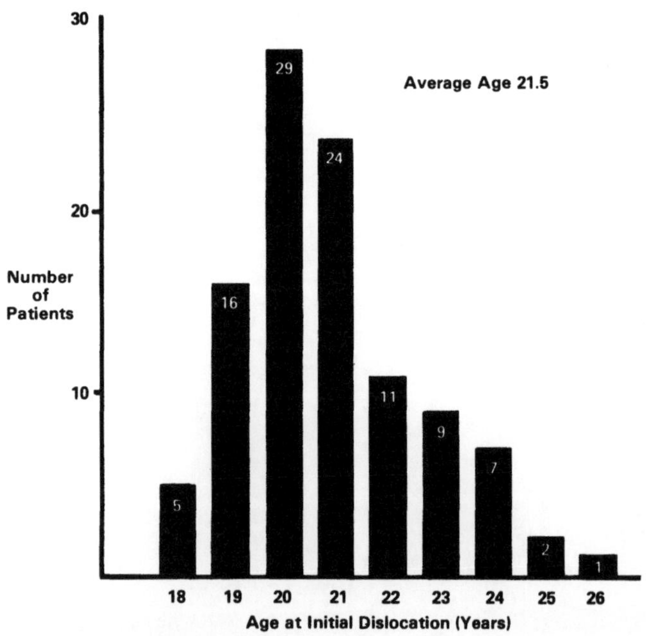

Fig. 1. Age at initial dislocation in 104 patients

Table 1. Follow-up of patients after shoulder dislocation

Year of dislocation	No. of patients followed-up	Year of dislocation	No. of patients followed-up
1952	1	1964	5
1953	0	1965	6
1954	2	1966	7
1955	0	1967	8
1956	2	1968	7
1957	3	1969	6
1958	3	1970	5
1959	4	1971	7
1960	5	1972	6
1961	4	1973	6
1962	5	1974	7
1963	5		

matic anterior dislocation in young males can be minimised by strict immobilisation for five weeks. Between 1952 and 1974, 212 University of Toronto students were treated for primary shoulder dislocation. All patients were males and all sustained thier dislocations during athletic activities, but owing to the long period of follow-up it was not possible to ascertain the exact mechanism of dislocation (direct blow versus twisting or forced abduction injuries). All were assessed at the University of Toronto Hart House Clinic. The arm was rested in a sling and swathe for five weeks. An exercise programme of six weeks was then instituted with an emphasis on no abduction past 90°. Exercises consisted of the "4*P*s": pendulum slings, wall pulleys, push-ups, and punching bag. Follow-up was obtained on 104 patients. Average age at time of dislocation was 21.5 years (Fig. 1). Average duration of follow-up was 13.1 years (Table 1).

Results

Patients were divided into two main groups (Fig. 2). In Group I, consisting of 86 patients (82.7%), there was no history of recurrence. They were further divided into subgroups: excellent (normal range and motion, no limitation of sports

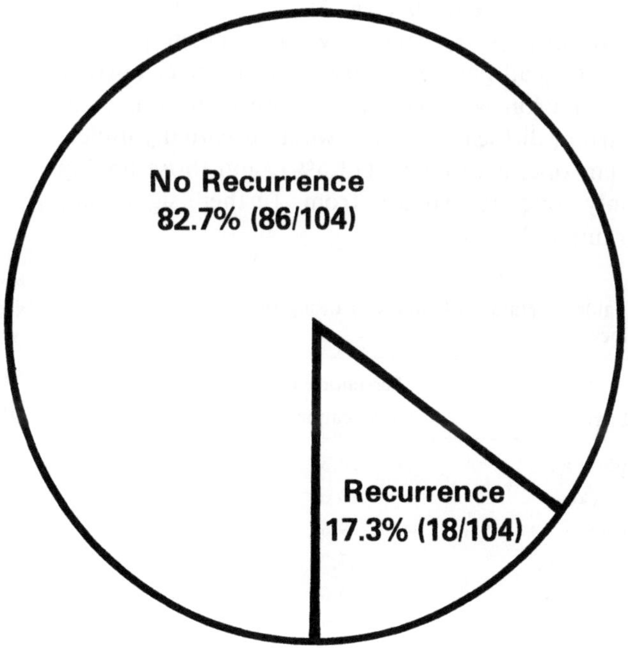

Fig. 2. Classification of patients according to results

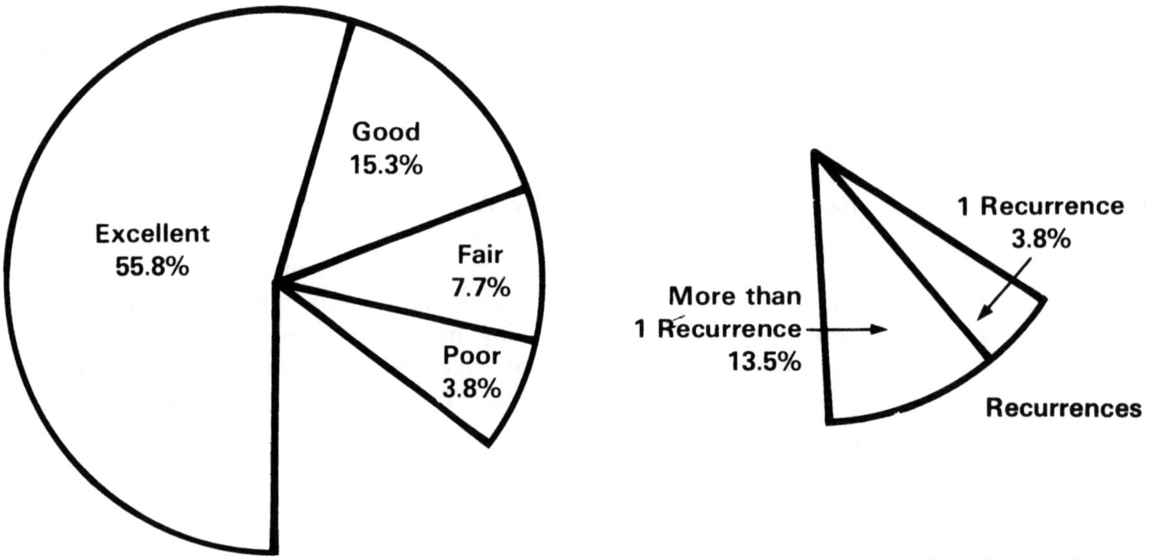

Fig. 3. Classification of patients' results according to groups

or occupation); good (approximately 25% limitation of external rotation with some limitation of sports but no occupational restriction); fair (50% limitation of external rotation with some need for adjustments in sports and heavy occupations). These first three subgroups were generally satisfied with their shoulders (Fig. 3). Patients were placed in the subgroup of poor if they had much limitation of motion, sports, and occupation and were generally dissatisfied and/or experienced apprehension with abduction and external rotation movements (Fig. 3).

In Group II, consisting of eighteen patients (17.3%) all gave a history of recurrence. Further subdivision was made into those going on to recurrent dislocation, all of whom eventually underwent operative repair (13.5%), and those having only one recurrence from further significant trauma (3.8%).

Table 2. Nature of injuries causing dislocations

Sport	Percentage of dislocations
Football	60.6
Hockey	10.6
Rugby	9.6
Wrestling	7.7
Basketball	3.8
Other	7.7

Football was the commonest provoking injury, causing 63 (60.6%) of the dislocations (Table 2). Other sports included hockey (10.6%), rugby (9.6%), wrestling (7.7%), basketball (3.8%), and an assortment of weight-training, boxing, martial arts, broomball, and water-polo injuries.

Table 3. Second dislocation provoked by significant trauma in four Group II patients who suffered only one recurrence

Age at 1st dislocation (years)	Age at 2nd dislocation (years)	Cause of 2nd dislocation
25	30	Fall from roof
23	30	Motor vehicle accident
22	24	Football injury
19	20	Football injury

Of the 18 patients experiencing recurrence, four sustained only a second dislocation provoked by significant trauma (Table 3). These occurred at 1, 2, 5, and 7 years respectively after initial dislocation. Although they were treated elsewhere with their second dislocation, each was immobilised for at least three weeks and none subsequently recurred. These four cases might almost then be regarded as a further instance of acute "primary" dislocation in that the provoking trauma was sufficiently violent to produce dislocation in a previously uninjured shoulder. In this case the overall recurrence rate, although stated as 17.3%, might also be regarded actually as less than this and closer to 13.5%, the number actually necessitating stabilisation.

Conclusions

Primary shoulder dislocation in young males has generally been considered of poor prognosis, going on to a high recurrence rate and inevitable operative repair. Our review of 104 males of average age 21 years has shown that with strict immobilisation for five weeks that the recurrence rate can be minimised to 17.3%.

It is therefore recommended that strict immobilisation following traumatic primary dislocation of the shoulder is worth while in reducing the necessity for surgical stabilisation and that a supervised rehabilitation programme can return the athlete to full capability without compromise in the vast majority of cases.

III.3. The Early Complications of Anterior Dislocation in the Middle Aged and Elderly Patient

J.R. Johnson and J.I.L. Bayley

Dislocation of the shoulder is often thought to be an injury of the young adult, but in reality as many primary dislocations of the shoulder occur after the age of 45 years as before [52]. However, the complications of anterior shoulder dislocation in these two groups are different. Under the age of 45 years the most common complication is recurrent instability, whilst in the over-45-year-old age group dislocation is more likely to be complicated by rotator cuff tear or fracture of the greater tuberosity. The explanation for this difference is that dislocation in a young person causes the anterior joint capsule to give way, whilst in the middle aged or elderly, the posterior supports fail leading to avulsion of the rotator cuff or fracture of the greater tuberosity. It is also in this latter group that nerve injuries are more likely to be encountered [32].

Dislocation with Fracture of the Greater Tuberosity

In a recent series at the Royal National Orthopaedic Hospital the incidence of greater tuberosity fracture after anterior shoulder dislocation was 24%, which is similar to the incidence of 30% quoted by Watson-Jones (1960) [66]. In most cases the tuberosity comes to lie in a perfect position when the dislocation is reduced, but in a few cases it is displaced beneath the acromion. Not uncommonly its presence there on an anteroposterior radiograph is obscured by the humeral head and the diagnosis is missed. Even if the displaced fragment is noted, our reliance upon radiographs causes us to neglect the soft tissues and we fail to realise that the tuberosity has been pulled medially by its attached segment of rotator

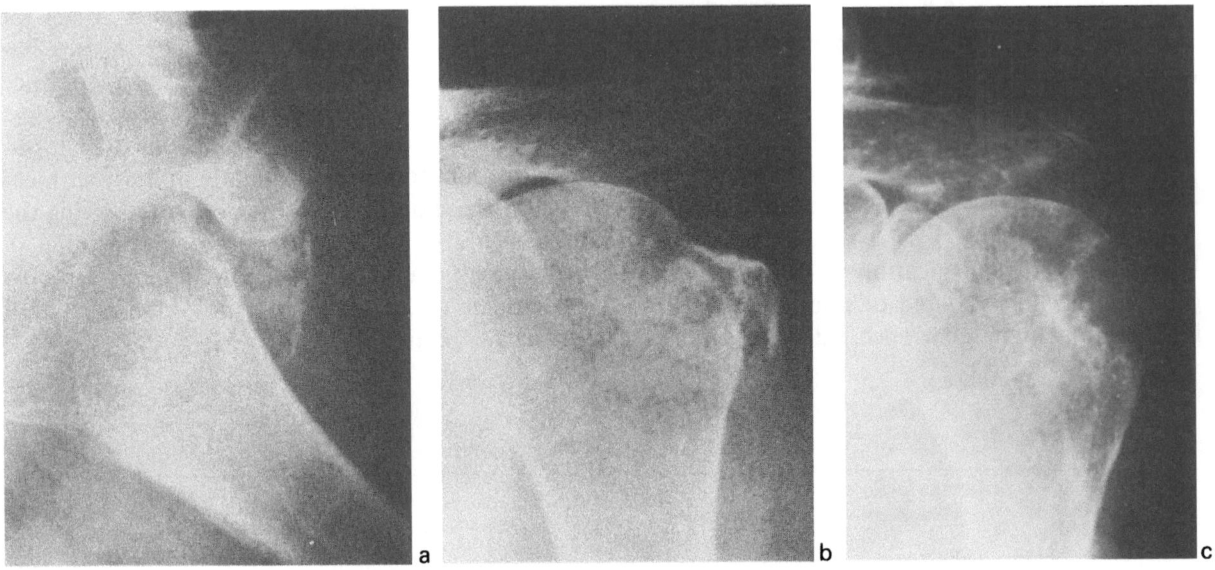

Fig. 1.a Anterior dislocation of the shoulder complicated by fracture of the greater tuberosity **b** Post-manipulation showing good alignment **c** After further dislocation and reduction the greater tuberosity fragment is medially displaced. Note the defect in the upper humerus from which the tuberosity has been avulsed

cuff. It should be emphasised that the visible avulsed fragment in fact represents the radiographic sign of a rotator cuff avulsion.

If the significance of the injury is appreciated, early open reduction and repair are easily accomplished, but failure to recognise the condition often leads to disastrous late results. McLaughlin [32] (1963) has shown that displacement of the greater tuberosity by more than one centimetre leads to a poor functional outcome.

During the past five years, six cases of neglected displaced tuberosity fracture following dislocation have been referred to the shoulder clinic at the Royal National Orthopaedic Hospital. A typical sequence of events is shown in Fig. 1 in which a 76-year-old woman suffered an anterior dislocation of the left shoulder. A post-manipulation radiograph showed good alignment of the fractured tuberosity, but unfortunately the shoulder redislocated and following further reduction the tuberosity remained widely displaced. The significance of this was not appreciated and at referral two years later the patient continued to complain of pain with considerable limitation of movement. An attempt was made to reconstitute the rotator cuff, as a result of which she obtained good pain relief with some improvement in range of active movement.

Nevertheless the outcome of late surgical intervention in these cases leaves much to be desired. The aim of operation in our patients was to relieve pain and in this we were largely successful but it is less easy to restore function because of dense scarring and retraction of the rotator cuff. The inevitable disability which ensues is the most dissatisfying when the excellent results which follow early repair are recalled.

Dislocation with Rotator Cuff Injury

Disinsertion or rupture of the rotator cuff without bone injury is often overlooked when it occurs with anterior dislocation. London [28] has drawn attention to the difficulties of diagnosis, and certainly the apparently normal plain radiographs may delude the unwary. Rotator cuff rupture should always be suspected in the middle-aged or elderly patient when recovery of active shoulder movement appears delayed. The diagnosis can be confirmed by arthrography and, if appropriate, surgical repair is undertaken.

Dislocation with Nerve Injury

Most articles on anterior dislocation of the shoulder make reference to associated peripheral nerve injury, in particular to lesions of the circumflex (axillary) nerve. However, there is little information on the incidence of this complication. Watson-Jones [66] suggests an incidence of 15%, a figure similar to that of Mumenthaler and Schliack [41]. More recently Pasila et al [46] in a series of 238 patients found 21% with nerve lesions of whom 9% had circumflex nerve palsies. Blom and Dahlback [6], in a series of 73 patients, found an incidence of 18% by the use of electromyographic (EMG) testing. This probably gives a more accurate figure for the incidence of the complication particularly as they found sensory loss to be a poor diagnostic sign. The brachial plexus may also be injured in dislocation of the shoulder. Sauer et al. [58] give an incidence of 5% in a large series of patients.

Being low-velocity injuries in continuity, most of these nerve palsies make a good functional recovery [36,58], and all of Blom and Dahlback's cases showed electromyographic evidence of regeneration.

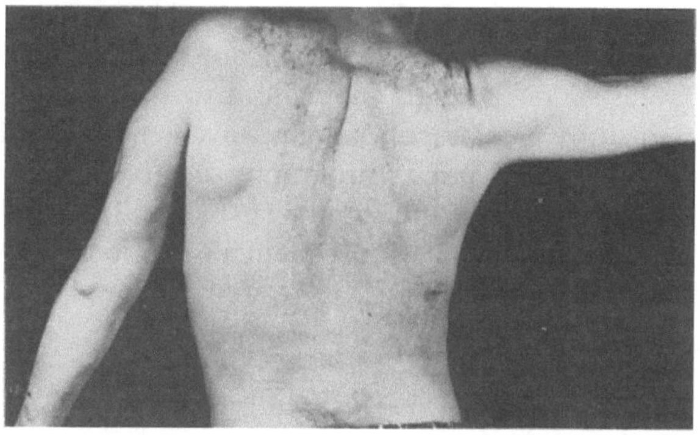

Fig. 2. Illustrative Case (GM). Loss of active elevation in abduction

Dislocation with Combined Rotator Cuff Rupture and Nerve Palsy

Although deltoid paralysis following anterior dislocation usually recovers, return of shoulder function sometimes does not. In Blom and Dahlback's series, in spite of electromyographic evidence of nerve regeneration, 60% of their patients continued to have reduced function after many months. To highlight one cause for this discrepancy we report here our experience with five such cases seen in a shoulder referral clinic in a recent two-year period (1978-79).

Illustrative Case (GE). This 54-year-old company secretary was assaulted three months prior to referral sustaining an anterior dislocation of the left shoulder complicated by circumflex nerve palsy. The dislocation was appropriately treated, but at presentation he continued to complain of pain and loss of active movement. On examination there was gross wasting not only of the deltoid but also of the spinati and loss of sensation in the circumflex nerve territory. Active abduction

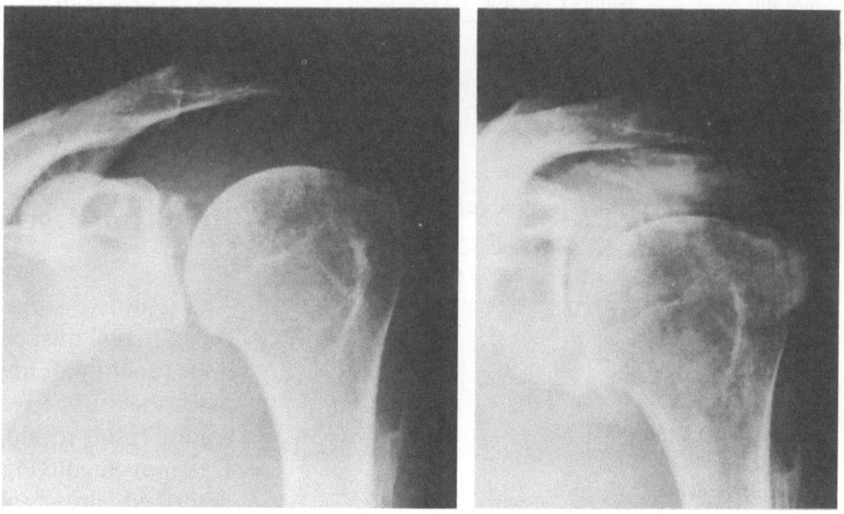

Fig. 3. Illustrative Case (GM). Arthrograph showing rotator cuff tear

was to 20° (Fig. 2). Electromyography confirmed denervation of the deltoid but not of the spinati. Eventual recovery of the deltoid was not accompanied by a corresponding improvement in shoulder function, and arthrography demonstrated a major rupture of the rotator cuff (Fig. 3). Repair was attempted, but subsequent disruption eventually led to arthrodesis.

Clinical Material

There were 4 males and 1 female. Their age at the time of injury ranged from 45 to 55 years with a mean of 51 years. The length of history from the time of injury to presentation at the shoulder clinic ranged from 3 months to 2 years with a mean of 9 months. The mechanism and type of injury is shown in Table 1, and Table 2 records the symptoms at referral.

Table 1. Circumflex palsy/rotator cuff rupture: mechanism of injury

	Mechanism	Injury
G.E.	Assault	Dislocation
G.L.	Fall	Dislocation + fracture of greater tuberosity
J.P.	Water-Skiing	Dislocation
K.C.	Fall from ladder	Dislocation
S.P.	Fall from ladder	Dislocation

Table 2. Circumflex palsy/rotator cuff rupture: symptoms at presentation

Symptom	Number of cases
Pain	4
Loss of Movement	5
Sensory Loss	3

Table 3. Circumflex palsy/rotator cuff rupture: signs at presentation

Signs	Number of cases
Wasting	
Deltoid	4
Spinati	4
Loss of Movement	
Abduction less than 45°	5
Sensory Loss	1
Circumflex nerve	

Although loss of active movement, particularly abduction, was a universal complaint, nearly all patients also experienced pain on movement. Signs at referral are summarised in Table 3. It should be noted that in 4 of the 5 cases there was wasting of the spinati muscles in addition to that of the deltoid. This was often marked and developed rapidly following injury. Its presence raised the possibility of either a traction lesion of the brachial plexus or of a double nerve injury. Active movement, particularly elevation in abduction, was always less than 45°. Objective sensory loss was found in only 1 case, although 2 other patients had noted subjective symptoms of hypoaesthesia over the outer aspect of the shoulder (Table 2).

Investigation

Supportive investigations included plain radiographs and when indicated, electromyography and arthrography. The latter was used in 4 cases, on each occasion demonstrating a rotator cuff rupture. Electromyography was performed on 4 shoulders and revealed total denervation of the deltoid in 1 and partial denervation in 3. In no instance was there evidence of denervation outside the territory of the circumflex nerve.

Indications for Surgery

Surgical repair of the rotator cuff was contemplated when recovery of shoulder function failed to parallel recovery of the deltoid. Operation was therefore deferred until the latter was well established. It became necessary in 4 of the 5 shoulders.

Results of Operation

The results of surgery were assessed by combining the patients' own evaluation in terms of pain relief and functional improvement with an objective assessment of active movement. Two patients with a good result regained a satisfactory range of pain-free movement (Fig. 4). The poor result has been described already (Illustrative Case) and was so

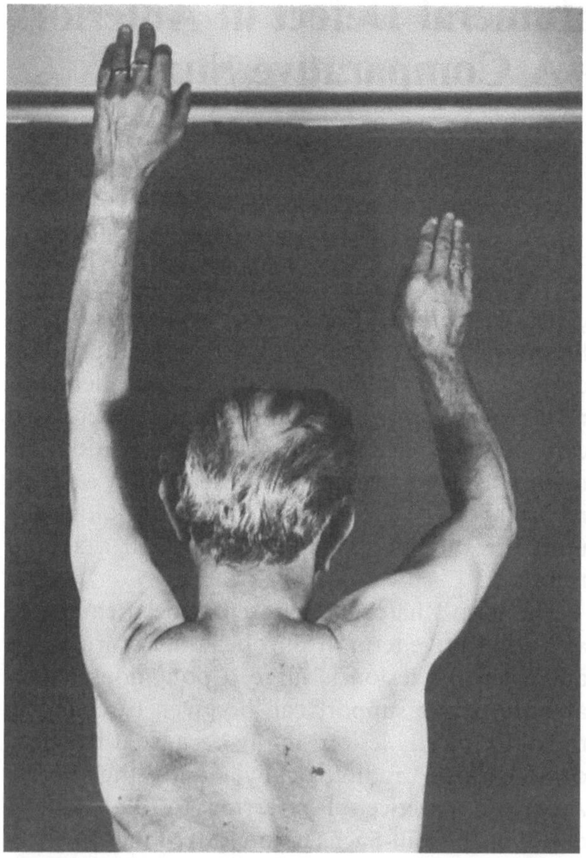

Fig. 4. Case No.5 (SP). Good result following rotator cuff repair. Note the transacromial scar

Table 4. Circumflex palsy/rotator cuff rupture: results of surgery

Results	Number of cases
Good	2
Fair	1
Poor	1

classified because the cuff repair failed. Arthrodesis gave him a useful shoulder and allowed him to resume his sport of hockey.

Summary and Conclusions

It is not generally appreciated that 50% of acute shoulder dislocations occur in patients over 45 years of age. In this group early complications differ from those encountered in the younger age groups.

Fracture of the greater tuberosity is a well-recognised complication in the older patient, but despite this we have treated six cases in whom the injury was missed or its significance not recognised. Early fixation of the displaced fragment gives a good functional result [4,32] whereas the results of late repair in terms of function leave much to be desired.

Rotator cuff rupture without tuberosity fracture is also well documented following dislocation. Reeves [49] found 27 cuff ruptures in 47 dislocations. A high incidence of suspicion in this group coupled with intelligent use of arthrography should allow the diagnosis to be made and some improvement of function can be expected from surgery in about 50% of cases.

The incidence of circumflex nerve palsy appears to be about 10%-20% [6,28,46,66]. Even in complete paresis spontaneous reinnervation may be expected up to one year after injury in most cases [3,6]. However, this is not always followed by restoration of shoulder function. Blom and Dahlback [6] found that 60% of their cases, most of whom were over 50 years of age, continued to suffer reduced active mobility of the shoulder. One cause of this discrepancy between recovering nerve function and failure to regain active movement may be an associated rotator cuff rupture. Ludin et al. [29] performed arthrography and electromyography on 13 patients suspected of having simple rotator cuff rupture and found that 8 patients showed evidence of a peripheral nerve lesion, 5 of which involved the circumflex nerve. Pasila et al. [46]) have reported a further 4 cases. We have seen 5 cases in the past eighteen months in which return of shoulder function failed to keep pace with deltoid recovery following circumflex nerve palsy secondary to anterior dislocation. The most noticeable physical sign was rapid and marked wasting of the spinati muscles in addition to the deltoid; a feature which may obscure the diagnosis of rotator cuff rupture by raising the possibility of a more extensive neurological injury. All the patients were over 45 years of age.

Arthrography and electromyography are useful investigations in these shoulders, both to exclude denervation of the wasted rotator cuff muscles and to reveal the underlying rupture which can itself be responsible for the marked wasting of the spinati muscles. Repair of the torn cuff is a worthwhile procedure which can restore function to a shoulder whose performance, would otherwise remain considerably reduced.

III.4. The Radiology of the Humeral Defect in Anterior Dislocation of the Shoulder — A Comparative Study

D.J. Stoker

The nature of the injuries sustained during anterior dislocation of the shoulder has, in general, been accepted for many years [7,11]. They include rupture or detachment of the anterior part of the capsule, usually close to its medial attachment, sometimes a separation of the glenoid labrum, and a depressed infraction of the cortex of the head and anatomical neck of the humerus, sometimes erroneously referred to as an avulsion fracture [16]. This paper is concerned with the radiological demonstration of this latter injury.

Early pathological observations were made in 1891 by Flower [13], who examined 41 specimens in museums in London, 32 of which were anterior (subcoracoid) dislocations. In this strange collection he observed the groove on the posterolateral aspect of the humerus between the articular part of the head and the greater tuberosity. He ascribed this to resorption of bone militated by changed pressure between the glenoid and the humerus.

In 1886, Francis Caird of Edinburgh read a paper before the Medico-Chirurgical Society of Edinburgh, published the following year [8], in which he stated that the defect sustained was an indentation fracture caused by the hard glenoid rim at the time of dislocation. He further stated that the true subcoracoid dislocation was *always* associated with an indentation fracture of the head of the humerus.

With the discovery of X-rays, successful attempts were made to demonstrate the defect radiographically [47]. However, the most comprehensive study was made by Hermodsson (1934) [19] and subsequently translated into English [40].

Although well described in the literature, the radiological evidence of the defect is often overlooked by orthopaedic surgeons and radiologists, mainly because unless it is very large, the humeral defect is not visible on routine anteroposterior and lateral projections of the shoulder.

Even now the designation of the lesion is not generally agreed. For years, in the European literature, it was merely described as "the typical defect". Some authors have called it the defect of recurrent anterior dislocation, a misnomer, as it can and does occur during a single dislocation; the main reason for its first identification in cases of recurrence is that it is not sought radiologically until the shoulder has been dislocated a second time.

The term "hatchet" defect has been employed as a descriptive term in European literature and is apt when the lesion is large. Eponymous names abound. Little support can be given to changing the name of any lesion simply because it has been demonstrated radiologically, and the North American practice of referring to the humeral defect as the Hill-Sachs lesion [20] cannot be justified on any ground.

If it is accepted as desirable that the defect should be demonstrated in support of a diagnosis, then it should be possible to demonstrate it in all cases [19]. In truth, in many cases of dislocation the facts are known and recorded, with radiological confirmation of anterior location of the humeral head. In others, the direction of the dislocation may be in doubt. It is also possible that the size of the defect reflects the degree of instability of the humerus.

Not all studies have approached the accuracy of Hermodsson's carefully planned demonstration of the defect in profile in two planes. Golding [14] recorded an accuracy of only 58%, using standard rotational projections.

Despite the accepted precision of Hermodsson's views, they are not easy to undertake or interpret. We therefore set out to evaluate and compare the two most popular views used at the Royal National Orthopaedic Hospital in the investigation of this injury.

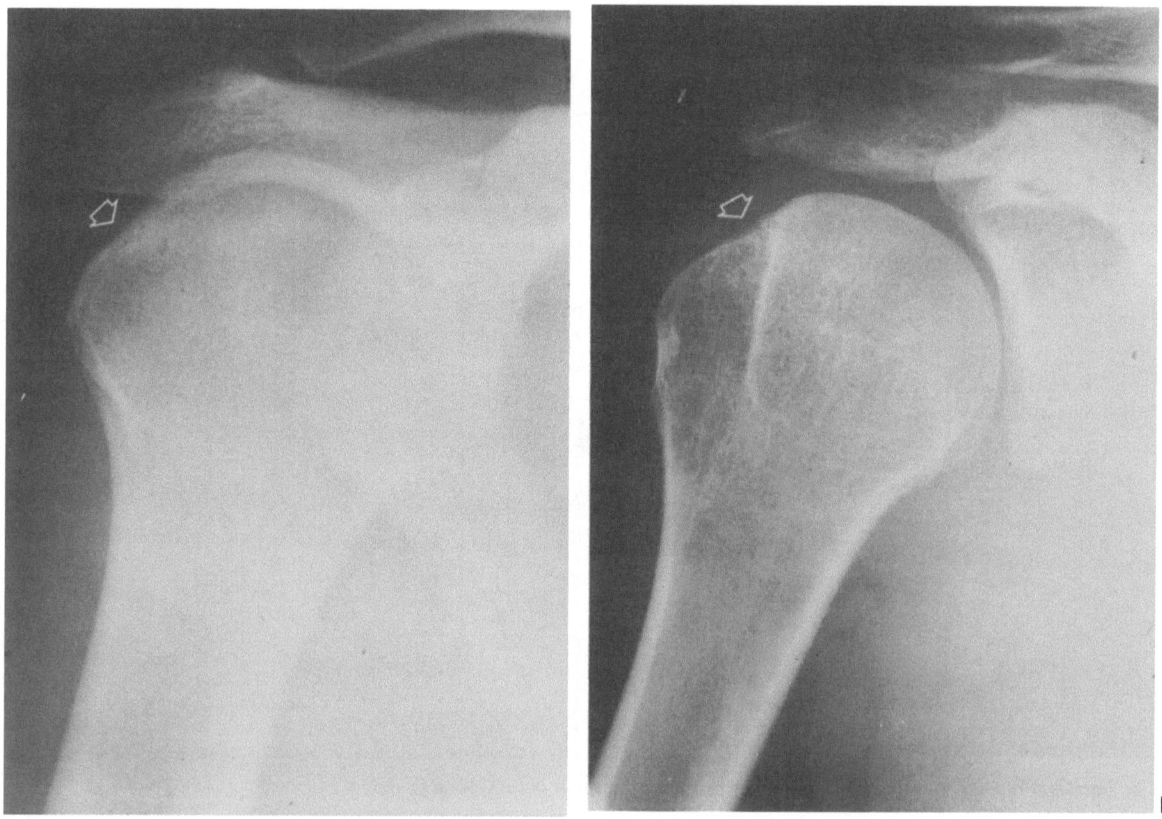

a b

Fig. 1. Humeral defects in 60° internal rotation projection: (a) small defect; (b) large defect

Material and Methods

Two series of X-ray films from 30 subjects were examined, 13 following anterior dislocation and 17 in whom no dislocation of the shoulder had been sustained. In one group a film in 60° of internal rotation and in the other a notch view (Stryker projection) was assessed. (The technique evolved from ideas expressed by Commander William S. Stryker, Medical Corps, United States Navy, in 1953. In their article describing the technique, Hall et al. [16] expressed a wish to avoid eponymous designation, but the term "Stryker view" has been in use at our hospital for many years and is unlikely to be abandoned at this time.) The projection is obtained with the patient lying in a supine position with his hand on the top of his head and the forearm and arm in the parasagittal plane. In this position the arm is found to be flexed slightly above 90°. The projection is slightly altered from the original description [16] by angling the tube 30° cephalad [62] and not 10°, in the belief that this improves visualisation of the notch defect and more readily distinguishes it from the normal depression of the anatomical neck. The projection demonstrates both the posterosuperior and anteroinferior aspects of the head and neck of the humerus.

The 60% internal rotation and notch views were assessed without knowledge of the subject's diagnosis and the presence or absence of a notch defect was recorded. These were initially graded as:

Grade I : erosion or roughening of cortex.

Grade II : small notch.

Grade III: large notch.

It became apparent on reviewing the results that erosion or roughening of the anatomical neck (so-called Grade I) was not directly related to anterior dislocation and was either a normal or a non-specific finding. Re-grading was therefore made only of a large or a small defect. Examples of these are shown for both projections in Figs. 1 and 2. The results of the assessment are shown in Table 1.

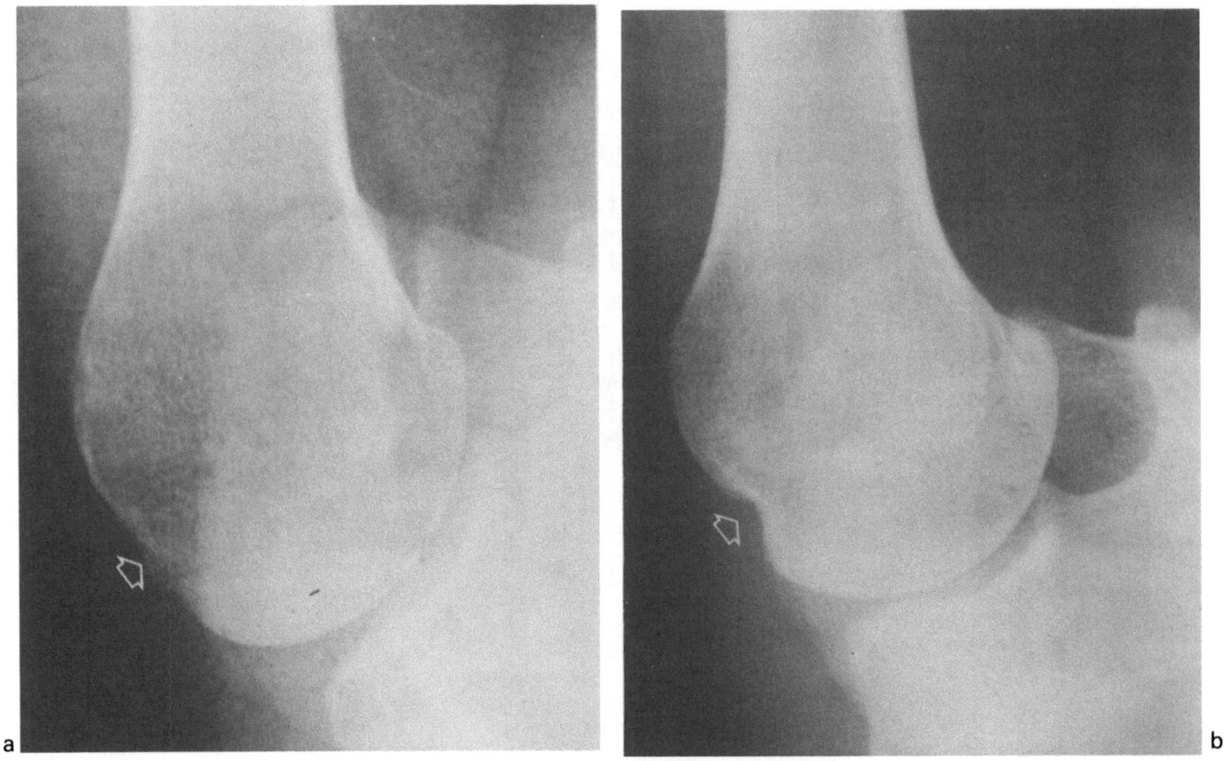

Fig. 2. Humeral defects in notch view (Stryker) projection **a** small defect; **b** large defect

Results

The findings indicate that in 60° internal rotation views no false positive results occurred, but in 5 of 13 (38.5%) the notch was not demonstrated. The one false positive finding in the Stryker views was considered to be due to erroneous interpretation of a subcortical cyst as a defect (not likely to be repeated since the problem has been defined) and 2 of 13 (15%) false negative results.

Taken as a single view, therefore, the notch or Stryker view is less likely to fail to demonstrate the humeral notch than the 60° internal rotation projection. It is also a projection which is easier for the radiographer to reproduce, as it does not require assessment of angles of rotation. It is clear from this study that, using either of the single views, it is not possible to detect the minor infraction from the normal roughening of the anatomical neck. To demonstrate defects in all cases, it seems necessary to obtain two tangential views of the notch, preferably at right-angles to one another [19].

Table 1. Results of radiological assessment

	60° internal rotation view	Notch view (Stryker)
Correctly diagnosed as normal	17	16
Correctly diagnosed as showing a notch	8	11
False positive	0	1
False negative	5	2

Summary

Despite historical evidence that a characteristic notch appears following anterior dislocation as a result of an indentation fracture of the posterosuperior aspect of the head of the humerus, this lesion often remains unrecognised because of radiological shortcomings. Using a single "notch" (Stryker) view, it was possible to demonstrate the lesion in 85% of cases in a random trial.

III.5. Technical Aspects of the Bristow Repair for Recurrent Anterior Shoulder Instability

B.E. Albrektsson, P. Herberts, L. Körner, C.R. Lamm and B.E. Zachrisson

The Bristow repair for recurrent anterior dislocation of the shoulder was first described by Helfet [18]. The operation is known to cause minimal postoperative loss of shoulder motion and has been used mainly in otherwise healthy athletes. The results have been rewarding [10,17,27] particularly when the main indication for repair has been post-traumatic shoulder instability [30]. The results of the Bristow procedure in spontaneous shoulder instability have however, been less predictable [10,27].

This paper reports our five-year experience with the operation which we have used in an unselected group of patients with anterior shoulder instability, i.e. post-traumatic as well as spontaneous dislocations. As might be expected, the results in the latter type are less satisfactory than in the post-traumatic group. The complications and recurrences will be discussed in relation to the technical aspects of the repair.

Material and Methods

From January 1975 through November 1979, 36 Bristow repairs were performed in our clinic on 34 patients. The results were followed up 6-60 months (mean 25.4 months) after operation. In one patient both shoulders were previously stabilised by other methods, and these two repairs were therefore not included in the review. Three cases were lost to follow-up for other reasons. In all, therefore, there were 31 shoulder repairs in 30 patients. The method of follow-up consisted of a detailed questionnaire, physical examination, and a radiographic assessment. Of the 30 patients, 21 were men and 9 women. The right shoulder was involved 18 times and the left side 13 times; there were 20 dominant and 11 non-dominant shoulders. Age at first luxation ranged from 14 to 40 years (mean 22.1 years), and at operation from 19 to 52 years (mean 27.6 years). To determine whether the instability was post-traumatic or spontaneous, we carefully investigated the force responsible for the primary dislocation in each patient (Table 1) as well as hereditary and constitutional factors. We considered falls, blows, and firm resistance to movements as adequate trauma for dislocation, but luxations after mere movement or occurring during sleep were judged to result from inadequate trauma. Six patients had close relatives with shoulder instability, 11 had dislocated another joint, and 12 had excessive hyperextension of knees and finger joints.

Table 1. Force responsible for first and subsequent dislocations

	Primary incident	Subsequent dislocations	Shoulders
Group A	Adequate	Inadequate	15
Group B	Adequate	Adequate	3
Group C	Inadequate	Inadequate	13
Total			31

Nineteen patients were not immobilised after the initial injury; the rest were immobilised in a Velpeau dressing for 2-4 weeks. Regardless of the initial treatment, 14 patients considered themselves stable after the first dislocation, while 19 never felt stable. None of these 19 primarily unstable shoulders experienced adequate trauma at redislocation. The frequency of subsequent episodes is summarised in Table 2 for the whole series.

Table 2. Number of dislocations before operation

Number of dislocations	Shoulders
More than 10	19
6–10	5
2–5	7
Total	31

At follow-up the patients were asked to grade their results as good, fair or poor. In addition an objective grading based on physical examination was performed [52]. Good results included not more than 25% limitation of outward rotation, freedom from pain, and ability to take part in sports or occupational activities without restriction. Fair results included a maximum of 50% limitation of outward rotation and 30% of flexion, and moderate restriction of sports and heavy work. Results graded as poor included shoulders which subsequently redislocated or which experienced persistent postoperative instability, pain, and severe limitation of activities or motion.

Radiographic follow-up included anteroposterior, lateral, oblique lateral, and modified axial projections. The two latter views were taken tangential to the base of the transplant and were used to achieve a clear picture of the union and position of the transposed coracoid [26]. The radiographic examination also included an assessment of passive stability under the image-intensifier with videotape record of the manoeuvre. At provocation the examiner rotated the arm fully outward in 90° of abduction. The provocation was discontinued if the patient felt pain or subluxation.

Surgery

At surgery, the procedure described by Collins and Wilde [10] was followed in most shoulders although in 8 cases the subscapularis was divided perpendicular to its fibres [30]. Inspection of the joint was reported in only 18 shoulders. The mean operation time was 89 minutes (standard deviation 28 minutes), and the average blood loss was 200 ml at surgery and 80 ml in the suction drainage bottle which was always used. Patients were confined to hospital for an average of 4.2 days and were immobilised postoperatively in a Velpeau dressing for a mean of 31 days (standard deviation 5.1 days).

The indications for repair as stated in the records were instability or recurrent dislocation in 29 shoulders and pain in 2 shoulders. The frequency of dislocation is shown in Table 2. Nine different surgeons performed the operations: Five performed three or more operations each; four performed only one each.

Table 3. Patient and examiner ratings at review

	Subjective (patient) assessment	Objective (examiner) assessment
Good	25 (80.6%)	22 (71.0%)
Fair	3 (9.7%)	5 (16.1%)
Poor	3 (9.7%)	4 (12.9%)
Totals	31 shoulders	31 shoulders

Results

The subjective (patient) and objective (examiner) postoperative ratings are given in Table 3. The incidence of redislocation or persistent instability was 5 of 31, (16.1%). All 5 patients with a recurrence or persistently unstable shoulder came from the spontaneously unstable group, i.e. they had not experienced adequate trauma at their first dislocation or later. Clinical features of the patients in which the procedure failed are given in Table 4.

Eight patients of 13 (61.5%) in the group with spontaneously unstable shoulders were stable after surgery. No patient achieving radiographically verified bony healing of a transplant in the proper position had any postoperative complaints of

Table 4. Features of patients with subsequent redislocation or persistent instability

Patients	Features
(1) Redislocation	Spontaneous instability including other joints. Musculocutaneous nerve damage at operation. Adequate violence at redislocation. Further bone block failed.
(2) Redislocation	Spontaneous instability including other joints plus general ligamentous laxity. Transplant migrated.
(3) Redislocation	Spontaneous instability including other joints plus general ligamentous laxity. Bony union of malpositioned transplant (too medially on scapular neck).
(4) Persistent Instability	Spontaneous instability with general ligamentous laxity. Transplant migrated.
(5) Persistent Instability	Spontaneous instability including other joints. Fibrous healing of transplant.

Table 5. Limitation of outward rotation at 90 degrees of abduction after operation

Limitation of movement (degrees)	Shoulders
0– 9	15
10–19	6
20–29	5
30–39	3
40–49	2
Total	31

Table 6. Radiographic evaluation of transplant

Radiological Status of Transplant	Shoulders
Bony Union	15
Fibrous Union	8
Transplant Migrated	6
Transplant Resorbed	1
Transplant Removed at Reoperation	1
Total	31

instability or pain, regardless of the type of preoperative instability.

Two patients had neural complications. In one the musculocutaneous nerve was partially trapped by a suture in the subscapularis. Neuritis with pain and paralysis developed postoperatively. After neurolysis most of these symptoms subsided. In the other the infraspinatus muscle atrophied postoperatively although the patient was symptom-free. The suprascapular nerve was probably damaged by a retractor during the exceptionally long operation (3 hours).

The postoperative limitation of outward rotation is shown in Table 5 and in most cases is negligible. In one patient in whom the subscapularis was divided perpendicular to its fibres and sutured with an overlap, the outward rotation was severely diminished.

Radiographic evaluation is summarised in Table 6. The best projections for examination of the transplant were the oblique lateral and the modified axial views. Bony union between coracoid and the collum scapulae occurred in 15 cases (Fig. 1): in 8 cases the union was judged to be fibrous (Fig. 2) because of the presence of a small gap between the transplant and the scapula; in 6 the transplant had migrated from its original position on the collum (Fig. 3), all 6 transplants having been broken during surgery. At follow-up 2 transplants were not radiographically visible; one had totally resorbed and the other had been excised in a previous reoperation for pain.

Nine screws were too short (did not engage the posterior cortex), and 3 were too long (passed the

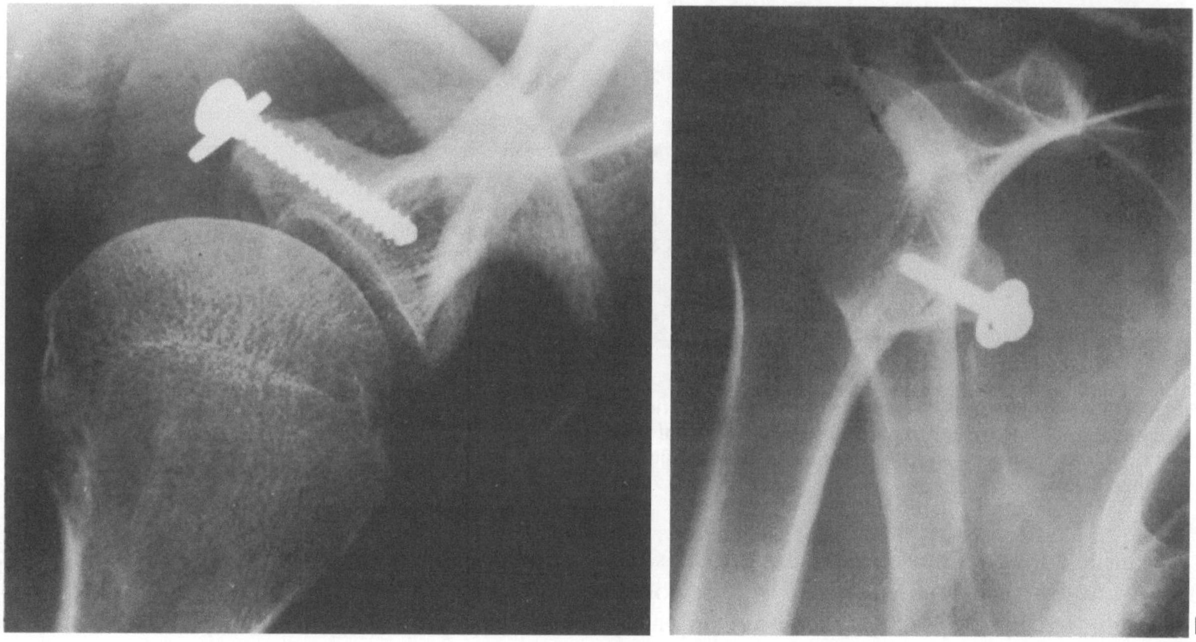

a b

Fig. 1. Modified axial (**a**) and oblique lateral (**b**) projection of a shoulder after the Bristow repair. The transposed coracoid has healed to the collum scapulae with bone

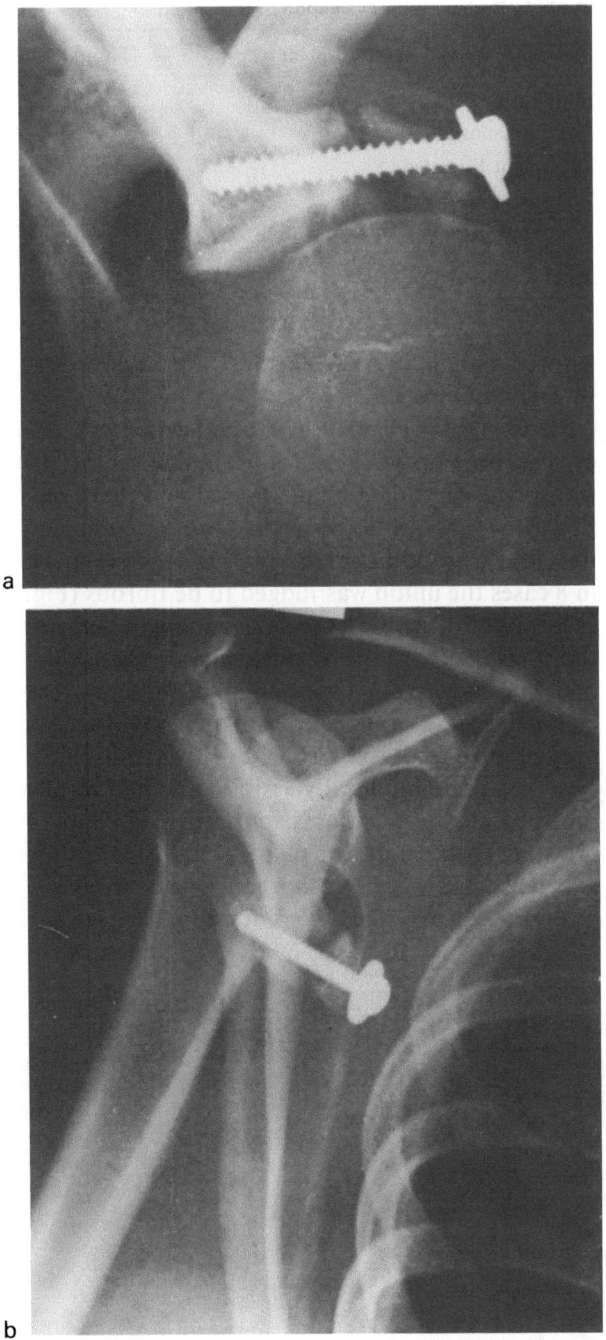

a

b

Fig. 2. Modified axial (**a**) and oblique lateral (**b**) projection of a shoulder after the Bristow repair. Note the radiolucent zone between the transplant and the scapula indicating fibrous healing

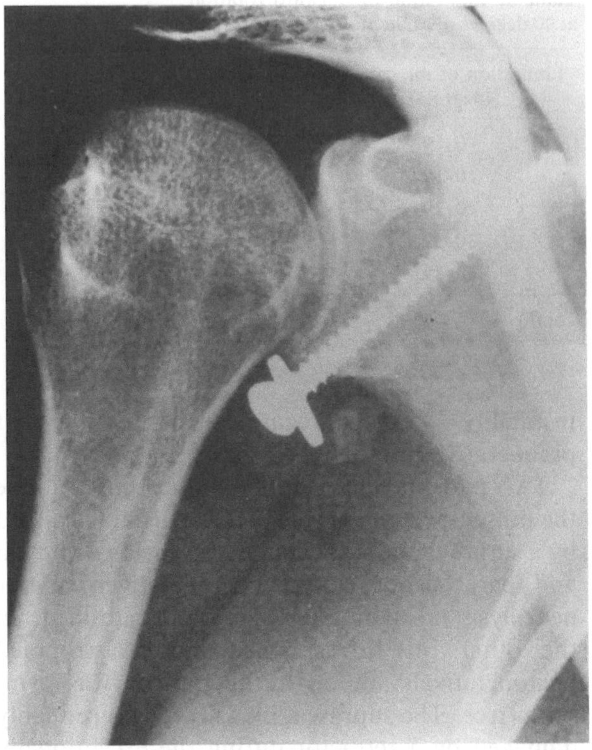

Fig. 3. Modified frontal projection of a shoulder after the Bristow repair. The transposed coracoid which was broken during surgery has migrated from the scapula because of the muscle forces acting on the transplant

Table 7. Complications after surgery

Complications	Shoulders
(Within three months)	
Superficial sepsis	3
Neurological deficit	2
Broken transplant	8
(After three months)	
Redislocation	3
Persistent instability	2
Pain	3
Severe limitation of movement	4
Severe keloid formation in scar	2
Total number of complications	27

posterior cortex by more than 5 mm). The short screws were frequently associated with osteolysis around their tips, especially when bony union did not occur. Mobility of the screw was seen in 3 cases, in one of which the transplant was also mobile. No definite subluxation or luxation could be diagnosed from the videotape recordings, even in patients judged as unstable. Table 7 summarises the local complications which were encountered. No systemic complications were reported.

Discussion

The Bristow repair has previously been reported to be a good method for dealing with post-traumatic shoulder instability in athletes [27]. The procedure is considered to be technically simpler than alternative repairs [17], and we have attempted to assess its suitability in other groups of patients. The high rate of recurrence reported here may seem discouraging but, as shown in Table 4, the failures occurred in the spontaneously unstable group in association with some kind of surgical error. Furthermore, bony healing of the transplant was always associated with a good result and should therefore be an aim of surgery, particularly when the Bristow repair is applied to spontaneously unstable shoulders. Technical aspects of the operation are thus of special importance in these patients as the tolerance for surgical error is lower when the instability is spontaneous.

In order to achieve bony healing it is important that the transplant is not broken during the operation. In our material, 8 transplants were broken, 6 of which migrated in spite of attempts to fasten them properly. One was resorbed and the other partly healed. If a transplant is broken, it is probably better to excise the bone and suture the conjoint tendon to the subscapularis according to the method originally designed by Rowley Bristow.

Bony healing also depends on adequate access to the anterior scapular neck. This can be difficult when the fibres of the subscapularis are split longitudinally. Proper positioning of the patient on the operating table with a pillow supporting the shoulder and the use of slender Hohman retractors inserted around the neck facilitate visualisation. The cortical bone should be carefully excised with a chisel. It is vital that the transplant is fixed with compression to the cancellous bone of the scapula and if AO-screws are used, the malleolar type with or without washers are preferable because they allow compression even if the drill hole in the transplant is only 3.2 mm. Larger-diameter drills might break the transplant. The length of the screw should be carefully measured, because if it fails to reach the posterior cortex, it cannot provide satisfactory compression.

Definite mobility of the transplant was shown in one case. The finding of osteolucency, especially in the presence of a short screw, probably indicates mobility of the transplant due to fibrous union. In our opinion, the snapping sensation associated with certain movements and reported by several patients can be caused by this type of transplant and screw instability. One patient with excessive snapping on abduction and outward rotation, who had a fibrous union and broad osteolysis around the screw, underwent screw extraction one year postoperatively. The snapping disappeared and the patient's condition improved.

To avoid the neurological complications which we encountered, one should proceed with great caution when dissecting the musculotendinous stalk of the transplant. For the same reason sutures in the subscapularis tendon should be applied with the utmost care and should not be used if the fibres have been split longitudinally. The reputation of the Bristow repair for causing only a small, if any, postoperative restriction of movement was confirmed in our material. However, overlapping of the subscapularis should be avoided, because it shortens the tendon and inevitably compromises outward rotation as seen in one of our patients. In the other patients with a more than 30° limitation of outward rotation, postoperative physiotherapy had been inadequate or the patient had been uncooperative.

The oblique lateral and modified axial X-ray projections proved valuable in determining the position and healing of the transplanted coracoid. With these views it was possible to obtain an excellent view of the base of the transplant and its relation to the nearby part of the scapular neck. The relation between the transplant and the scapula was obscured in the routine views. Radiography, furthermore, gave exact information of the size of the transplant and the position of the screw as well as the other bony structures in the operated region. Examination under the image-intensifier supplemented the radiographic assessment but proved unreliable in the determination of anterior instability.

Conclusions

The Bristow procedure is simpler to perform than are other types of repair for shoulder instability. The technical failures in our material occurred in the first or second patient operated on by each surgeon. Therefore it is our opinion that if the Bristow repair is to be successful it must be carefully performed by a surgeon with a thorough knowledge of the possible pitfalls. This is particularly so in the spontaneously unstable shoulder, but properly performed, the repair gives a rapid postoperative recovery and excellent results even in this group.

III.6. Results of the Bristow Repair: Sports Participation After Surgery

C. Akermark, L. Hovelius, P. Herberts, T. Wredmark, B. Gustafsson, L. Körner and E. Berg

Anterior shoulder dislocation is a relatively common injury in many sports, but publications on the exact incidence of dislocation [amongst sportsmen] are scarce. In a study of Swedish ice-hockey players in the top league [21] the incidence was found to be 8%, and the incidence in a randomly selected Swedish population has been reported to be 1.7% [22]. The subsequent rate of recurrent dislocation is high in athletes, especially in contact sports and activities involving arm elevation above shoulder level.

As reported by Collins and Wilde [10] most of the operative techniques in use today for the treatment of recurrent dislocation of the shoulder share one disadvantage, i.e. limitation of external rotation. This is usually less disabling than expected in common sports, but in racket and throwing activities even a slight limitation of external rotation may prevent return to athletic activity. In 1958 Helfet [18] was the first to describe the Bristow procedure, and he reported that most of his cases recovered a full range of motion. Good results with a modified Bristow technique have also been reported by Allman [1] and by Collins and Wilde [10], who had no redislocations in 50 cases. Sweeney et al. [63] reported a recurrence rate of 3% in 97 operated cases, and Lombardo et al. [27], in a report on 51 cases, had a redislocation rate of 2%. They stated, however, that "Of those individuals involved competitively in athletics at the onset of their disability, none returned to their original level of performance".

The purpose of this report is to present some preliminary results of the modified Bristow repair in 80 patients active in competitive or recreational sports.

Material and Methods

Patients from four different hospitals are included in this study. Questionnaires were distributed to 82 patients operated on before November 1979. Two patients could not be located, so 80 patients with involvement of 81 shoulders were included in the study; 61 shoulders were in males and 20 were in females. The mean observation time was 17.5 months (range 6-59 months) and the mean age at surgery was 26.2 years (range 16-40 years). The left shoulder was operated on in 35 patients, the

Table 1. Type of athletics

Competitive athletes		Recreational athletes	
Ice hockey	8	Badminton	9
Soccer	7	Running	6
Handball	5	Swimming	5
Rugby	2	Alpine skiing	4
Bandy	2	Soccer	4
Other	7	Other	22
Totals	31		50

right in 44 and both in one patient. In 44 shoulders the dominant side was involved, in 37 the non-dominant. Thirty-one shoulders were required for competitive sports and the remaining 50 for different recreational sports as shown in Table 1.

The operative procedure used has been described by Haley and House [15] and by others [10,30]. Through a longitudinal, deltopectoral incision, the tip of the coracoid process is osteomised. The subscapularis muscle is split longitudinally, and in some cases an additional superior transverse transection is used. In a few cases it was split tranversely. The coracoid tip with the attached conjoined tendon is then passed over the inferior part of the split subscapular muscle and attached with a screw to the anterior part of the neck of the scapula.

Results

After operation the disability caused by pain or limited range of motion, if present, was judged by the patient himself to be of minor importance in normal daily activities. Pain during athletic activity was reported in 26 shoulders; 50 were pain-free. Three patients (3 shoulders) did not return to athletics postoperatively and could not comment, and information from 2 patients (2 shoulders) was missing.

Table 2. Limited range of post-operative motion as graded subjectively by patients

Severe	4
Moderate	30
Minimal	13
Total	47

In 47 shoulders (58%) there was a complaint of some limitation of mobility after operation. This limitation was of varying degree (Table 2): it was experienced as very disturbing in athletic activity in 2 shoulders, moderately disturbing in 24 and not disturbing in 18. The 3 patients who did not return to athletics also lost movement but clearly they could not relate it to their sporting ability. Table 3 summarises the ability of the athletes to take part in their main sport before and after the surgical repair. In 63 shoulders (78%) the patient had to give up athletics preoperatively; 18 (22%) were able to continue until the operation. After operation all 18 shoulders (the majority being in ice-hockey and soccer players) allowed return to pre-injury sport as did 54 of those which would not allow participation preoperatively. Of the 9 who could not return, 6 were involved in racket and throwing sports, 2 were soccer players and 1 was a weightlifter. Five of these suffered a recurrence of instability (2 subluxed and 3 dislocated).

Table 3. Patients' ability to participate in their main sport before and after surgical repair

Ability	Before surgery	After surgery
Yes	18 →	72
	54 ↗	
No	63 → 9 →	9

Table 4. Ability to return to pre-injury athletic performance in all athletes and in various subgroups

		Return to pre-injury athletics	
Group[a]	No.	No.	Percentage
I	81	72	90
II	44	39	89
III	21	18	86
IV	31	28	90

[a] I. All athletes; II. Athletes operated on dominant side; III. Racket and throwing athletes operated on dominant side; IV. Competitive athletes

In Table 4 the ability to return to pre-injury athletic performance is presented for four different groups of athletes. There were no major differences between the groups.

Postoperative redislocation occurred in 3 of 81 shoulders (3.7%). This failure rate is comparable to results reported by others. The cases were as follows: a 23-year-old competitive handball player who redislocated in his car 6 months after operation when abducting his arm to put on his seatbelt; a 27-year-old recreational badminton player who redislocated while scratching her neck 8 months after surgery; and a 30-year-old competitive soccer player who sustained a redislocation in a fall from height on to his outstretched arm 13 months after operation.

The overall subluxation rate was 8.6% (7of 81 shoulders). Five occurred during athletics. In spite of subluxation 2 patients graded the operative result as excellent, 4 as good, and 1 found it fair. Only 2 subluxators were unable to pursue their sporting activities.

The results of operation as assessed by the patients themselves are presented in Table 5. Excellent or good results were reported in more than 90% in all athletes as well as in the subgroups listed in Table 4. We did, however, find differing results among the four hospitals. Possible explanations for this will be discussed in due course, but in essence the results concerning recurrence of instability, ability to return to athletics, and patients' assessment were broadly similar in three hospitals (59 patients) and throughout were better than those from the fourth hospital (22 patients).

Discussion and Conclusions

The purpose of this study was to present the preliminary results of the modified Bristow repair in athletes. Our experience is that this operative technique is effective in recreational or competitive sports, and results are obtained even in the critical group of racket or throwing athletes with dominant-side involvement. Almost 90% of athletes in this group and 90% in the competitive group could return to their preinjury sport after surgery, in spite of loss of mobility which was subjectively present in 58% of our cases. These results agree with earlier findings that limited external rotation does not affect return to sporting activity in most cases [10] but conflict with the statement by Lombardo [27] cited earlier in this report.

Table 5. Results of the operation assessed by the patient

	No.	Percentage
Excellent	51	63.0
Good	23	28.4
Fair	4	4.9
Poor	3	3.7
Total	81	100.0

Of all patients 91% assessed the operative results to be excellent or good. It must be emphasised, however, that a mean observation time of 17.5 months is not long enough, and a longer follow-up is planned which will probably give more reliable information in this respect.

The discrepancy between the results from the four hospitals has been mentioned and in this respect some variations in practice might be of importance. These were as follows:

(1) In one hospital the subscapularis was incised without entering the joint in the majority of cases; in the other three the joint was regularly opened and the necessary repair performed.

(2) The shoulder was immobilised for four weeks after surgery in one hospital and for two to three weeks in the others.

(3) Nine different surgeons, some junior, performed the operations (22) in one hospital whereas only one or two experienced surgeons did all the operations (59) in the others. In this respect the modified Bristow procedure cannot be regarded as technically more demanding than other operations but to judge from our preliminary results it is advisable that it should be performed by an experienced surgeon. When thus performed very good results can be obtained even in athletes active in shoulder demanding sports.

According to our experience to date, therefore, young athletes who have had two to three recurrent anterior dislocations and who strongly wish to return to athletic activities (including those which place the shoulder at high risk) may be offered surgical repair with a high chance of returning to the sport of their choice.

III.7. Posterior Glenoid Osteotomy for Posterior Dislocation of the Shoulder

Harry H. Kretzler, Jr and Daniel J. Scott, Jr

In this chapter our combined series of posterior dislocations of the shoulder, treated by osteotomy of the glenoid, is presented. We are well aware of the controversy surrounding surgery for this condition, and we are in full accord with Rowe [55] that these patients require careful evaluation before surgery is recommended. Because no two surgeons can collect a large series of their own, we are indebted to many other orthopaedic surgeons for allowing us to include their cases in this report.

Classification and Material

The classification of posterior dislocations of the shoulder has always been somewhat confusing, and in this chapter they are simply classified according to occurrence and aetiology (see Table 1). We have done osteotomies in all categories, to a total of 100 operations on 92 patients (8 were bilateral dislocators). There were 71 males and 21 females.

Table 1. Classification of posterior dislocation of the shoulder

Acute Traumatic	
Chronic Traumatic	
Recurrent Traumatic	Involuntary
Recurrent Neurological	or
Recurrent Idiopathic	Voluntary

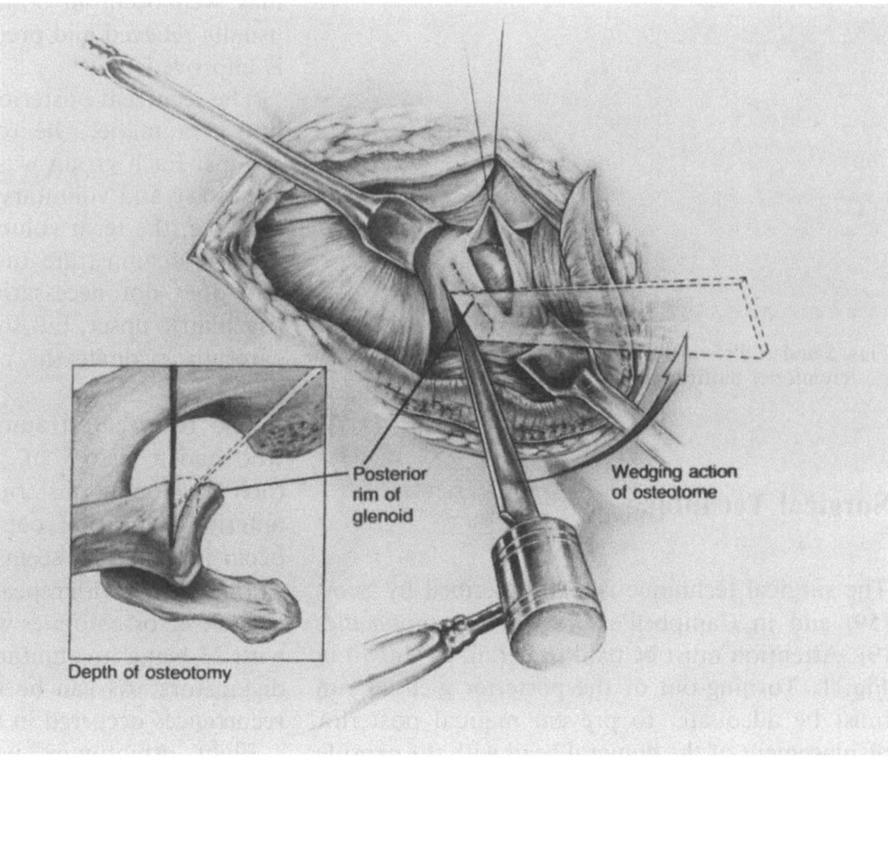

Fig. 1. Surgical technique. Note the depth of osteotomy and use of an osteotome to turn out the posterior glenoid rim which is maintained by a wedge bone graft from the angle of the acromion

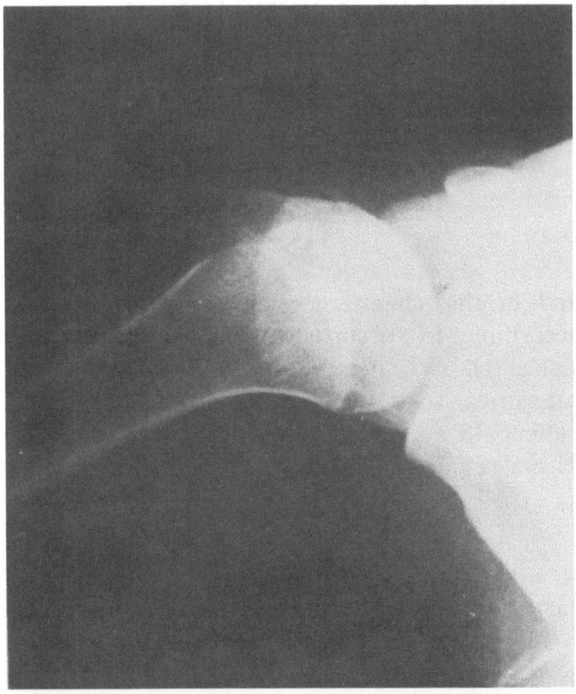

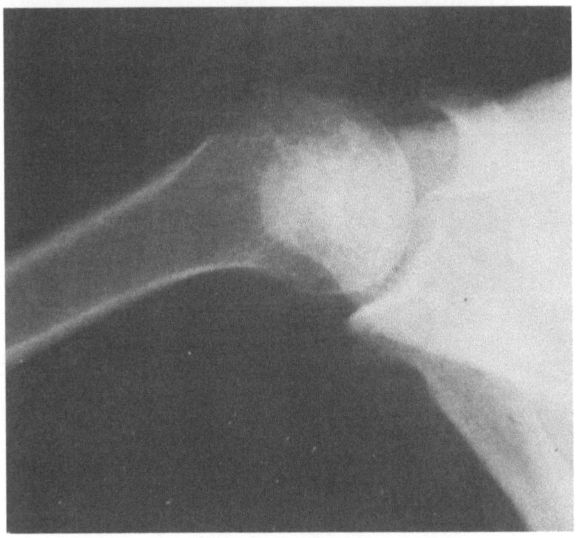

Figs. 2 and 3. Pre- and postoperative radiographs. Note the posteroinferior buttress provided by the osteotomy

Surgical Technique

The surgical technique is well described by Scott [59] and in Campbell's *Operative Orthopaedics* [9]. Attention must be paid to detail, as shown in Fig. 1. Turning-out of the posterior glenoid rim must be adequate, to prevent manual posterior displacement of the humeral head with the capsule open. The inferior corner of the glenoid neck must be free to rotate outward to give support in this area (Figs. 2 and 3).

Clinical Material

One hundred osteotomies have been collected, and their distribution is seen in Table 2. Two were done for an acute dislocation, with a fracture of the humerus that compromised closed treatment of the dislocation; 3 were done for chronic, traumatic, unreduced dislocations; 42 were done on patients in the recurrent, traumatic category; 8 were done for recurrent dislocations due to a neurological cause; and 45 were done on recurrent, idiopathic dislocators. The youngest patient was aged 9 years and the oldest 70 years. Altogether 40 surgeons were involved.

A chronic, traumatic dislocation is one in which the shoulder has been out for at least four weeks. It requires open reduction and is often unstable because of the humeral head defect and/or erosion of the posterior glenoid rim. Either a McLaughlin [31] subscapularis transfer into the defect, or a posterior glenoid osteotomy can be used to achieve stability. Limitation of motion may well occur in both procedures, but pain is usually relieved and preoperative range of motion is improved.

The recurrent posterior dislocators were divided into traumatic, neurological and idiopathic groups. Each group was then subdivided into involuntary and voluntary (Tables 1 and 2). In this instance, the term voluntary means the patient is able to demonstrate the dislocation on demand and does not necessarily connote emotional or psychiatric upset, but should alert the surgeon to carefully evaluate the patient before recommending repair.

The recurrent, traumatic patients were those who had a history of trauma which resulted in their developing posterior dislocations. Unlike an anterior dislocation, complete dislocation may not occur initially, but seems to develop over a period of time, often with repeated episodes of trauma. A total of 42 osteotomies were done in this category, with 23 being involuntary and nineteen voluntary dislocators. As can be seen, the majority of the recurrences occurred in the voluntary group.

Eight osteotomies were done for recurrent,

Table 2. The results of glenoid osteotomy according to group

Groups	Involuntary		Voluntary	
	Operations	Recurrence	Operations	Recurrence
Acute Traumatic	2	–	–	–
Chronic Traumatic	3	–	–	–
Recurrent Traumatic	23	1	19	3
Recurrent Neurological	7	2	1	–
Recurrent Idiopathic	10	–	35	7
Total Number of Shoulders	45	3	55	10

Table 3. Advantages of posterior osteotomy glenoid

(1) Provides bony support.
(2) Maintains articular cartilage contact.
(3) Changes no muscle groups.
(4) Causes minimal loss of motion.
(5) Useful in all groups.
(6) Compatible with contact sports.
(7) Compatible with other procedures.

neurological dislocations. This group comprised 2 bilateral cerebral palsy athetoids, 2 cerebral palsy hemiplegics, 1 brachial plexus injury, and 1 cerebrovascular accident. Except for the 1 athetoid, who recurred bilaterally in 6 months, the procedure gave stability to the shoulders of these patients. The other athetoid is now 15 years postoperative.

The recurrent, idiopathic dislocators have no history of trauma, and are frequently seen at an early age. Some may be able to dislocate their shoulders anteriorly, inferiorly, and posteriorly at will. It is this group, particularly, that must be carefully evaluated before recommending surgery. A total of 45 osteotomies were done on patients in this category, with the only recurrences being in the voluntary group – 7 out of 35.

The evaluation and non-operative care of voluntary dislocators was well discussed by Rowe et al. [55]. We agree that a muscle-strengthening programme and careful evaluation should precede surgery on any patient who dislocates posteriorly and particularly on the idiopathic voluntary dislocator. However, one may not need to rule out surgical repair if the patient cooperates in the presurgery exercise programme and seems genuinely desirous of preventing future dislocations.

Discussion

The success of an operation may be judged in many ways. Does the procedure correct the problem? Does it interfere with function? Does it stand the test of time? Can it be performed by many surgeons? We feel that the posterior glenoid osteotomy fulfills these criteria in correcting posterior dislocations of the shoulder. In addition, we feel there are some specific advantages of the glenoid osteotomy when compared with other procedures, and these are listed in Table 3.

III.8. Anteversion of the Shoulder — A Rare Clinical Sign

N.J. Barton

In 1971 I saw three patients in whom the prominent point of the shoulder was directed forwards instead of laterally as in the normal person (Fig. 1), and since then I have come across two more patients with a similar abnormality. I call this anteversion of the shoulder, by which I mean of the whole shoulder girdle as opposed to simple anteversion of the neck of the scapula or humerus.

In the first patient the abnormality is bilateral (Fig. 2) and was first noticed in a school clinic when he was aged five. I have followed him up for six years and he has never suffered much disability. Very detailed examinations have been made, but the essential finding, is that there is congenital absence of the trapezius. This reveals the rhomboids, which seem normal, as do all the other muscles in the region. Our interpretation is that lack of trapezius action has allowed the scapulae to be drawn forwards round the side of the chest so that they lie at an angle of 60° to the coronal plane (Fig. 3), compared to the normal 25° to 45°. This interpretation is supported by another patient aged 38 who has anteversion of the right shoulder due to paralysis of the lower two-thirds of the trapezius, following an operation in Australia in 1977 for excision of a fibro-

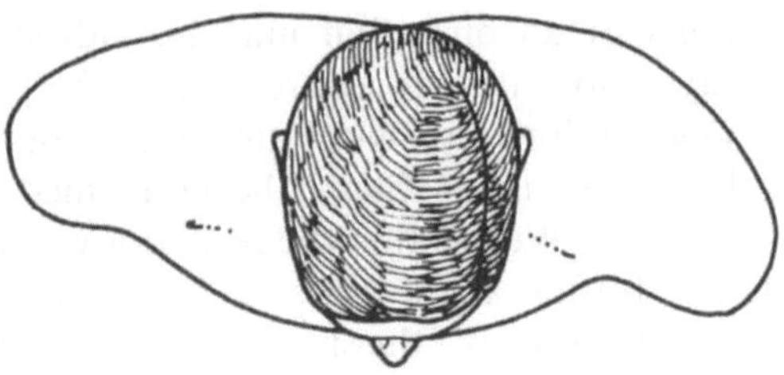

Fig. 1. Unilateral anteversion of the shoulder girdle complex

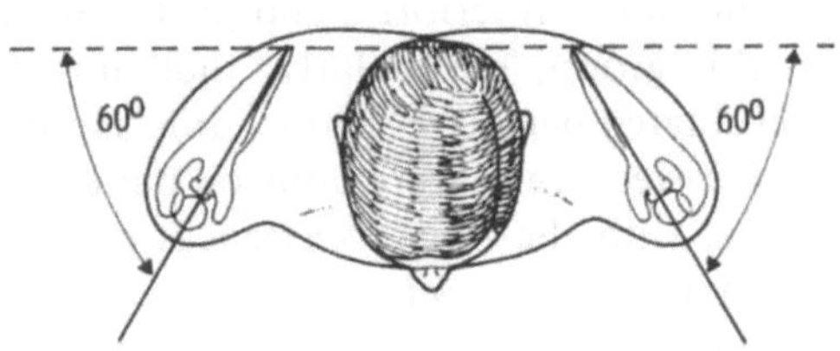

Fig. 3. Bilateral anteversion of the shoulder: the scapulae lie at an increased angle of 60° to the coronal plane

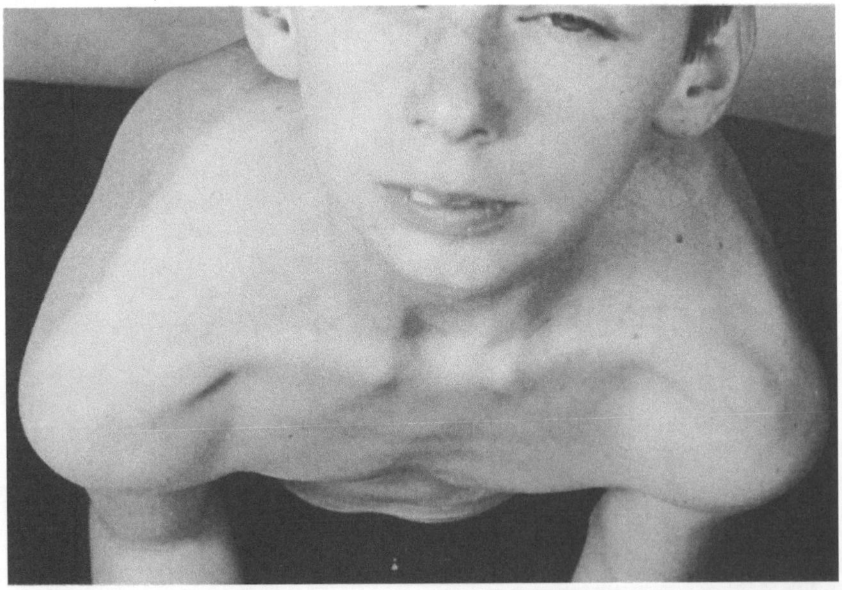

Fig. 2. Case Number 1: Bilateral anteversion of the shoulder girdle with absence of trapezius

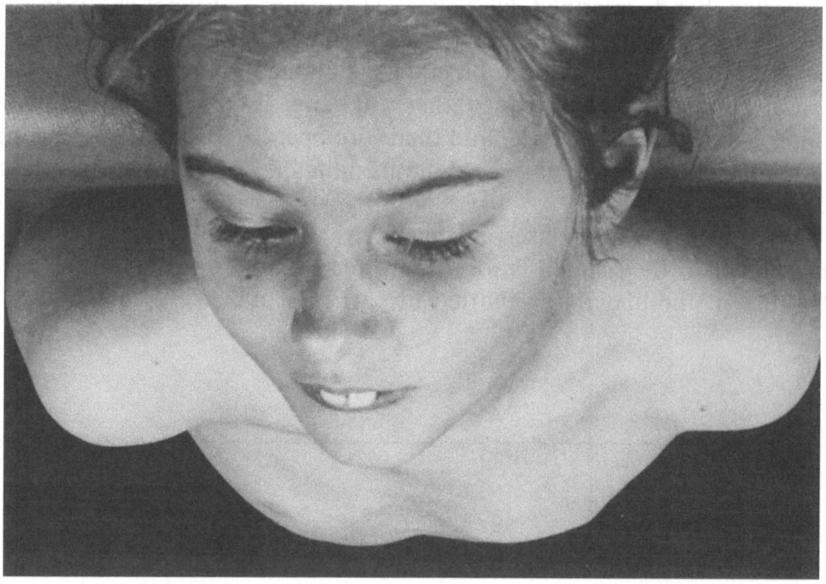

Fig. 4. Case Number 4: Unilateral anteversion of the right shoulder girdle with absence of pectoralis major (sternal head)

xanthoma of the upper part of the scapula.

The third patient has a Sprengel's shoulder. Robinson et al. [50] pointed out that in Sprengel's deformity there is not only elevation of the scapula but also "the clavicle is shorter than normal", and to obtain complete correction it is not enough to lower the scapula; it is also necessary to lengthen the clavicle. They recommend subperiosteal excision of the middle third of the clavicle, chopping it up into small fragments or morsels, and putting the bits back inside the periosteal tube.

The fourth patient is a puzzle. She has congenital absence of most of the pectoralis major on the right side, with only part of the clavicular head present, and pectoralis minor also seems to be absent. The lack of these muscles naturally creates a hollow in front of the right shoulder, now concealed by her developing breasts, which creates an illusion of anteversion, but I am satisfied there is also actual forward inclination of the point of the shoulder, as shown in Fig. 4, taken when she was younger. I cannot explain this. If absence of trapezius leads to anteversion, then absence of pectoralis ought to lead to retroversion. She has been followed up from the age of 3 to 14. She has full shoulder movements but slightly altered rhythm, with delay in scapular rotation during abduction. There is no disability, and she is fully active in sports.

In the last patient I am also unable to explain the deformity and have to resort to calling it *idiopathic*. It was causing no symptoms, but I noticed it in a 32-year-old man whom I was examining for backache. The left shoulder was displaced forwards, and he said he had been born with it like this. He stood with a slight thoracolumbar scoliosis, convex to the left but not enough to displace the scapula, and the scoliosis was not a structural one, and corrected on bending forwards. The left clavicle was 14 cm long, compared to 18 cm for the right clavicle. Glenohumeral abduction was to 80° but total elevation to 100°.

In 1975 Salter and Kay [57] described a familial deformity which they called congenital forward fixation of the scapula, causing an "extremely narrow and sloping appearance of the shoulders, which were rigidly fixed in the extreme forward position". This seems to be a more severe deformity than in my patients. It is due to a rare Mendelian autosomal dominant gene with 88% penetrance, causing an abnormal fibrous band from the base of the coracoid process to the anterior end of the first rib. Such a band occurs normally in the duck-billed platypus. In Salter's patients excision of the band was said to allow passive correction of the deformity, whereas if it was left until adult life, it became partly ossified, like an omovertebral bone.

Wilkinson [68], of Southampton, has operated on several patients with anteversion of the shoulder, some due to Sprengel's deformity and some idiopathic, but has been unable to find the tethering band described by Salter. He recommends lengthening of the clavicle by a method similar to that used by Robinson and has obtained good correction. He stresses that the aim is improvement in appearance, and therefore operative correction should only be done in unilateral cases.

Wilkinson has also observed that forward displacement of the scapula is sometimes due to deformity of the underlying thorax, in particular a funnel-chest: in such cases one cannot, of course, rectify the situation by operating on the shoulder girdle.

In none of my own patients has the deformity or disability been enough to justify exploration, but I wish to draw attention to this uncommon physical sign, and to suggest that there may be several different causes, some of which we do not yet understand.

III.9. Reflections on Dislocation and Recurrent Instability of the Shoulder

Anthony F. DePalma

Dislocation of the shoulder is an entity that has claimed the attention of practitioners of medicine for many centuries: as pointed out by Hovelius (Chapter III 1), Hippocrates was keenly aware of the disorder and proposed a method of treatment. Yet, despite the fact that this disorder has been studied and recorded for many centuries, there is still a great lack of knowledge as to its natural history and genetic background. If indeed there is one. There is much disagreement as to the responsible aetiological factors, the associated pathologic changes in the glenohumeral joint, and the prognosis and the treatment.

The preceding chapters on recurrent instability consist of contributions by a group of internationally recognised experts in the field of shoulder disorders. There is no doubt that they have provided some significant new information based on carefully planned prospective and retrospective studies; it is also true that some of the presentations again interjected disagreement in areas of prognosis and treatment.

Dr L. Hovelius' study of the incidence and prognosis of shoulder dislocations (Chapter III.1) provides statistics which give us a clearer view of the natural history of this disorder than we had in the past. That the incidence of shoulder dislocation in the general population is 1.7% is new and revealing, and the statistics of the sex ratio in three age groups of primary dislocations reveals that between the ages of 21 and 30 the male : female ratio is 9:1 and that it drops to 2:1 in the age group 31 to 40. That age is an important factor in recurrence of a primary dislocation is an established fact, but the many studies on the incidence of recurrence are at great variance. Dr Hovelius' study provides interesting and necessary information in this area. In the age group under 20 only 20% achieve a cure; between 21 and 30, 60%; and between 31 and 40, 80%. Finally, this study again emphasises the futility of immobilisation of primary dislocation. My own experience leans in support of this concept.

Dr Stoker's presentation on the radiology of

recurrent anterior dislocation (Chapter III.4) and on the techniques employed and the interpretations reveals the radiological peculiarities of recurrent anterior dislocation, facilitates making a positive diagnosis, and further emphasises the many new radiological tools at our disposal to study the disorders of the shoulder joint. As has been shown by Mr Johnson in Chapter III.3 on rupture of the rotator cuff associated with anterior dislocation, only arthrography of the impaired shoulder will definitely establish the diagnosis. It becomes obvious that the use of such tools becomes mandatory in order to make a correct diagnosis and institute early and affective treatment.

Mr Johnson's observation (Chapter 111.3) that 50% of acute dislocations occur after the age of 45 years is not generally appreciated. Although the complications associated with acute dislocation which he describes are well known, often their recognition is missed or their significance underestimated. In fact, all acute dislocations in this age group should be considered as being complicated by a rupture of the rotator cuff until proven otherwise. If a fracture of the greater tuberosity is present and medial displacement of the fragments persists after reduction, this situation is comparable to a rupture of the cuff and must be treated as such. Since the number of persons in the age category over 45 years is steadily increasing, the complications recorded by Mr Johnson are timely and worthy of emphasis. These are: rupture of the rotator cuff with or without fracture of the greater tuberosity; neural damage (injury to the circumflex nerve (18%), the brachial plexus (5%)); and neural damage associated with a rupture of the cuff. Early electromyographic studies will establish the diagnosis of neural damage and are far more important than clinical assessment of neural impairment. Also arthrographic studies will establish the diagnosis of a complete tear of the cuff. Although these important points have been emphasised by Mr Johnson, there is one point in the treatment of combined lesions (rupture of the cuff and circumflex nerve damage) with which I disagree. Mr Johnson prefers to wait until the neural damage has recovered fully (which may be up to one year) before repairing the cuff. My experience indicates that the results are better if a ruptured cuff is repaired as soon as the diagnosis is made. This is true with or without neural complications.

The contributions of Dr Herberts (Chapter III.5) and of Dr Akermark (Chapter III.6) emphasise some important features of this procedure. On the other hand, the results attained are in disagreement with most of the observers who have published their results. There is no dispute with the opinion that the Bristow operation is one of the few operations which, properly performed, has few recurrences in the category of post-traumatic recurrences and that it is associated with minimal limitation of external rotation. However, I must take issue with the opinion that in spontaneous recurrences a cure will be effected if the technique is properly performed and union of the graft is achieved. This has not been my experience in spontaneous recurrences nor the experience of others. We have had failures in this group when all the conditions specified by Dr Herberts have been met. Also, this operation as described by Dr Herberts is not a simple procedure, for the margin for technical error is great (adequate exposure, properly prepared graft site, adequate fixation of graft, proper placement of graft, proper length of screw, etc.).

In view of the high incidence of complications reported in Chapter III.5 one wonders whether the procedure should be given such a high preference over other procedures. Of 31 operations the complications listed are: (*a*) within 3 months—superficial infections, 3; neurological deficits, 2; broken transplants, 8; (*b*) after 3 months—reluxation, 3; instability without reluxation, 2; pain, 3; severe restriction of motion, 4; and severe keloid formation, 2.

The results attained by Dr Akermark and his group certainly deserve commendation. He reports that 90% of all competitive athletes returned to pre-injury performance and 86% of athletes participating in throwing sports returned to pre-injury performance. These results are at variance with most of the series of cases reported in America and abroad.

Dr Kretzler and Dr Scott (Chapter III.7) deserve much credit in being able to assemble a series of 100 cases of posterior dislocations of the shoulder; this is a remarkable feat requiring many hours of work. Their cases fall into all categories of posterior dislocation, 45 being in the involuntary category and 55 in the voluntary category. All cases were treated by a posterior glenoid osteotomy . The incidences of recurrence were 3 in the involuntary group which comprised 45 shoulders and 10 recurrences in the voluntary group in which there were 55 shoulders. Seven of these 10 recurrences were in patients classified as recurrent idiopathic posterior dislocations of which there were 35. Considering the difficulties posterior dislocations pose when stabilisation is attempted, I consider that the above results speak well for this procedure. Although my personal experience is far from that reported in this series my results with posterior glenoid osteotomy support their observations.

References

1 Allman F (1974) Presentation, The American Academy of Orthop Surg, Committee on Sports Med, Course on Athletic Injuries of the Upper Extremities, Eugene, Oregon
2 Allman F (1975) Symposium on Sports Injuries to the Shoulder. Contemp Surg 7: 88
3 Assmus H, Meinel A (1976) Schulterverletzung und axillarisparese. Unfallheilkunde 79: 183-187
4 Baker DM, Leach RE (1965) Fracture dislocation of the shoulder— report of three unusual cases with rotator cuff avulsion. J Trauma 5: 659-664
5 Bankart ASB (1928) Dislocation of the shoulder joints. Robert Jones birthday volume. A collection of surgical essays. London, Oxford University Press
6 Blom S, Dahlback LO (1970) Nerve injuries in dislocations of the shoulder joint and fractures of the neck of the humerus (a clinical and electromyographic study). Acta Chir Scand 136: 461-466
7 Broca A, Hartman H (1890) Contribution à l'étude des luxations de l'épaule. Bull Soc Anat Paris 5me série 4: 312-336, 416-423
8 Caird FM (1887) The shoulder joint in relation to certain dislocations and fractures. Edinburgh Med J 32: 708-714
9 Campbell's Operative Orthopaedics (1971) 5th Edit. The CV Mosby Co, St Louis pp 468-470
10 Collins HR, Wilde AH (1973) Shoulder instability in athletics. Orthop Clinics N Amer Vol 4: No 3, 759-774
11 DePalma AF (1950) Surgery of the shoulder. JB Lippincott Co, Philadelphia
12 Ehgartner K (1977) Hat die Dauer der Gipsfixation nach Schulterluxatimen linen Einfluss auf die Näuftigkeit der habitullen Schulterluxatimen? Arch Orthop Unfall-Chir 89: 187-190
13 Flower WH (1861) On the pathological changes produced in the shoulder joint by traumatic dislocation as derived from an examination of all the specimens illustrating this injury in the Museum of London. Trans Path Soc London 12: 179-200
14 Golding FC (1962) The shoulder—the forgotten joint. Brit J Radiol 35: 149-158
15 Haley PH, House JH (1974) Recurrent anterior dislocation of the shoulder. Minnesota Medicine, Nov 1974: 882-885
16 Hall RH, Issac F, Booth CR (1959) Dislocations of the shoulder with special reference to accompanying small fractures. J Bone Jt Surg 41-A: 489-494
17 Halley DK, Olix ML (1975) A review of the Bristow operation for recurrent anterior shoulder dislocation in athletes. Clin Orthop Rel Res 106: 175-179
18 Helfet AJ (1958) Coracoid transplantation for recurring dislocation of the shoulder. J Bone Jt Surg 40-B: 198-202
19 Hermodsson I (1934) Roentgenolische Studien über die traumatischen und habituellen Schultergelenkverienkungen nach von und nach unter. Acta Radiol Supp 20: 1-173
20 Hill HA, Sachs MD (1940) The grooved defect of the humeral head. A frequently unrecognised complication of dislocations of the shoulder. Radiology 35: 690-700
21 Hovelius L (1978) Shoulder dislocations in Swedish ice-hockey players. Amer J Sports Med 6: 373-377
22 Hovelius L (1980) Incidence of shoulder dislocation in Sweden (To be published)
23 Hovelius L, Eriksson K, Fredin H, Hagberg G, Lind B, Thorling J, Weckström J (1980) Prospective multicentre study on treatment and prognosis of primary shoulder dislocation (In progress)
24 Hovelius L, Thorling J, Fredin H (1979) Recurrent anterior dislocation of the shoulder. Results after the Bankart and Putti-Platt operations. J Bone Jt Surg 61-A: 566-569
25 Kazar B, Belovszky E (1969) Prognosis of primary dislocation of the shoulder. Acta Orthop Scand 40: 216-224
26 Lamm CR, Zachrisson B (1980) Personal Communication
27 Lombardo SJ, Kerlan RK, Jobe FW, Carter VS, Blazina ME, Shields CL (1976) The modified Bristow procedure for recurrent dislocation of the shoulder. J Bone Jt Surg 58-A: 256-261
28 London PS (1971) Treatment and after care for dislocation of the shoulder. Physiotherapy 57/1: 2-6
29 Ludin HP, Haertel M, Meyer RP, Noesberger B (1975) Die Kombination der traumatischen ruptur der rotatorenmanschette mit nervenläsionen. Dtsch Med Wschr 100: 142-148
30 May JV (1970) A modified Bristow operation for anterior recurrent dislocation of the shoulder. J Bone Jt Surg 52-A: 1010-1016
31 McLaughlin HL (1952) Posterior dislocation of the shoulder. J Bone Jt Surg 34-A: 584-590
32 McLaughlin HL (1963) Dislocation of the shoulder with tuberosity fracture. Surg Clin North Am 43/6: 1615-1620
33 McLaughlin HL, Asherman EG (1951) Lesions of the musculotendinous cuff of the shoulder. J Bone Jt Surg 33-A: 76
34 McLaughlin HL, Cavallaro WU (1950) Primary anterior dislocation of the shoulder. Amer J Surg 80: 615-621
35 McLaughlin HL, McLellan DI (1967) Recurrent anterior dislocation of the shoulder. A comparative study. J Trauma 7: 191-201
36 McManus F (1976) Brachial plexus lesions complicating anterior fracture dislocation of the shoulder joint. Injury 8/1: 63-66
37 Morrey BF, Janes JM (1976) Recurrent anterior dislocation of the shoulder. J Bone Jt Surg 58-A: 252-261
38 Moseley HF (1961) Recurrent dislocation of the shoulder. E & S Livingstone Ltd p 120
39 Moseley HF (1928) Recurrent dislocation of the shoulder. Montreal. McGill University Press
40 Moseley HF, Overgaard B (1963) Hermodsson's roentgenological studies of traumatic and recurrent anterior and inferior dislocations of the shoulder joint. E & S Livingston, Edinburgh
41 Mumenthaler M, Schliack H (1965) Läsionen peripherer nerven. Georg Thieme Verlag Stuttgart
42 Neer CS (1979) Personal Communication
43 Neer CS, Welsh RP (1977) The shoulder in sports. Orthop Clin North Am 8: 583-591

44 Oster A (1967) Recurrent anterior dislocation of the shoulder treated by the Eden-Hybbinette operation. Follow up on 78 cases. Acta Orthop Scand 40: 43-52
45 Palmer I, Widén A (1948) The bone block method for recurrent dislocation of the shoulder joint. J Bone Jt Surg 30-B: 53-58
46 Pasila M, Jaroma H, Kiviluoto O, Sundholm A (1978) Early complications of primary shoulder dislocations. Acta Orthop Scand 49: 260-263
47 Perthes G (1906) Uber operationen bei habitueller Schulterluxationen. Dtsch Z Chir 85: 199-227
48 Post M (1978) The shoulder. Lea & Febiger, Philadelphia p 439
49 Reeves B (1969) Acute anterior dislocation of the shoulder. Ann Roy Coll Surg Eng 44: 255-273
50 Robinson RA, Braun RM, Mack P, Zadek R (1967) The surgical importance of the clavicular component of Sprengel's Deformity. J Bone Jt Surg 49-A: 1481
51 Rowe CR (1956) Prognosis in dislocations of the shoulder. J Bone Jt Surg 38-A: 967-977
52 Rowe CR (1963) The results of operative treatment of recurrent dislocaiton of the shoulder. Surg Clin N Am 43: 1667-1670
53 Rowe CR (1979) Personal Communication
54 Rowe CR, Patel D, Southmayd WW (1978) The Bankart procedure. A long term end result study. J Bone Jt Surg 60-A: 1-16
55 Rowe CR, Pierce DS, Clark JG (1973) Voluntary dislocation of the shoulder. J Bone & Joint Surg. 55-A: 445-460
56 Rowe CR, Sakellarides HT (1961) Factors related to recurrences of anterior dislocation of the shoulder. Clin Orthop 20: 40-48
57 Salter RB, Kay GD (1976) Congenital foreward fixation of the scapula. J Bone Jt Surg 58-B: 132-3
58 Sauer G, Fasol P, Sandbach G (1975) Zur prognose der nervenlasionen nach verrenkungen und verrenkundgsbruchen der Schultersowie frakturen des oberarmhalses. Hefte Unfallheilkel 126: 176-8
59 Scott DJ (1967) Treatment of recurrent posterior dislocation of the shoulder by glenoplasty. J Bone Jt Surg 49-A: 471-476
60 Sisk TD, Boyd HB (1974) Management of recurrent anterior dislocation of the shoulder. Du Toit type of staple capsulorraphy. Clin Orthop 103: 150-156
61 Skogland LB, Sundt P (1973) Recurrent anterior dislocation of the shoulder. The Eden-Hybbinette operation. Acta Orthop Scand 44: 739-747
62 Stripp WJ (1977) In: Murray RO, Jacobsen HG The radiology of skeletal disorders, 2nd Edit Churchill Livingstone, Edinburgh p 1980
63 Sweeney HJ, Mead NC, Dawson WJ, Fitzsimmons P (1975) Fourteen years experience with the modified Bristow procedure for recurrent anterior dislocation of the shoulder. Read at the annual meeting of The American Academy of Orthop Surg San Franc Calif
64 Watson-Jones R (1948) Recurrent dislocation of the shoulder. J Bone Jt Surg 30-B: 6-8
65 Watson-Jones R (1955) Fractures and joint injuries, Vol 2 4th Edit, E & S Livingstone, London
66 Watson-Jones R (1960) Fractures and joint injuries, Vol 2, 4th Edit, E & S Livingstone, Edinburgh, London
67 White M (1929) Some later results of dislocation of the shoulder. Trans Roy Med Chir Soc Glasgow 1927-1928, 22: 243-248
68 Wilkinson JA (1980) Personal Communication

Section IV. The Frozen Shoulder

Moderator—Mr. B.F. Reeves

IV.1. Pathomechanics of the Frozen Shoulder and the Effect of the Brisement Force

Bo J. Lundberg

Since its recognition more than a century ago by Duplay [15] no other shoulder disorder has so intrigued the mind as the condition named by Codman (1934) [11] the frozen shoulder. Many structures and theories have been implicated to explain the predominant symptoms of stiffness and pain, but Neviaser [31] must be credited with todays most likely theory of pathomechanics. By observing shoulders at operation he described a restrictive process of the capsule, probably of inflammatory origin. Further evidence was adduced by Kessel [20], who described some degree of obliteration of the inferior joint recesses at arthrography in three patients with the frozen shoulder syndrome. He found no support for the theory that adhesions exist between the synovial membrane and the head of the humerus nor did he find a connection with bicipital tenosynovitis. The presence of restriction and later improvement in all planes of passive mobility is best explained by a capsular cause, and the incremental relationship of joint volume to range of movement adds further evidence to the central role of the capsule.

Cinearthrography is a useful way of illustrating and confirming the suggested mechanism. The following account reviews a film based on this technique which contains sequences of normal and frozen shoulders. In addition to demonstrating the capsular mechanism the work also aimed to study the dynamics of the sudden release of a frozen shoulder subjected to forced manipulation under general anaesthesia.

Material and Methods

Three shoulders with normal mobility were injected intra-articularly with contrast medium under local anaesthesia; 6 with varying degrees of restricted mobility, 5 primary frozen shoulders and 1 secondary to a fracture of the proximal humerus [26] had the same procedure under general anaesthesia. The patients lay supine with the involved shoulder under the X-ray tube, and the sequence of events was recorded by a movie camera via an amplifier screen. The actual field was bordered by shields of lead. Under this rather restricting arrangement the pattern of the joint's movement was studied. The investigation was completed by manipulation under muscle relaxation with the contrast medium still visible in the shoulder. It was carried out by elevation and outward rotation of the patients arm. The force was applied at the elbow using the humerus as a lever. The manipulation was completed by an inward rotation which was not forced if the tissues offered resistance.

Results

The joint capacity of the three shoulders with normal mobility was 15 ml or more. Characteristic of these cases were the spacious joint recesses, especially the axillary (Fig. 1a) and the unlimited glenohumeral action (Fig. 1b). The first case of primary frozen shoulder was in a 63-year-old woman whose joint capacity was 12 ml. Her shoulder mobility was moderately restricted so that full elevation of the humeral head under the acromion could not be achieved. The axillary recess was somewhat reduced in size.

The second case of primary frozen shoulder was also in a 63-year-old woman. Her shoulder joint had a volume of 8 ml with an obliterated inferior joint recess (Fig. 2a,b). During cinearthrography the joint was stretched to the point of shoulder release when at the moment of snapping, an increased glenohumeral angle appeared with a jump. Instantly contrast became visible escaping from the joint inferiorly followed by further effusion in that region (Fig. 2c,d).

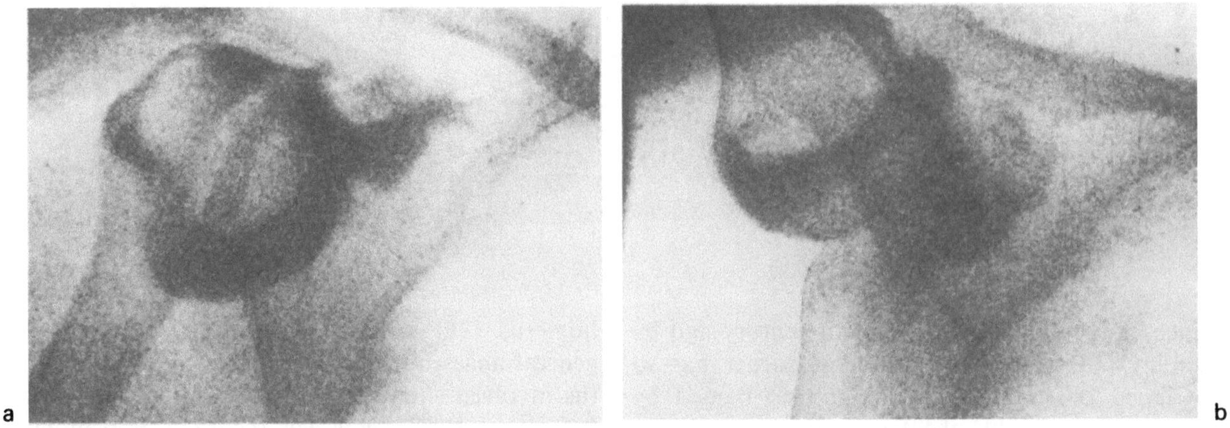

Fig. 1. Cinearthrography of a normal shoulder joint. **a** Note the spacious axillary joint recess. **b** The position of full elevation

The frozen shoulder of a man aged 49 years was the third case, having a joint capacity of 6 ml and no axillary recess at all. There was no gleno-humeral mobility, only scapular rotation. Despite repeated attempts at manipulation, no increase in movement could be achieved and there was no leakage of contrast.

The following two patients, both women aged 52 years, with joint volumes reduced to 8 and 5 ml respectively, had similar cinearthrograms to the second case. There was simultaneously a sudden release of the joint with a jump, a snapping sound and leakage of contrast in the axillary region (Fig. 3a-d). In these three cases contrast at the humeral

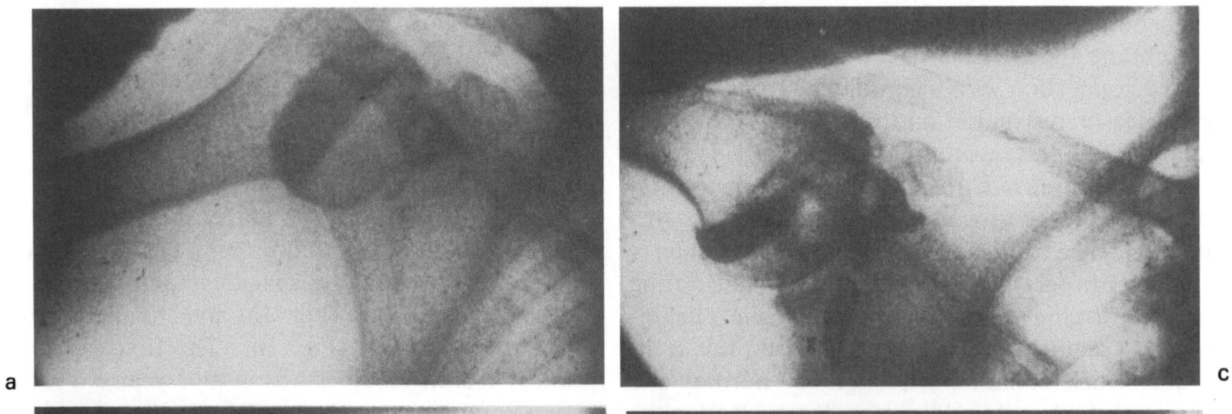

Fig. 2. Primary frozen shoulder: Case Number Two. **a** The obliterated inferior joint recess. **b** Prior to release at manipulation, under general anaesthesia. **c** The first sign of contrast escaping the joint after brisement. **d** Further contrast effusion visible. O: separation of contrast from the humerus which may indicate capsular tearing at this site. Z: contrast outside the joint after brisement

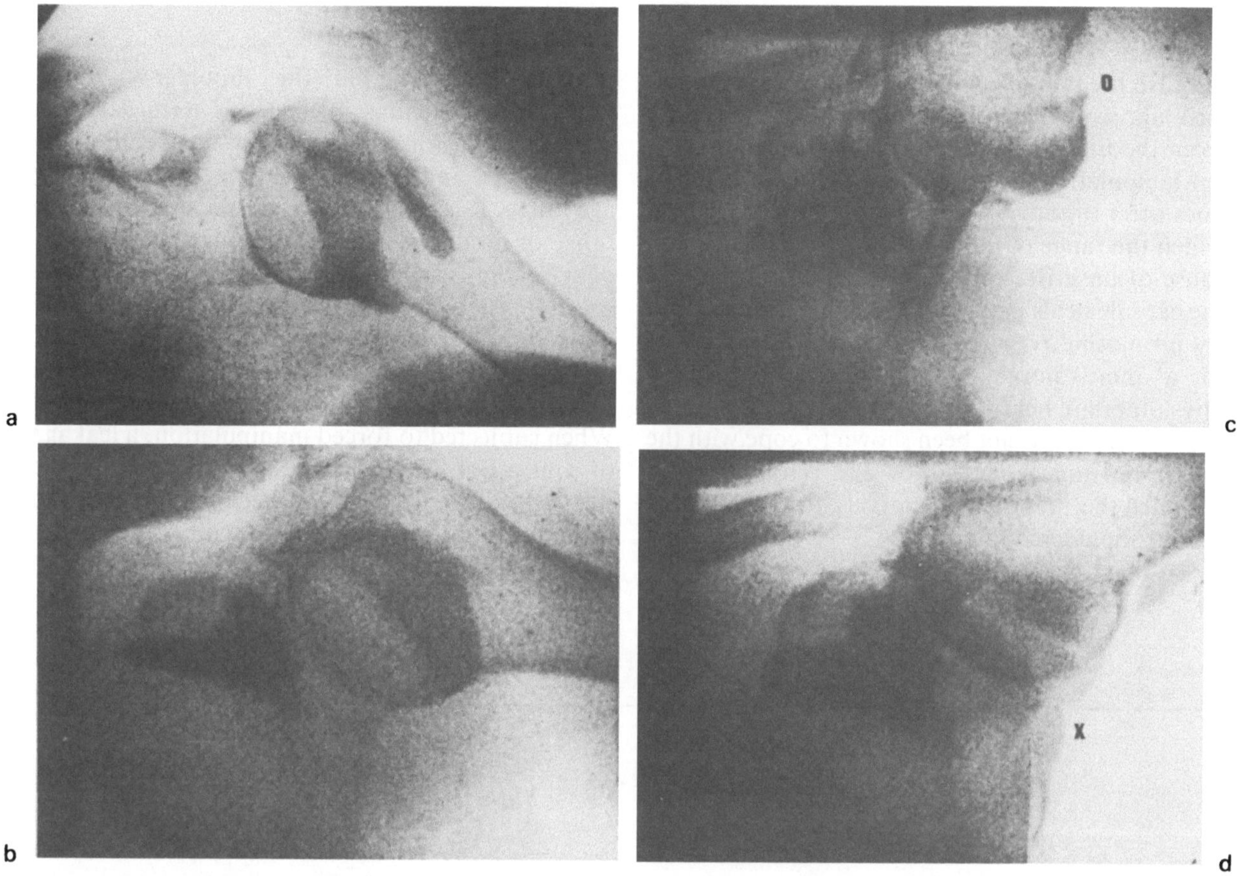

Fig. 3. Primary frozen shoulder, Case Number Four. Note similar sequence to Fig. 2. O: separation of contrast from the humerus which may indicate capsular tearing at this site. X: contrast outside the joint after brisement

insertion of the obliterated axillary recess was seen to separate from the line of the humeral neck (Fig. 2b and 3c) when force was applied for manipulation. This separation, which increased prior to the sudden release of the joint and escape of contrast, accords with the theories of capsular change and indicates capsular tearing at this site.

In the last case, a woman aged 60 with a frozen shoulder secondary to a fracture of the neck of the humerus three months earlier, joint capacity was 7 ml. The cinearthrographic picture did not differ; the resistance gave away with force, but without any visible jump. The contrast absolutely exploded in a cascade round the neck of the humerus.

None of the frozen shoulder cinearthrograms showed any irregularities in the contrast or any other signs indicating intra-articular adhesions.

Comments

The aetiology of the frozen shoulder is still obscure, but its well-delineated course makes the disorder a well-defined clinical entity. All cases recover spontaneously in due time, which seems surprising when the long-standing structural changes visualised in this study are borne in mind. As joint function is completely restored, it seems unlikely that the joint surfaces suffer from intra-articular adhesions, since this would leave lasting dysfunction. The capsular thickening consists histologically of fibrosis and fibroplasia [31,13,26]. There is reason to believe that the unavoidable capsular tearing at manipulation includes not only the axillary recess but also extends forwards and backwards so that a broad communication to the periarticular structures is created. The effect is similar to synovectomy. Not only is mobility through that measure improved, but also the pain-relieving effect [10] is sometimes striking, which could be explained by the release from the iron grip of the retracted capsule.

Manipulation is an optional procedure, but it does offer the advantage of shortening the time in which the range of motion is decreased. The main cause of unsatisfactory results appears to be that the capsule heals in the original state of retraction. By promoting regeneration of the synovial tissue to a more normal state, adjuvant intensive physiotherapy helps to prevent such relapse. Such therapy alone has not been shown to cope with the tough resistance offered by the retracted joint capsule, the predominant target structure of the frozen shoulder.

Summary

Stiffness and pain in the shoulder, without noticeable exogenous influence is termed frozen shoulder. The disease occurs almost entirely in middle-aged individuals within a rather narrow age range. It is self-limiting, and in all cases a free range of motion is restored although the duration of symptoms varies considerably. Still in many respects mysterious, the retracted condition of the joint capsule evidently causes the restriction of motion. By means of cinearthrography in six frozen shoulders this becomes clearly visible. When subjected to forced manipulation, a leakage of contrast in the region of the axillary recess was regularly demonstrated which coincided with the instantaneous increase of mobility—a further proof of the role of the capsular changes.

IV.2. Immunological Studies in the Frozen Shouder

Adam Young

The aetiology of the frozen shoulder is not known. Macnab [27] advanced the view based on experimental and clinical observation, that the condition is due to an autoimmune response to alteration of the collagen in chronic rotator cuff degeneration. Confirmatory evidence for an immunological basis for the condition has been found in only a few studies.

There have been reports of an association with autoimmune diseases particularly thyroid disease [30] and diabetes [5], but firm statistical evidence is lacking. The finding of an increased prevalence of the histocompatibility antigen HLA-B27 in 38 patients with frozen shoulder suggested a genetically linked immune disorder [7]. This antigen is known to be associated with the chronic inflammatory and familial condition ankylosing spondylitis [4]. Later studies to investigate an imunological aetiology showed reduced lymphocyte function as measured with lymphocyte transformation tests and a relative deficiency of one immunoglobulin class, IgA (but not IgG or IgM) in 25 patients with frozen shoulder [8]. Since IgA production and lymphocyte function are closely related to effective thymic control, it was suggested that these patients had a deficiency of the cellular immune system. The latter may predispose patients to autoimmune disease [1], and it was proposed that an autoimmune inflammatory reaction followed supraspinatus tendon degeneration patients with a pre-existing deficiency of cellular immunity. This is in keeping with experiments on rabbit tendons which suggest a type IV autoimmune reaction [27].

To test the autoimmune hypothesis we performed some studies using immunological parameters currently regarded as markers of diseases related to autoimmunity and immune dysfunction. Apart from one retrospective study all the investigations were carried out prospectively on 50 consecutive patients who fulfilled the following minimal diagnostic criteria of frozen shoulder:

(a) *Spontaneous* onset of pain localised to the shoulder region, the pain increasing in severity and usually worse at night.

(b) Limitation of *all* shoulder movements by at least 50%.

(c) No clinical or radiological identifiable lesion of the shoulder.

A control group, which was age- and sex-matched, consisted of 50 patients with degenerative disease of the lumbar spine.

Clinical Studies

Retrospective Survey

The case notes of all patients with a diagnosis of frozen shoulder who attended a rheumatology clinic over a five-year period were examined. The prevalence of other medical conditions in 180 patients was obtained. However, it must be stressed that in this small study, the diagnostic definition of frozen shoulder was variable and did not necessarily conform to the criteria given above. Only three diseases appeared to be more prevalent than expected: thyroid disease, diabetes, and cervical spondylosis. However, when compared to an age- and sex-matched control group, the figures for both thyroid disease and diabetes were not statistically significant at a level of $P = 0.02$ (Table 1).

Table 1. Prevalence of thyroid disease and diabetes in frozen shoulder and control patients (retrospective study)

	Expected	Controls ($n = 200$)	Frozen Shoulder ($n = 180$)
Autoimmune Thyroid Disease	0.5%–2.5% [25]	4%	8.3% ($P = 0.02$)
Diabetes	1.5%–5.0% [29]	3%	7.2% ($P = 0.02$)

Prospective Survey

A thorough history was therefore taken from each patient in the prospective study of 50 patients with particular attention to previous known immunological disorders, both in the patient and in first- and second-degree relatives. The patients were questioned in detail concerning childhood infections, frequency of upper respiratory infections, influenza, allergies and hypersensitivity reactions, as well as previous and current medication. All patients were clinically examined by the same physician to exclude other medical conditions claimed to be associated with the frozen shoulder.

Of the 50 patients there were 23 women and 27 men with a mean age of 51 years. We found no genetic linkage; a positive family history of this condition is unusual and was only present in one of our patients. Only autoimmune thyroid disease was more prevalent (8%) than expected, but when compared to the control group (4%) it did not achieve statistical significance ($P < 0.05$). There was no association with previous or current medication. Although the numbers were small for such a study, at least the patients included were a clearly defined homogeneous group compared to the patients in the retrospective survey.

Laboratory Data

Histocompatability Antigens (HLA System)

Tissue typing was performed on all fifty patients. The prevalence of the HLA-B27 locus antigen was 6% which is similar to that found in the normal population [19].

Serology

The following investigations were performed on all fifty patients:

1. Autoantibody screening for:
   (a) Organ-specific antibodies to thyroid and gastric parietal cells.

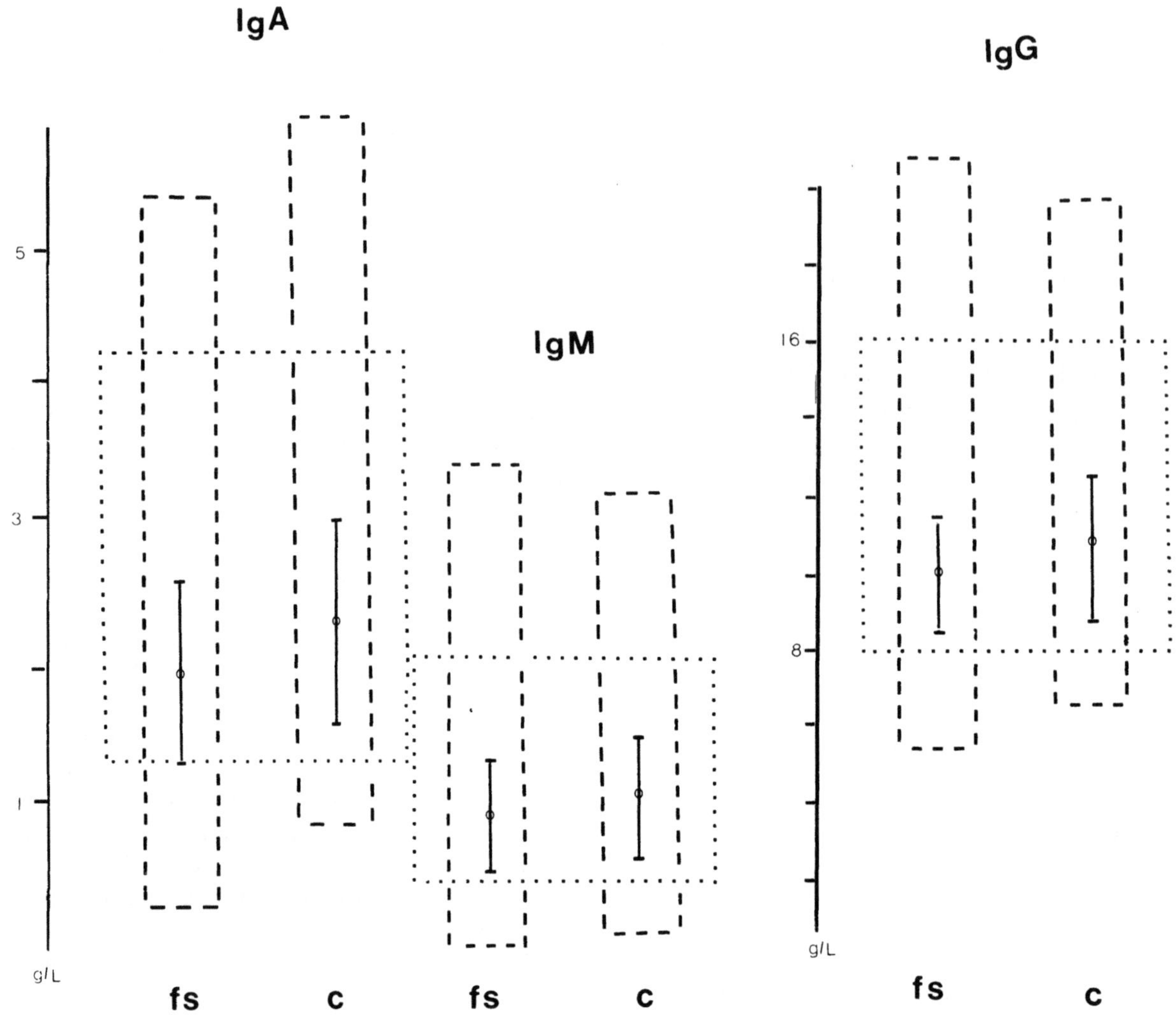

Fig. 1. Immunoglobulin levels in 50 patients with frozen shoulder compared with 50 age- and sex-matched controls

I = mean and standard deviation [ ] = scatter [ ] = normal laboratory range fs= frozen shoulders c= controls

(b) Non-organ-specific antibodies to nuclear material, mitochondria, smooth muscle, collagen, cartilage, and rheumatoid factors.

2. Immunoglobulins: immunoelectrophoresis, quantitative estimations of IgA, IgG, IgM.
3. Immune complexes and complement estimations.

(2 and 3 were performed on a laser nephelometer PDQ using rabbit antisera according to Hyland manufacturers.)

Thyroid antibodies were detected only in those patients with thyroid disease. Rheumatoid factor (both latex and SCAT after Roitt and Doniach) [37] was found in significantly raised titres in 6%, which was only slightly higher than in the control group (4%) and did not reach statistical significance ($P > 0.05$). None of our patients had clinical rheumatoid arthritis. The remaining organ- and non-organ-specific antibodies were not found in our patients.

Quantitative estimations of the immunoglobulin classes IgG, IgA and IgM were similar to the control group (Fig. 1). These figures did not reach statistical significance (Student's t distribution between control and frozen shoulder of each immunoglobulin class gave $P > 0.05$). Five patients with frozen shoulder had depressed IgA levels, three of whom also had abnormally low IgG and IgM concentrations. This compares with two controls who had depressed levels of all three immunoglobulin classes. Selective IgA deficiency occurs in 1 in 500 [18] in the normal population and an association has been found with some autoimmune disorders [2], but the significance of relative depressions of IgA as in our patients is uncertain. This group clearly need to be followed up.

Haematology

1. Full blood count and differential white cell count.
2. Erythrocyte sedimentation rate (ESR).

None of the patients had unusual differential counts nor significantly raised ESR.

Conclusions

Thus, there was no statistically relevant clinical or laboratory evidence from our studies to corroborate an immune-deficient or autoimmune state which may pre-exist and predispose to frozen shoulder. The effect of the early use of steroid treatment found in some studies and discussed below would lend support to an immune disorder, although its purely anti-inflammatory action cannot be discounted. Clearly, an immune disorder may exist, but present-day laboratory methods lack sensitivity for its detection. Alternatively, immune dysfunction may develop following the condition, and further studies are planned to repeat the investigations in a follow-up group of patients.

IV.3. Arthroscopic Examination of the Shoulder

A.M. Wiley

In 1934, Burman et al. [9] published articles on arthroscopy of the knee and also described the examination of other joints. In 1972 we undertook examination of the shoulder of cadavers with a Watanabe-21 arthroscope, using a Tungsten light source, and found that the joint was easy to enter through a posterior approach. Subsequent anatomical dissections around the instrument showed penetration of the infraspinatus. Examination was facilitated by distraction of the joint, and it was shown that seven-eighths of the shoulder joint could be examined, especially when the humerus was rotated inwards and outwards during distraction. In succeeding years we examined the interior of "frozen" shoulders. These patients were undergoing distension of the shoulder joints under anaesthetic, a procedure known as brisement, and we asked each patient whether we could examine the interior of the joint at the same time. We used a 3.8 mm Storz fibro-optic arthroscope with a 2.7 mm telescope: angle of vision was 30° and the field of vision 90°. A light source was provided by a standard cold light fountain. Photography was possible using the Storz Endocamera,

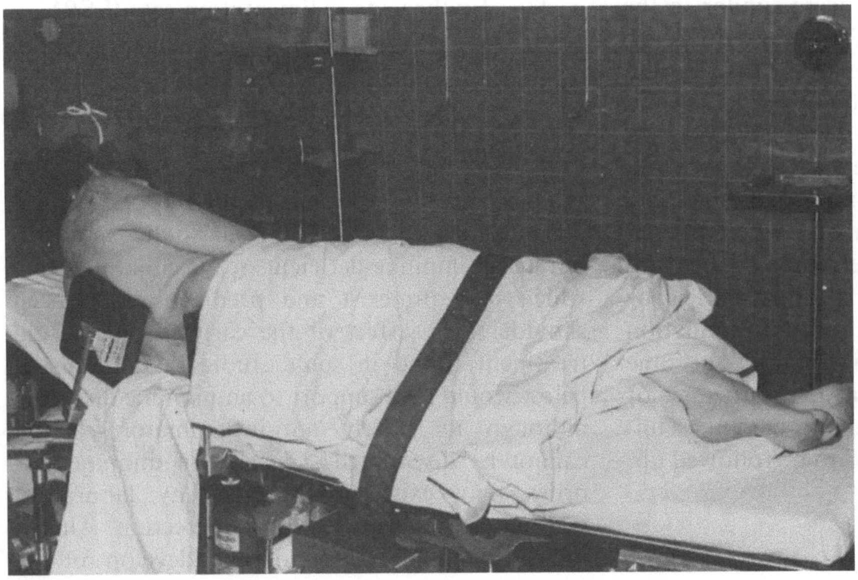

Fig. 1. Position of patient for posterior insertion of shoulder arthroscope

synchronised with a flash through an electronic flash generator.

The findings in these patients have caused us to review the pathology of frozen shoulder. We noted obliteration of the subscapular bursa in many patients and were suprised that the infraglenoid recess showed little evidence of involvement when seen from the inside. The arthrographic appearances must be due to some extra-articular contracture.

Following the success of these examinations through the 3.8 mm Storz sheath, we subsequently carried out 120 successful shoulder arthroscopies for poorly diagnosed shoulder conditions and have now had an opportunity to review the place of the arthroscope in the diagnosis and management of such conditions [42].

Technique of Instrumentation

Arthroscopy has been performed under anaesthesia in all but two patients, in whom local anaesthesia with infiltration permitted us to insert the instrument, but the discomfort to the patient and the difficulty in distracting and rotating the humerus led us to prefer general anaesthesia. The patient is placed upon his side with the affected shoulder uppermost. Chest supports prevent the patient from rolling from side to side on the operating table. The patient's flank is flexed to facilitate viewing of the interior of the joint when the instrument is introduced. From the posterior aspect of the shoulder (Figs. 1 and 2) the patient's humeral head is grasped between finger and thumb just below the angle of the acromion. Initially a size 18-gauge needle is inserted into the shoulder joint just over the tip of the thumb and the needle insinuated into the shoulder joint, a manoeuvre assisted by distraction of the joint. The joint is irrigated and joint fluid, if any, can be examined (in this fashion we detected two patients with postoperative sepsis, unsuspected on clinical and preoperative radiological examinations). The capacity of the shoulder joint can be estimated; it is normally 35 cc but is usually restricted when significant pericapsulitis exists. The needle is extracted leaving the joint distended, and the arthroscope is inserted through a fresh puncture at the same site. It is usual to nick the skin to allow the sharp pointed trocar to be inserted. The instrument is inserted in the same direction, with the same force, and under the same circumstances, as is the irrigation needle. It will be appreciated that irrigation is carried out through the arthroscope and not through a separate needle. It is quite feasible for the surgeon to examine the joint standing or sitting, and apart from the moment of insertion and subsequent examination of the humeral head, it is not necessary for the assistant to keep distracting the shoulder joint. A successful insertion of the instrument is immediately apparent when turning on the cold light source.

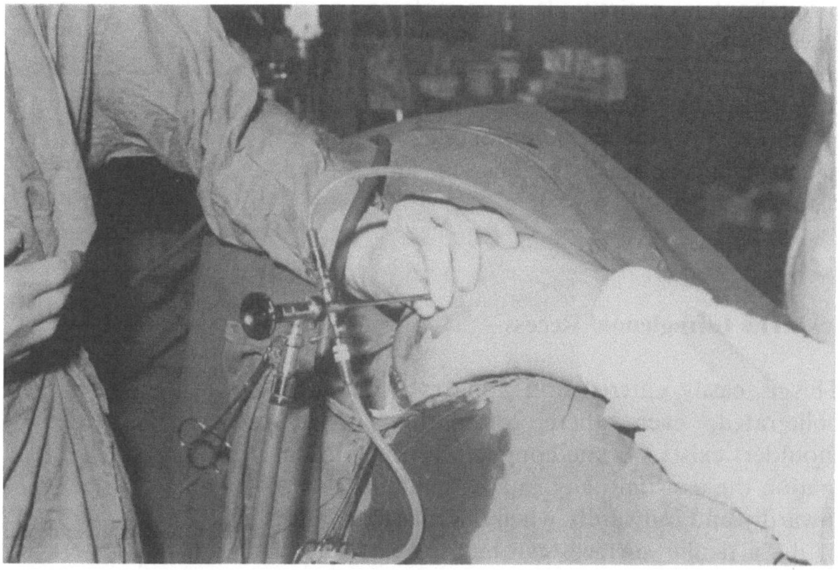

Fig. 2. Arthroscope inserted. Assistant distracts humerus

Extra-articular instrumentation will reveal imperfect soft-tissue cleavage planes while intra-articular appearances are quite striking. It has been usual to examine the joint in three directions: (a) supraglenoid, (b) midfield, and, (c) infraglenoid recess.

(a) The Supraglenoid View

Figure 3 shows the structures which can be visualised. The rotator cuff is clearly outlined, as is the long head of the biceps, its origin from the supraglenoid tubercle, and often its synovial sheath and point of exit at the biceps groove (Fig. 4). The head of the humerus can be seen and, if present, a Hill-Sachs humeral head defect. It is felt that many patients with even one dislocation demonstrate ulceration or indentation corresponding with this lesion.

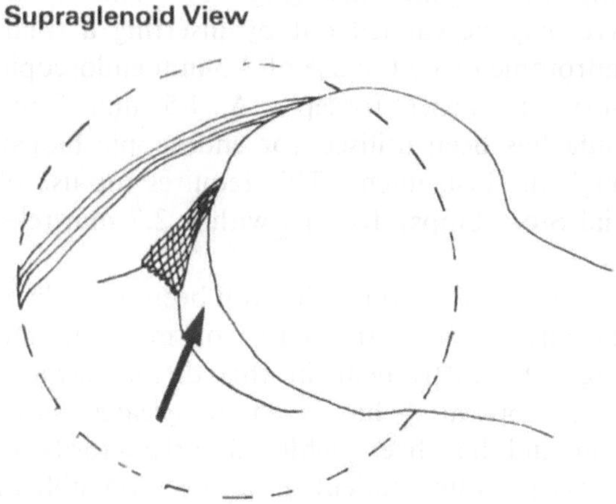

Fig. 3. Diagram to show inspection area during arthroscopy of shoulder

(b) The Midfield View

Examination of the midfield is assisted by distraction of the humerus. The labrum can be seen

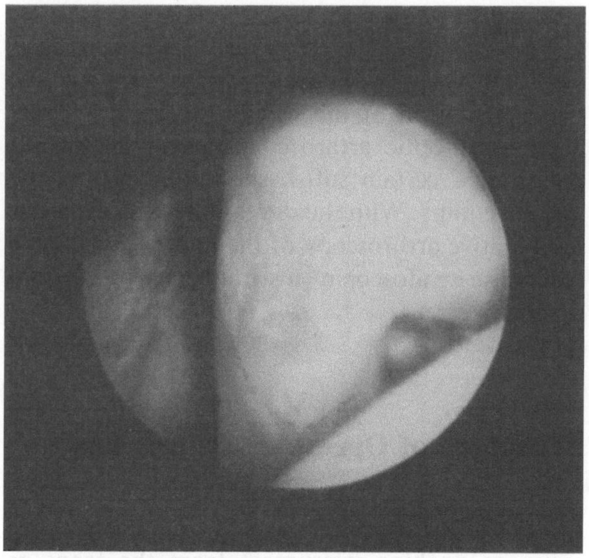

Fig. 4. Interior of shoulder, showing biceps arising from supraglenoid tubercle

throughout its entirety. It is possible to see disinsertion of the labrum and also possible to detect capsular tearing. The instrument is advanced through to the front of the joint in this field. The examiner will note the anterior glenoid humeral ligament and above it the opening into the subscapular bursa.

(c) The Infraglenoid Recess

This is easily entered and appears infrequently obliterated, even where pericapsulitis (frozen shoulder) exists. At the completion of the examination the assistant may rotate the humeral head inwardly and outwardly when degenerate changes of the articular surfaces can be assessed. The instrument is then extracted. It has been the practice to use a Steri-strip to close the very small skin incision.

In 120 cases only one patient had undue discomfort and significant postoperative symptoms. In this case a good deal of extracapsular irrigation fluid was inserted in error in the belief that the joint was accepting irrigation fluid. This patient developed swelling of the axilla, which resolved within a few hours without any sequelae. Patients were able to leave the hospital on the same day and resume a regime appropriate with the diagnosis.

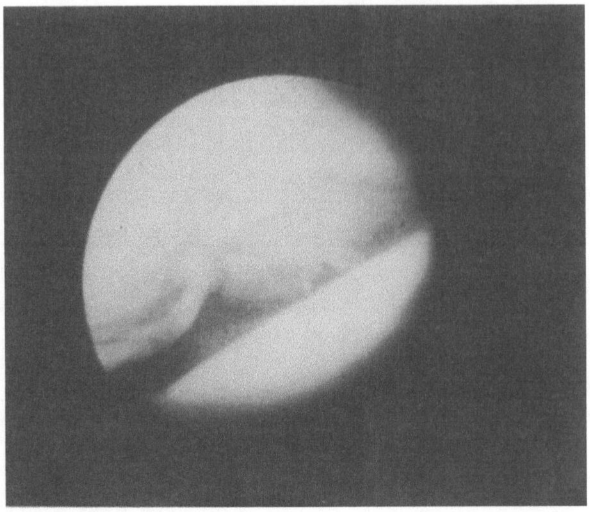

Fig. 5. Incomplete tear of rotator cuff as seen through the arthroscope

Operative Arthroscopy

Instrumentation of the shoulder with a 3.8 mm Storz fibro-optic arthroscope has invited manipulation of certain soft-tissue lesions within the shoulder joint. With the development of expertise in operative arthroscopy of the knee we were able to utilise endoscopic instruments for certain manoeuvres.

Technique of Operative Arthroscopy

Lesions of the shoulder may be manipulated by inserting a probing instrument from the front or from the rear. Anterior instrumentation has taken the form of attempts to divide the coracoacromial ligament under direct vision with the arthroscope in the subacromial bursa. The development of haemorrhage from the small vessel in the coracoacromial ligament has made this procedure less than satisfactory. Most endoscopic operative procedures have been carried out by bimanual manoeuvres from the posterior route. The surgeon inserts the endoscopic instruments under direct vision from the rear of the shoulder. It is possible to insert a Dandy hook to outline the size and edge of a rotator cuff tear; an estimate of the extent and duration of the tear is thus provided. It is also possible to debride the undersurface of the rotator cuff where an incomplete lesion exists, resulting in impingement symptoms (Fig. 5). This manoeuvre may be carried out by inserting a small chondrotome or by the use of 3.3 mm endoscopic scissors or basket forceps. A 4.5 mm Storz cannula has been utilised for endoscopic biopsy through the instrument. This requires the use of special Storz biopsy forceps with a 2.7 mm telescope.

At the time of writing it has not been possible to adapt any other instruments for manipulation through the instrument in this direct fashion. Bimanual operating has given the greatest satisfaction and has been achieved satisfactorily in eight cases. In two patients it has been possible to divide a stenosing condition of the long head of the biceps tendon using an arthroscopic approach.

Experiences with Soft-Tissue Lesions of the Shoulder

Using the arthroscope inserted in the fashion described, it has been possible to examine degenerative arthritis of the shoulder, complete and incomplete lesions of the rotator cuff (some producing impingement syndrome), instability of the shoulder, specific arthritis of the shoulder, and abnormalities of the biceps tendon.

Degenerative Arthritis of the Shoulder

This presents a striking appearance through the arthroscope. Debris, ulceration and chronic synovitis have been identified and, indeed, expected. We were struck by the dense adhesions, sometimes with associated obliteration of the biceps tendon in this condition, and speculate on the role of this finding upon the patient's symptomatology. It should be possible to relieve this by endoscopic surgery combined with debridement.

Rotator Cuff Lesions

Complete tears of the rotator cuff have been estimated for size and duration. Whilst much information about such a lesion can be obtained from a shoulder arthrogram, arthroscopy can, in addition, indicate whether the lesion is a fresh one, show the extent of it, and warn the surgeon to prepare suitable instruments and make surgical decisions accordingly.

Instability of the Shoulder

For us, the recognition of a Bankart lesion has made it mandatory to employ a Bankart repair, whereas capsular loosening may be treated satisfactorily by Putti-Platt operation or similar method. A loose labrum without dislocation was encountered in two patients, one being treated subsequently by endoscopic surgery.

Specific Arthritis

In four patients the diagnosis of specific arthritis was made by endoscopy and biopsy. One patient suffered from rheumatoid arthritis, the shoulder joint being the first affected by the disease. Another developed leukaemic arthritis, where again the shoulder joint was the area first affected. Two patients had infective arthritis following earlier shoulder surgery, aspiration and examination providing this diagnosis.

Abnormalities of the Biceps Tendon

In a number of patients it was possible to see a loose and ruptured biceps tendon which was symptomatic. Several patients were found to have stenosing, adhesive bicipital tendonitis, the symptomatology of which is as yet ill defined.

Arthroscopy in Subsequent Assessment of Rotator Cuff Repairs

In 15 patients it has been possible to examine the integrity of a rotator cuff repair. In 6 of these the repair was less than perfect or had given way in the postoperative period. Five of these patients demonstrated a slow and imperfect result of surgery, for which an explanation was clear through the arthroscope. One patient subsequently underwent further repair, with good result, and another underwent two subsequent repairs. It is felt that arthroscopy of the shoulder may provide valuable information about the effectiveness and efficiency of many rotator cuff repairs.

Accuracy of Arthroscopy

In 15 instances it was possible to follow arthroscopy of the shoulder by an open operation and exploration: in 14 of these the arthroscopic findings were verified; in one patient a rotator cuff tear was suspected at arthroscopy but could not be found at open operation.

Complications of Arthroscopy

In the first 25 patients we experienced one complication, scoring of the humeral head, which did not produce any significant symptoms. There were no infections and one extra-articular instillation of irrigation fluid produced temporary brachial paraesthesiae.

Conclusions

1) Experience with shoulder arthroscopy using a fibro-optic instrument has proved useful in diagnosing specific forms of arthritis.

2) This technique assists in the assessment of rotator cuff tears, complete or incomplete, and in the planning of approaches for surgical repair.

3) Endoscopic shoulder surgery is clearly possible and may be indicated in the débridement of the rotator cuff, in the release of bicipital tendonitis, removal of loose bodies and fragments.

4) Arthroscopic examination of the shoulder has a low morbidity. In common conditions, such as the frozen shoulder, distension of the joint preceding the instrumentation has resulted in early resolution of the patient's symptoms.

IV.4. Treatment of the Frozen Shoulder by Manipulation: A Pilot Study

J.I.L. Bayley and Lipmann Kessel

The term frozen shoulder is frequently misused to label a wide variety of shoulder disorders. As a consequence of overdiagnosis the true incidence of the condition is obscured, and there is considerable blurring of the clinical parameters which constitute the syndrome.

Broadly, two distinct entities exist. The first is a phenomenon in which shoulder movements become limited either as a result of some readily diagnosed intrinsic disorder or from disuse following injury. The second has been called idiopathic or primary frozen shoulder, and its exact cause remains unknown. Diffuse pain develops spontaneously or follows some minor abuse and rapidly escalates until it is severe and constant. Movement becomes progressively limited until, in the worst cases, there is little or no free glenohumeral excursion. In the ensuing weeks pain gradually subsides, and thereafter movement slowly returns over a period as long as twelve to eighteen months. In this type of frozen shoulder there is no clearly identifiable intrinsic clinical or radiographic cause, although several medical conditions are said to occur more frequently in patients with the disorder. These include ischaemic heart disease and diabetes mellitus.

It is important that in the present state of our knowledge the term frozen shoulder should be reserved for this circumscribed group of patients.

As intimated, the condition tends to be self-limiting and the majority of shoulders eventually regain full function. However, resolution may take many months, during which time disability can be considerable. The aim of treatment must therefore be to so compress the natural cycle as to reduce the period of disability to a minimum. To this end a variety of treatments have been advocated. Lee et al. [22] compared regimes involving an exercise programme with a regime of analgesics alone. They found patients treated with exercise fared the best, but the addition of various adjuvants such as infra-red heat therapy or local steroid injection to the exercise programme did not materially influence the result. More active methods of treatment include manipulation of the shoulder under general anaesthesia [24] and hydrostatic distension of the joint either to the point of capsular rupture [33] or just short of it [28].

In this chapter our preliminary experience of a prospective double-blind trial which attempts to compare a regime involving manipulation of the shoulder under general anaesthesia with or without a short course of an oral steroid will be reported.

Material and Methods

All patients satisfied the basic criteria outlined above for a diagnosis of frozen shoulder. Accurate measurement of shoulder movement is difficult, and to avoid the danger of drawing false conclusions from minor improvements in mobility it was stipulated that patients should have lost 50% or more of their normal movements as judged by reference to the unaffected side. In practice this meant that in most shoulders preserved movement consisted largely of scapulothoracic excursion.

The basic treatment regime consists of rest in a broad arm sling for two weeks followed by admission for manipulation at which time the glenohumeral joint is also injected with 25 mg hydrocortisone acetate in 10 ml 0.5% Bupivacaine. Outpatient physiotherapy starts the following day, and pain and mobility are monitored at regular intervals until full recovery.

The method of manipulation deserves comment: it has long been used by the senior author (LK) and has proved to be safe and reliable. In contrast to other methods the long lever arm of the humerus is avoided; rather the scapula is manipulated on the humerus and in such a way that the applied force is concentrated at the shoulder, thus reducing the dangers of humeral fracture. The operator stands at the appropriate side, facing the patient's head. The upper humerus is grasped firmly by the hand opposite to the side to be manipulated—right hand for left shoulder and vice versa. The patient's flexed forearm rests comfortably in the crook of the operator's elbow. After abducting the arm to its full available excursion the operator places the flat of his free hand over the broad mass of the acromial arch. The manipulation is performed by a sharp downward thrust on the acromion against the platform of the immobilised humerus and is usually accompanied by a palpable and audible tearing of the shoulder capsule. Thereafter the joint can be put through a full excursion in all planes with a minimum of effort.

Patients were allocated at random to one of two groups. The same basic regime described above was followed in each patient. In Group A an oral steroid was prescribed in the form of prednisone 5 mg three times daily for two weeks prior to manipulation and, in diminishing dosage, for two weeks thereafter. Patients in Group B received an oral placebo according to the same programme. At no time were the patient or medical staff directly concerned with assessment aware of the allocation.

In the three years 1977 to 1979, 32 patients were admitted to the trial. They formed part of the clinical group undergoing immunological investigation the results of which are reported in Chapter IV.2. One patient suffered sequential bilateral frozen shoulders, and of the 32 patients 5 were excluded from analysis for reasons of insufficient information: 3 were in Group A and 2 in Group B. Therefore 28 shoulders in 27 patients were available for study: 12 in Group A and 16 in Group B. The clinical material is summarised in Table 1, from which it may be seen that the two groups were of broad similarity.

Table 1. Clinical material

	Group A	Group B
Males	5	8
Females	7	8
Age range (years)	46–70	40–63
Average age (years)	53	53
Left shoulder	9	10
Right shoulder	3	6

Results

The outcome of treatment in both groups was assessed in relation to several parameters: ease of

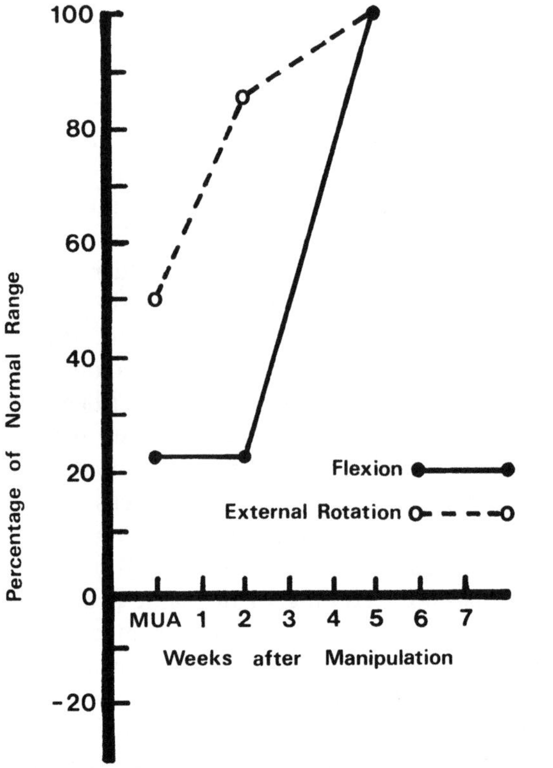

Fig. 1. Dramatic response to manipulation under anaesthesia (MUA) (Case no. 15)

manipulation, the effect of duration of symptoms, pain response, and the rapidity with which shoulder movement was regained. By and large patients fell into two distinct groups in their response to manipulation; those achieving a dramatic restoration of mobility over only a few weeks and those in whom movement returned more slowly. Examples of each group are illustrated in Figs. 1 and 2. Five shoulders required a second manipulation: 2 in Group A and 3 in Group B.

Ease of Manipulation

Under anaesthetic shoulders either "gave" suddenly with only moderate force or they exhibited a plastic resistance which was difficult to overcome. Occasionally quite major force was required before sudden release of the joint, and in this respect an advantage of the manipulative technique is that it obliges the operator to work harder by depriving him of the long lever arm of the humerus so that he is much more aware of the force he is exerting. Furthermore, as his hands are

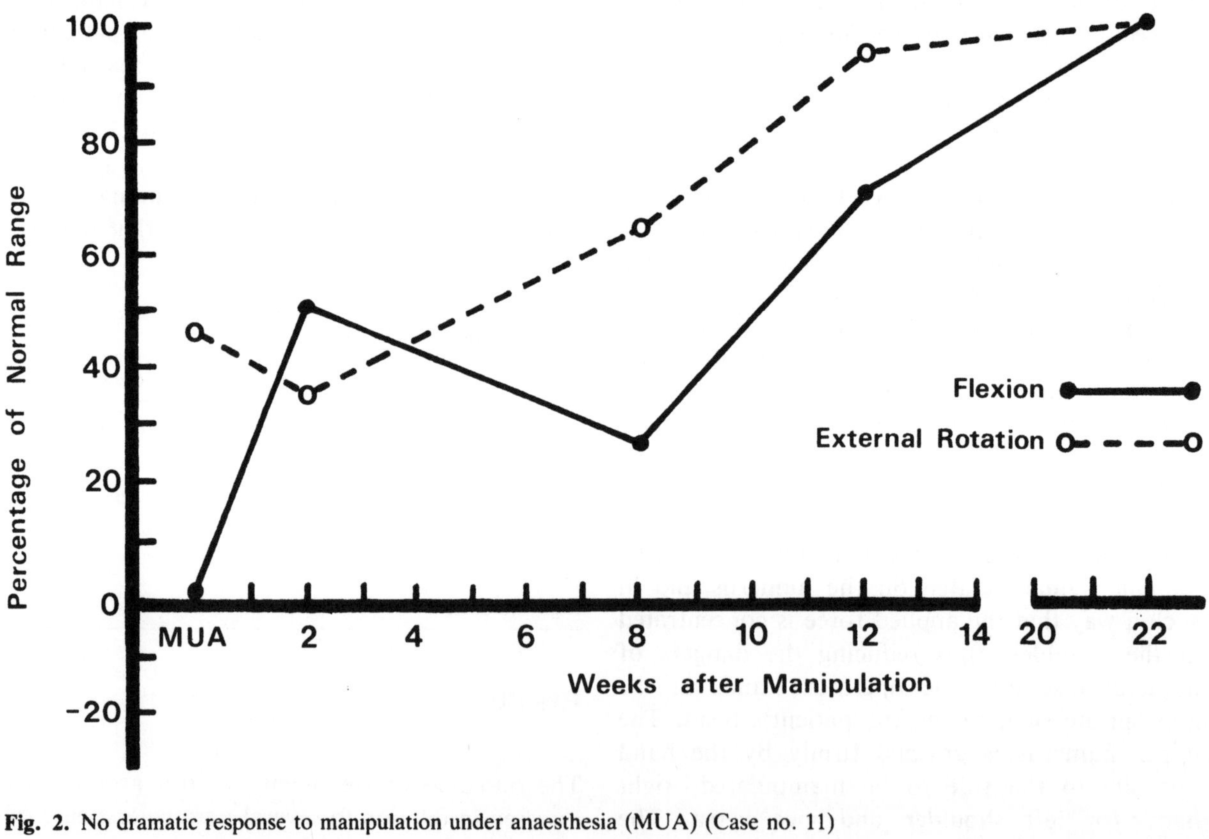

Fig. 2. No dramatic response to manipulation under anaesthesia (MUA) (Case no. 11)

closer to the shoulder than in other methods, the operator has a finer sense of how the joint is responding to the applied force.

In the final analysis oral steroids had no effect on the ease with which manipulation freed a shoulder, three-quarters of the joints in each group giving way with only moderate force. Nor was there a clear correlation between ease of manipulation and the ultimate result; difficult manipulation sometimes gave good results and vice versa.

Duration of Symptoms

We attempted to assess the effect that length of history exerted on the outcome of treatment: 17 shoulders were seen within 6 months of the onset of symptoms; in 11 the shoulder had been affected for 6 to 18 months. One would expect a shoulder frozen for six months or longer to have entered the phase of resolution and that its response to treatment might be enhanced. This was not borne out in practice: patients with longer histories nevertheless continued to complain of severe pain at referral and, on average, mobility at presentation did not vary significantly with duration of symptoms. Nor did the outcome of treatment depend on the length of history (Table 2) even when Groups A and B are analysed separately.

Table 2. Effect of duration of symptoms

Response to Manipulation	Duration of Symptoms	
	Under six months	Over six months
Good	7 (41%)	5 (45%)
Poor	10 (59%)	6 (55%)

The Influence and Response of Pain

Spontaneously reducing pain might suggest resolution of the disease process and persistence of severe pain should equate with continuing disease activity, therefore the outcome of treatment might be expected to vary with pain intensity at presentation. This does not appear to be the case, however, for although the numbers in this series are small, patients with only moderate pain did not enjoy an increased incidence of dramatic response to manipulation, nor was there a significant difference in this respect between patients receiving steroids or placebo.

When considering the effect of manipulation on pain, about half the patients (15) reported that the manoeuvre exacerbated their pain but in only 4 shoulders was this of longer duration than a few hours or days. Oral steroids did not confer increased protection against pain exacerbation, but whatever its intensity at presentation, as a rule, pain ceased to be a problem within a few weeks of manipulation regardless of its duration beforehand.

Restoration of Movement

The normal range of shoulder movement varies with the individual, particularly in external rotation. For this reason absolute values have little meaning as a guide to progress, and where possible we prefer to express values as a percentage of the unaffected side. Equally, as previously stated, it is difficult to measure shoulder movement accurately, and we have chosen a rather gross end-point to treatment which equates with our criteria for entry to the trial. Thus, when better than 80% of normal movement is achieved we judge the shoulder to have reached the end point because our experience has shown that such a shoulder rapidly gains full mobility.

Although movement in each plane was recorded separately, we found the most useful indices of progress to be external rotation and elevation in flexion. The former is the most resistant to treatment and the latter is most useful for function. In general abduction recovers in parallel with flexion. Movements have been tabulated at 6, 12, and 18 weeks after manipulation (Figs. 3 and 4).

When studying elevation in flexion (Fig. 3) it will be seen that by 6 weeks 7 of 12 shoulders (60%) in the steroid group had achieved better than 80% of normal mobility whilst in the placebo group only 3 of 16 shoulders (15%) had done so. The discrepancy lessens with time but marginally remains by the eighteenth week (60%; 50%). In the case of external rotation (Fig. 4) a similar pattern emerges, with 6 of 12 shoulders (50%) in the steroid group reaching the end point by the sixth week against only 2 of 16 shoulders (12%) in the placebo group. Again the gap closes but is still visible by the eighteenth week (60%; 40%).

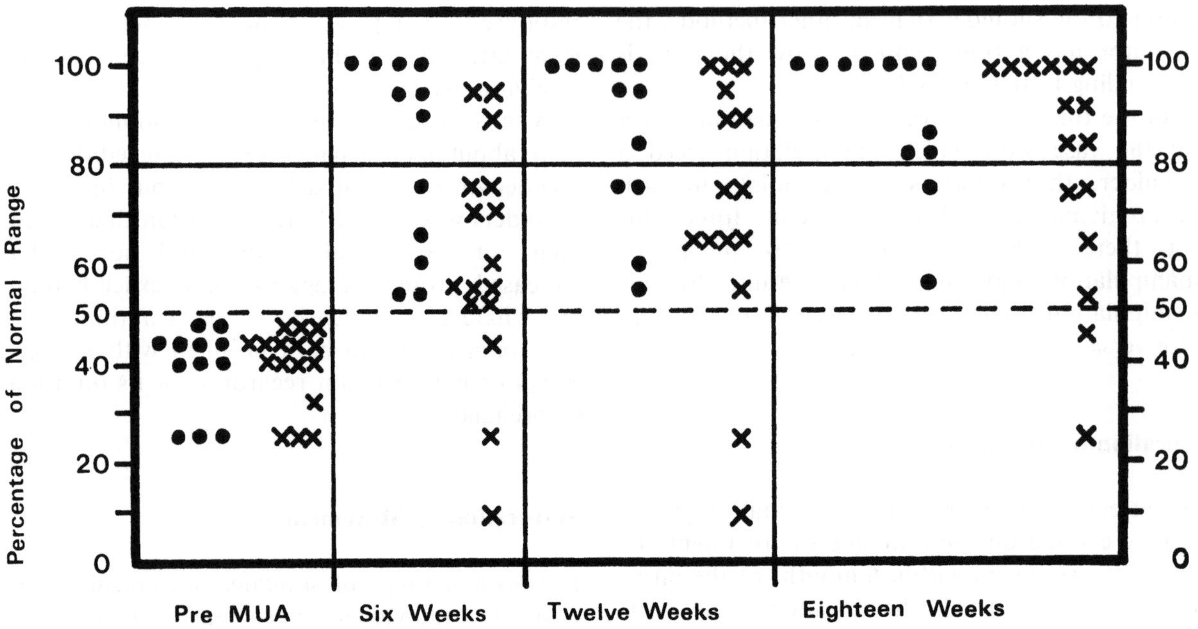

Fig. 3. Frozen shoulder: elevation in flexion before and after manipulation under anaesthesia (MUA) ●, steroid group; X, placebo group

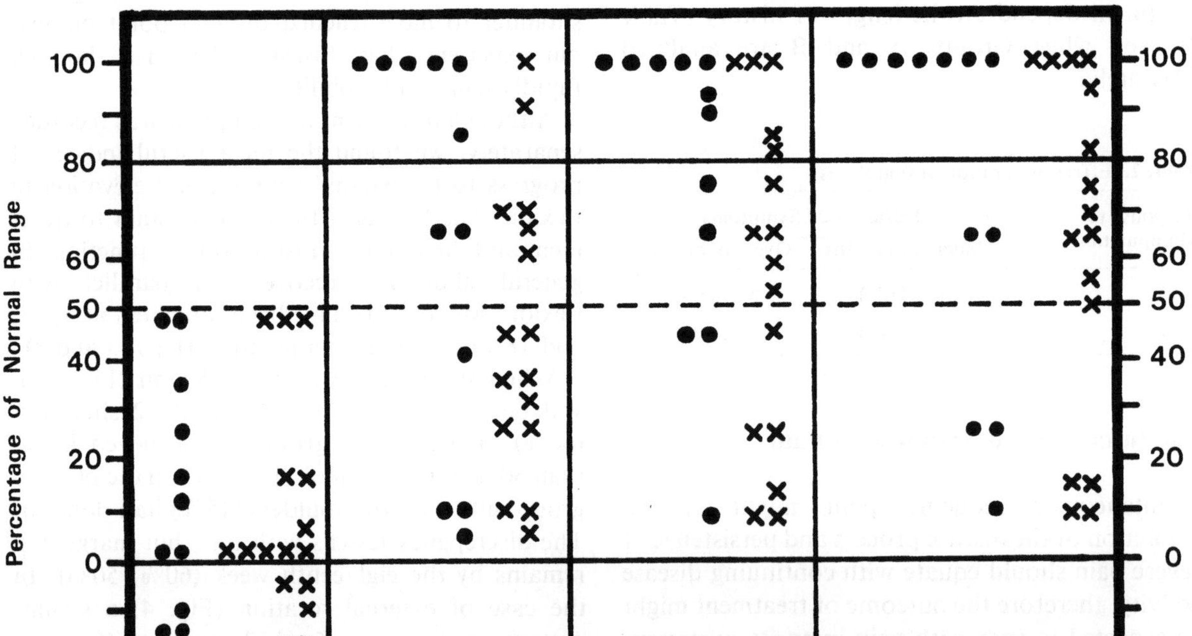

Fig. 4. Frozen shoulder: external rotation before and after manipulation under anaesthesia (MUA) ●, steroid group; X, placebo group

Conclusions

The value of a short course of an oral steroid as an adjunct to manipulation of a frozen shoulder has not been proven in this trial because the numbers are not yet large enough to allow valid statistical analysis. Certainly oral steroids do not appear to confer any advantage in protection against post-manipulation pain exacerbation. Nevertheless a trend has emerged which hints at a more rapid return of movement in the steroid group.

Our provisional opinion is that manipulation under general anaesthesia followed by physiotherapy is a useful mode of treatment for frozen shoulders and the addition of a short course of an oral steroid may be a useful adjuvant to this treatment. By these means it would appear that in a large majority (80%) disability can be reduced from eighteen months to eighteen weeks and in a high proportion (60%) to as little as six weeks.

IV.5. Distension Arthrography of the Shoulder Joint

M.W.J. Older

The frozen shoulder is a unique entity within the musculoskeletal system and is a common cause of chronic invalidism in our society.

We believe that the main cause lies in the fixator tendons of the capsule. Simmonds [39] drew attention to the supraspinatus component of the rotator cuff. He submitted that the basic lesion was cell death, and this has recently been confirmed by Macnab [28]. The underlying basic pathological lesion is focal cell death which evokes an inflammatory response causing rotator cuff tendonitis. When the degenerative changes spread to involve all the tendons diffuse capsulitis results and is characterised by a well-known cycle of events: increasingly severe pain during the inflammatory stage and limitation of movement by muscle spasm. Later the pain becomes less severe, but the stiffness persists by contracture of the capsule. This is the clinical syndrome known as frozen shoulder.

Treatment in the initial irritative phase is usually by rest in a sling and analgesia. As the severity of the pain decreases physiotherapy in the form of active exercises is recommended. There is still debate about the efficacy of local and systemic steroids [6,8,15] although Roy and Oldham [38] suggest that the frozen shoulder is the result of a neglected painful shoulder and recommend early treatment with steroid injections.

Manipulation of the shoulder has been advocated, but since its description by Duplay in 1872 [15] its role has been controversial. Proponents claim that rapid return to normality can be obtained but opponents decry the method, claiming the tissues are grossly torn and that manipulation results in further scarring, not to mention the danger of fracture.

In the chronic phase, treatment varies from masterly inactivity to open operation with resection of the subscapularis tendon and the underlying capsule.

Codman [11] stated that the prognosis is excellent and that given time recovery is full. Grey [17] recently reported that of 25 patients with idiopathic frozen shoulder treated with only reassurance, simple analgesia and hypnotics, all 25 had returned to normal within two years. He concluded that in the great majority of these patients the condition is self-limiting, symptoms subside and full shoulder movement returns.

Simmonds [39], however, reported that the shoulder returned to normal in only one-third of his patients. Others agree that there is a small group of patients who reach a plateau of recovery and are left with permanent painful restriction of shoulder motion despite conventional therapy. We also recognise this minority group, and it is in these time-expired patients that we have found hydrostatic distension to be helpful. We think this is best done using the technique of arthrography under fluoroscopic control, immediately followed by a programme of intensive physiotherapy.

Arthrography of the shoulder was first employed by Oberholzer [32], using air as the contrast medium, but although a number of authors have since demonstrated arthrography to be a useful diagnostic investigation it is still not widely performed. However Preston and Jackson [34] have shown that the double contrast technique can be informative. Shoulder arthrography as a therapeutic procedure was first reported by Andren and Lundberg [3], who treated 64 rigid shoulders in patients with rotator cuff ruptures, fractures and frozen shoulders. Follow-up was short and the results mixed, although Preston and Jackson [34] recorded three patients with capsulitis who experienced considerable relief from the procedure.

Reeves [35] has reported favourable results in two patients treated with serial distension, and DePalma [14] has suggested that before manipulation one should distend the joint with saline under pressure until free flow is established. Simon [40] claims excellent results for a method of infiltration under general anaesthesia in which the joint is distended with a fluid mixture of lidocaine and triamcinolone until rupture occurs and is then manipulated. Conti [12] reports treating the frozen shoulder using all modes, arthrography via an arthroscope, distension with saline, incision of the capsule then a steroid injection and finally passive manipulation with traction. He claims a cure in three weeks.

For patients who have reached a plateau of recovery Macnab [28] recommends hydraulic distension of the glenohumeral joint. Saline is injected under pressure until the patient experiences significant discomfort. Then the joint is aspirated, and the injection concluded by instilling hydrocortisone.

The first distension arthrogram was performed by McIntyre in 1972. In 1976 we presented data on the first six patients treated by arthrographic distension [33] and a further report was made in 1978 [23]. We concluded that distension arthrography was a useful mode of treatment for patients with painful stiff shoulders who had failed to respond to conventional therapy. Encouraged by our early results, we have continued to use this procedure and we report here our experience to date.

Technique

Distension arthrography is performed in hospital under full aseptic conditions, usually with local analgesia and light sedation, but general anaesthesia may be given to the particularly apprehensive person.

The patient is positioned supine. Under fluoroscopic control the anteroinferior part of the glenohumeral joint is identified and a 5 cm 18 gauge needle inserted through the skin towards the joint, infiltrating the tissues with local anaesthetic as the needle is advanced. A 10 cm 22 gauge needle with trocar is inserted through the first needle into the joint space and connected by an extension tube to a 50 ml syringe containing 68% sodium iothalamate (Conray 400). Sodium iothalamate is used in preference to the diatrizoate derivatives because it is less irritant chemically.

To confirm that the needle is in the joint space 1 ml of contrast material is injected. The physician then manually injects contrast medium, and as the joint distends and resistance increases further force is needed. The physician watches this distension of the joint under fluoroscopic control until he sees the contrast medium suddenly leave the joint space. When this occurs, resistance usually ceases and no further fluid is injected.

Under local analgesia distension arthrography may be very painful, and some patients experience the sensation that "something has given way". As soon as possible after the procedure the patient starts a course of intensive physiotherapy in which the physiotherapist will apply ice packs and commence active assisted exercises. Appropriate anal-

Table 1. Clinical data: 1972-1979

	Number of Patients
Diffuse rotator cuff tendonitis	40
Stiffness from neglect	7
Postoperative stiffness	5
Rheumatoid arthritis	4
Post-traumatic reflex dystrophy	2
Total	58

gesics are provided to increase the patient's participation in the exercise programme.

Results

During the period 1972-1979 we treated 58 patients with distension arthrography for a variety of conditions as shown in Table 1. Forty patients had a frozen shoulder due to a diffuse rotator cuff tendonitis, and their age range and sex ratio are shown in Table 2. To assess the usefulness of hydrostatic distension we examined patients at least a year after the arthrogram and determined the degree of pain and range of motion.

Table 2. Diffuse rotator cuff tendonitis (capsulitis)

Sex	Number of Patients
Male	24
Female	16
Total	40
Age range (years)	25-68

Table 3 shows that in those patients with capsulitis about half the patients had completely recovered a full range of painless motion in the shoulder joint and there was some improvement in a further 25%, so that three-quarters of the patients had been helped and were able to return to full activity. A quarter were unchanged, with the same level of discomfort and disability after the distension as before.

When a new technique is successful there is always a tendency to use it to treat other conditions. We successfully treated 7 patients who had developed a painful stiff shoulder due to neglect associated with conditions outside the shoulder joint. Of these, 3 had thoracotomies and the other 4 either serious forearm fractures or multiple injuries and prolonged intravenous therapy. There was rapid relief of pain in all cases and a return to full mobility of the glenohumeral joint. Two patients with post-traumatic reflex dystrophy were treated: one obtained complete relief of pain, and the other improved the range of motion.

Table 3. Diffuse Rotator Cuff Tendinitis: Results of Distension Arthrography (one year follow-up)

	Number of Patients
Range of motion	
Full	18
Limited – no disability	12
– continuing disability	10
Pain Relief	
– complete	21
– partial (no disability)	9
– no change (disabled)	10
Total	40

In 5 patients with postoperative stiffness of the shoulder there was only marginal improvement in 2, one after a Putti-Platt and the other a fracture of the greater tuberosity. Distension arthrography made no contribution to the rehabilitation of two patients with open reduction and internal fixation for fractures of the humeral neck. The only success in this group was the fifth patient, previously reported by the authors [33], who had stiffness after repair of a complete tear of the supraspinatus tendon. His recovery after distension was so good that he successfully completed a degree course in physical education.

In patients with rheumatoid arthritis and stiff painful shoulders, distension only made the pain worse and gave no improvement in mobility, and we consider our attempts to treat rheumatoid patients in this way have failed.

Discussion

In our study of patients with frozen shoulders we found that the arthrographic picture of capsulitis is a joint of low capacity with small synovial recesses and, initially, non-filling of the bicipital tendon sheath. This accords with the findings of others [34,35,40].

It is interesting to speculate on what occurs when the capsule is distended. In the majority of patients, when the soft tissues "give", the contrast medium is seen to pass medially. This may be through the subscapularis bursa and would accord with the views of Wiley and Older [41], who in arthroscopic examination of patients with a frozen shoulder found the subscapularis bursa to be an important factor in the capsulitis. However, there is also a point of apparent disagreement between arthrographic and arthroscopic findings. Arthrograms show little or no axillary recess, whereas Wiley and Older found no evidence on arthrography (IV3) of any contracture or pathology in this region. Further work is required to elucidate the part played by the subscapular and axillary recesses in capsulitis.

We would stress that we have not used distension arthrography for all patients presenting with a frozen shoulder. We have deliberately used it only to help the time-expired group who have proved resistant to other forms of therapy and in whom no further spontaneous improvement could be expected.

Our data suggests that for 'time-expired' patients with a frozen shoulder arising from a diffuse rotator cuff tendonitis our treatment will cure 50% of patients and improve a further 25%. It is also very helpful in patients with stiffness due to neglect, but it has no place in the treatment of patients with a frozen shoulder of other aetiology, and in some conditions such as rheumatoid arthritis can make the condition worse.

Whatever its role, from our experience, distension alone does not relieve pain or result in an increased range of movement, but seems to free the glenohumeral joint thus helping the patient to cooperate more enthusiastically with the exercise programme.

Distension arthrography is easy to perform, and although patients may have some pain during the procedure there are no serious complications.

References

1 Allison AC, Denman AM, Barnes RD (1971) Cooperating and controlling functions of thymus—derived lymphocytes in relation to autoimmunity. Lancet 2: 135-140

2 Amman AJ, Hong R (1971) Selective IgA deficiency: presentation of 30 cases and a review of the literature. Medicine 50: 223-236

3 Andren L, Lundberg BJ (1965) Treatment of rigid shoulders by joint distension during arthrography. Acta Orthop Scand 36: 45-53

4 Brewerton DA, Hart FD, Nicholls A, Caffrey M, James DCO, Sturrock RD (1973) Ankylosing spondylitis and HL-A27. Lancet 1: 904

5 Bridgeman JF (1972) Periarthritis of the shoulder and diabetes mellitus. Ann Rheum Dis 31: 69-71

6 British Medical Journal (1976) Shoulder cuff lesions. Brit Med J 1: 672-673

7 Bulgen DY, Hazleman BL, Voak D (1976) HLA-B27 and frozen shoulder. Lancet 1: 1042-1043

8 Bulgen DY, Hazleman BL, Ward M, McCallum M (1978) Immunological studies in frozen shoulder. Ann Rheum Dis 37: 135-138

9 Burman MS, Finkelstein H, Mayer L (1934) Arthroscopy of the knee joint. J Bone Jt Surg. 16: 255

10 Charnley J (1959) Periarthritis of the shoulder. Postgraduate Med J 35: 384

11 Codman EA (1934) The shoulder. Thomas Todd Co. Boston

12 Conti V (1979) Arthroscopy in rehabilitation. Orthop Clin N Am 10: 709-711

13 DePalma AF (1952) Loss of scapulohumeral motion (Frozen Shoulder) Ann Surg 135: 193

14 DePalma AF (1973) Surgery of the shoulder. 2nd Ed. JB Lippincott Co. Philadelphia

15 Duplay S (1872) De la péri-arthrite scapulo-humérale et des raideurs de l'épaule qui en sont les conséquence. Arch Gen Med 20: 513

16 Ganda SP, Soelaner SS (1977) Genetic, acquired and related factors in the aetiology of diabetes mellitus. Arch Int Med 137: 461-469

17 Grey RG (1978) The natural history of idiopathic frozen shoulder. J Bone Joint Surg 60-A: 564

18 Hobbs JR (1968) Immune imbalance in dysgammaglobulinaemia type IV. Lancet 2: 110-114

19 Joint Report from the Sixty International Histocompatability Workshop Conference (1976) II Typing for HLA-D (CALL & MLC) determinants. In: Histocompatibility testing (1975) Ed. Kissmeyer—Nielsen F. Copenhagen Munksgard

20 Kessel L (1950) Arthrography of the shoulder joint. Proc Roy Soc Med 43: 418

21 Lancet Injecting the painful shoulder (1976) Lancet 1: 27

22 Lee M, Haq AMMM, Wright V, Longton EB (1973) Periarthritis of the shoulder: a controlled trial of physiotherapy. Physiotherapy Vol 59, No 10: 312-315

23 Lloyd GJ, McIntyre JL, Older MWJ (1978) The treatment of shoulder stiffness by hydrostatic manipulation. J Bone Jt Surg 60-B: 440-441

24 Lloyd-Roberts GC, French PR (1959) Periarthritis of the shoulder, a study of the disease and its treatment. British Med J (i): 1569-1571

25 Logan WPD, Cushion AA (1958) Morbidity statistics from general practice, Vol 1 (General) HM Stationery Office London

26 Lundberg BJ (1969) The frozen shoulder. Acta Orthop Scand (Suppl) 119

27 Macnab I (1973) Rotator cuff tendinitis. Ann Roy Coll Surg Eng 53: 271-287

28 Macnab I (1979) Rotator cuff tendinitis. Recent advances in orthopaedics. McKibbin B (Ed). Churchill Livingston pp 89-109

29 Malins JM (1978) In "Clinical diabetes mellitus" Eyre & Spottiswoode, London

30 Meulengracht E, Schwartz M (1952) The course and prognosis of periarthrosis humeroscapularis with regard to cases of general symptoms. Acta Med Scand 143: 350-360

31 Neviaser JS (1945) Adhesive capsulitis of the shoulder. J Bone Jt Surg 27: 211

32 Oberholzer J (1933) Die Arthropneumoradiographie bei habitueller Schulterluxation. Roentgen Praxis 5: 589-590

33 Older MWJ, McIntyre JL, Lloyd GJ (1976) Distension arthrography of the shoulder joint. Can J Surg 19: 203-207

34 Preston BJ, Jackson JP (1977) Investigation of shoulder disability by arthrography. Clin Radiol 28: 259-266

35 Reeves B (1966) Arthrographic changes in frozen and post traumatic stiff shoulders. Proc R Soc Med 59: 827-830

36 Richardson AT (1975) The painful shoulder. Proc R Soc Med 68: 731-736

37 Roitt IM, Doniach D (1969) Manual of autoimmune serology. WHO Geneva

38 Roy S, Oldham R (1976) Management of painful shoulder. Lancet 1: 1322-1324

39 Simmonds FA (1949) Shoulder pain with particular reference to the frozen shoulder. J Bone Jt Surg 31-B: 426-432

40 Simon WH (1975) Soft tissue disorders of shoulder. Orthop Clin N Am 6: 521-539

41 Tunbridge WMG, Evered DC, Appleton D, Browis M, Clark F, Grimley Evans J, Young E, Hall R (1976) The prevalence of thyroid disorders in an English community. Robbins J et al Ed. Thyroid research Amsterdam—Exerpta Medica p 520-522

42 Wiley AM, Older MWJ (1980) Shoulder arthroscopy. Investigations with a fibro optic instrument. Am J Sports Med 8: 30

Section V. Prosthetic Replacement

Moderator—A.W.F. Lettin

V.1. The Shoulder Joint in Rheumatoid Arthritis

J.F. Crossan and R. Vallance

Introduction

In the last decade total replacement of the shoulder joint has become a surgical reality which will have a bearing on the management of pain in the severely damaged joint in rheumatoid arthritis. Little has been written on the natural history of the shoulder in this disease in which considerable destruction of the shoulder may occur before onset of significant pain. The anatomical derangements thus produced may lead to technical problems in joint replacement not encountered in degenerative arthritis. The purpose of this study is to review the clinical and radiological presentation of rheumatoid arthritis in the shoulder and to discuss the natural history of the changes which occur.

Clinical Presentation

Rheumatoid arthritis rarely presents initially with pain in the shoulder joint. However, shoulder pain often occurs within the first year or two of onset of the disease process. Characteristically such patients have several episodes of shoulder pain early in the disease and subsequently may suffer only from intermittent discomfort. The majority

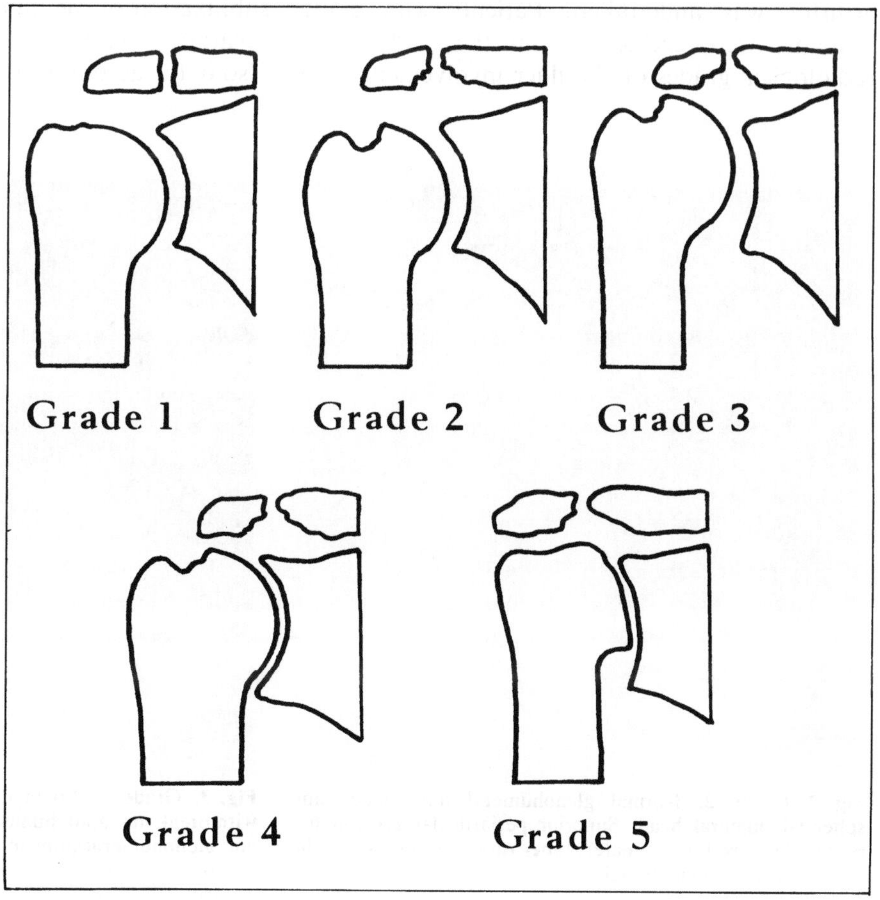

Fig. 1. Grade 1, normal. Grade 2, normal glenohumeral articulation with periarticular erosions. Grade 3, proximal subluxation of the humeral head with similar erosive changes and a preserved glenohumeral joint space. Grade 4, loss of glenohumeral joint space with spherical humeral head, and periarticular erosions. Grade 5, partial destruction of humeral head and glenoid fossa with loss of sphericity in the humeral head

of patients retain satisfactory shoulder function following these acute episodes, although in a small number of patients relentless destruction of the joint occurs over a period of a few months. Such patients characteristically have aggressive changes in other joints.

In the early stages of the disease, pain may be referred to the deltoid muscle mass and has the characteristics of pain originating from the rotator cuff. Only a small number of patients will indicate the acromioclavicular joint as the source of their pain. In the later stages of the disease pain may be referred to the coracoid process where clinical examination reveals the presence of marked tenderness. This feature has been noted to occur in patients suffering from irritative lesions of the glenohumeral joint from other causes [42].

Radiological Grading

A radiological study of 100 shoulder joints in 50 hospitalised patients with seropositive rheumatoid arthritis was undertaken. Patients with acute synovitis were excluded from the study. Five radiological grades of shoulder involvement were observed (Fig. 1). The radiological features associated with each grade are described below:

Grade 1 (11%). No abnormal radiological features are noted in this group of shoulders.

Grade 2 (35%). The humeral head retains its sphericity, and the glenohumeral joint space remains normal. Erosions are frequently seen at the superior periarticular margin of the humeral head, and similar lesions are also present anteriorly or posteriorly in many shoulders (Fig. 2). Erosions are often present in the acromioclavicular joints and their overall distribution is shown in Table 1.

Table 1. Distribution of erosions in grade 2 shoulders

Humeral head alone	9
Acromioclavicular joint alone	6
Both	20

Grade 3 (16%). The humeral head retains its sphericity with apparent preservation of the glenohumeral joint space (but with proximal subluxation of the humerus). Erosive changes are invariably present in the humeral head and often also in the acromioclavicular joint (Fig. 3). In half

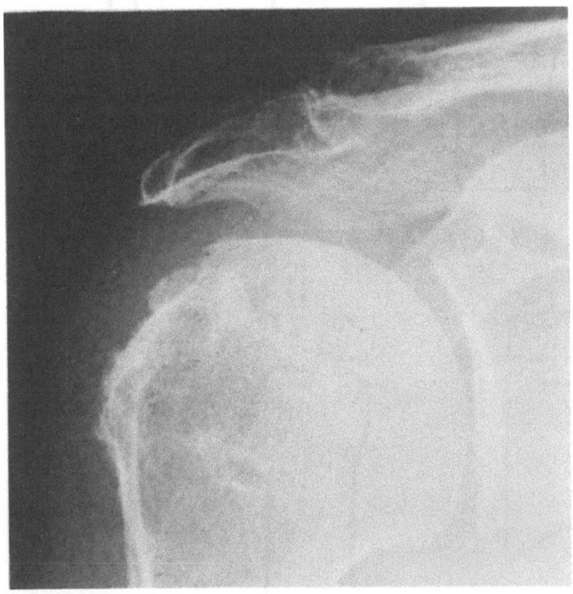

Fig. 2. Grade 2. Normal glenohumeral joint space and spherical humeral head. Superior periarticular erosion has partly destroyed the greater tuberosity. No break in the normal scapulohumeral arch

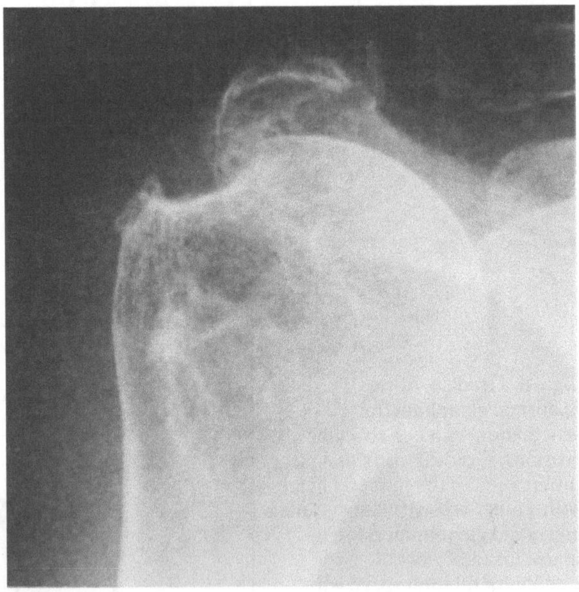

Fig. 3. Grade 3. Proximal subluxation of the humeral head with break in scapulohumeral arch. Humeral head is spherical and glenohumeral joint space retained. Superior and inferior periarticular erosions in the humeral head. Early erosion of clavicular side of acromioclavicular joint

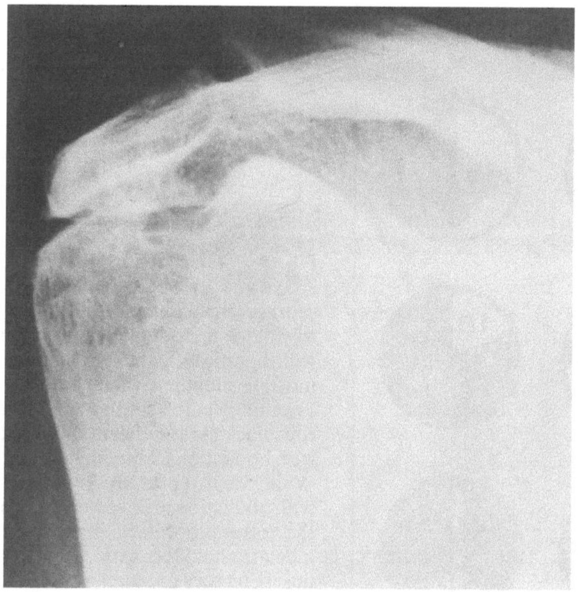

Fig. 4. Glenohumeral joint space reduced but humeral head remains spherical. Proximal subluxation of humeral head and large superior periarticular erosion

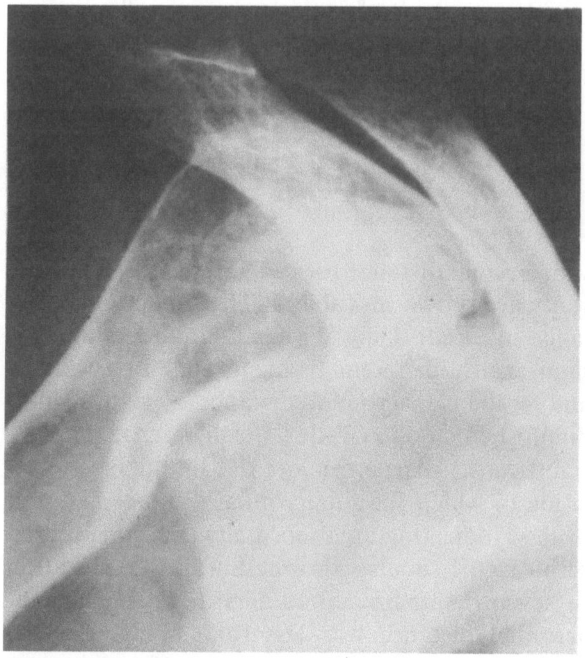

Fig. 5. Cross destruction of both the humeral head and glenoid fossa. Bone loss has contributed to gross medial displacement of the humeral head. Note profound osteoporosis

of these shoulders there is erosion of the greater tuberosity of the humerus.

Grade 4 (16%). The humeral head retains its sphericity, but the glenohumeral joint space is markedly reduced. Erosive changes are invariably present in the humeral head at the periarticular margin and often also in the acromioclavicular joint (Fig. 4). In many of these shoulders there is proximal subluxation of the humeral head.

Grade 5 (22%). These shoulders represent end-stage disease in which distortion of the humeral head and glenoid fossa has occurred. Glenohumeral joint space is reduced, the subacromial distance is considerably diminished, and there is often considerable erosion of the glenoid fossa. The combination of bone loss from both sides of the glenohumeral articulation frequently produces medial displacement of the humeral head which often comes to lie beneath the acromioclavicular joint (Fig. 5).

Correlation of Clinical Features with Radiological Grade

The clinical features of each shoulder were recorded. Three parameters were chosen to illustrate the extent of clinical involvement (Fig. 6). Grade 1 shoulders produced no pain and no significant limitation of movement or of function. One quarter to one third of shoulders of Grades 2, 3 and 4 produced pain requiring the use of analgesics. In end-stage disease more than half had pain requiring the use of analgesics. In the presence of normal rotation in the shoulder joint, abduction and flexion to 90° allows an adequate range of movement for personal hygiene. The ranges of flexion invariably equalled or somewhat exceeded the ranges of abduction. Rotational movements were significantly limited only in those shoulders in which disabling pain was present or in those shoulders with severe glenohumeral disease. Limitation of abduction below 90° was uncommon in Grades 2, 3 and 4 but occurred in the majority of end-stage shoulders. An assessment of overall function was made using the numerical scale devised by Neer [45]. This assessment takes into account the presence of pain, range of movement, the ability to perform certain tasks and the anatomical structure of the shoulder joint. Unsatisfactory function was rare in Grade 2, but

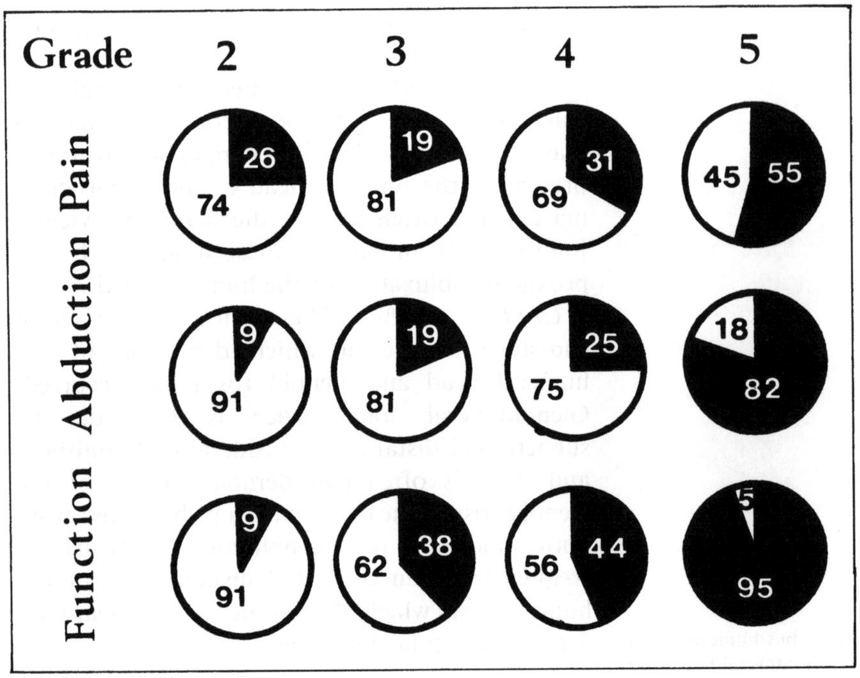

Fig. 6. Clinical features of Grade 2, 3, 4 and 5. Figures in the circles represent percentages. In the top row block areas indicate shoulders with significant pain. White areas indicate shoulders which are essentially painfree. In the middle row black areas indicate shoulders with abduction less than 90°. White areas represent shoulders with abduction in excess of 90°. In the bottom row black areas indicate shoulders with unsatisfactory function on Neer's assessment system. White areas represent shoulders with satisfactory function

was present in more than one-third of shoulders of Grades 3 and 4. In end-stage disease shoulder function was almost invariably severely compromised.

Significance of Subacromial Distance

It is often difficult to assess rotator cuff function clinically in the patient with rheumatoid arthritis and plain radiographs yield little information regarding the presence or absence of rotator cuff tears. Arthrography was not performed in the patients studied, but previous studies using arthrography have demonstrated rotator cuff tears in up to 25% of painful rheumatoid shoulders [21]. However, it is difficult to assess the size and therefore the significance of rotator cuff defects using arthrography.

In degenerative disease of the shoulder, the subacromial distance has proved to be of some value in assessing the presence of rotator cuff tears which are invariably present when the subacromial distance is less than 6 mm [15,24,65]. The converse, however, is not true and values in the normal range of 7-14 mm may be associated on occasions with large tears. The mean values of subacromial distance for each grade in the present study are shown in Table 2. The subacromial distance in Grade 1 and Grade 2 shoulders are not significantly different from normal. In Grades 3 and 4 the subacromial distance is significantly diminished, and in Grade 5 the difference is highly significant. The percentage of shoulders in each grade in which the subacromial distance is 6 mm or less, indicating an abnormally thin or ruptured rotator cuff, is also shown. Surgical exploration of seven rheumatoid shoulders in which the subacromial distance was less than 6 mm demonstrated the presence of a rotator cuff tear in only one shoulder. In the remaining shoulders the rotator cuff was attenuated and of poor quality. Similar observations have been made by Cruess

Table 2. Subacromial distances according to grade

Grade	Mean subacromial distance (mm)	Subacromial distance less than 6 mm (%)
1	8.7	0
2	8.8	11.4
3	6.2	50.0
4	6.0	43.8
5	4.1	86.4

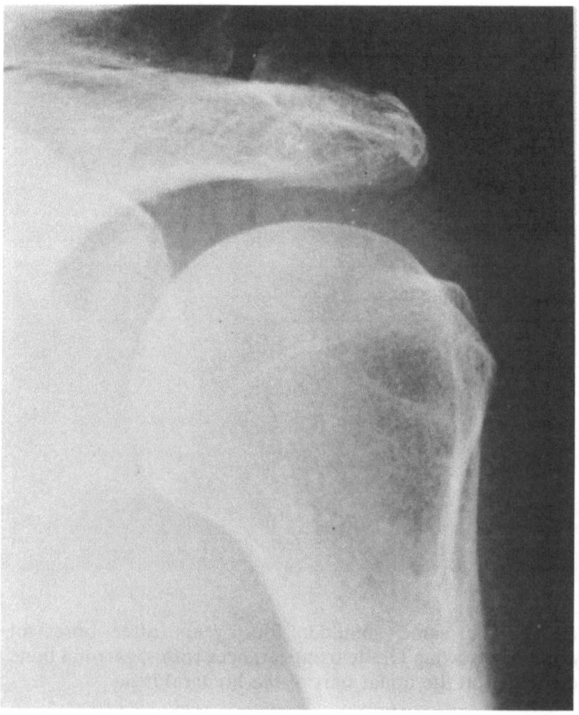

Fig. 7. Radiograph of rheumatoid patient with acute onset of shoulder pain. Normal radiological appearances

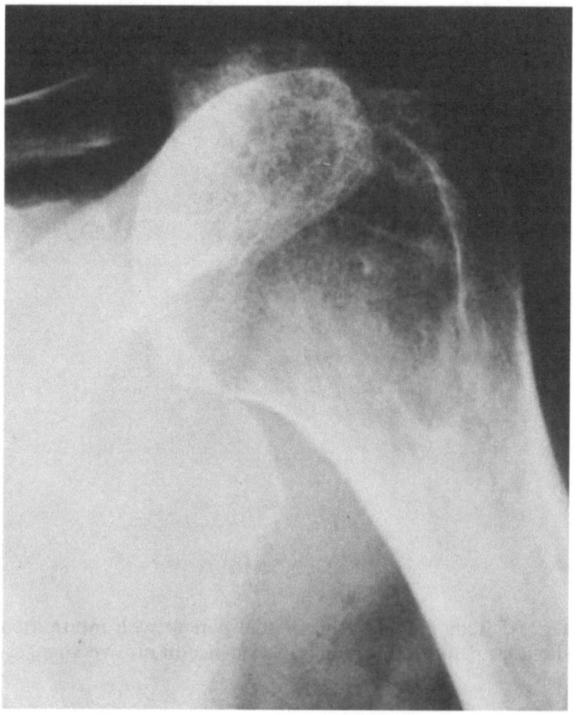

Fig. 8. Radiograph of same shoulder 4 months later showing severe proximal subluxation of the humeral head and early erosive changes at the superior periarticular margin of the humeral head and in the acromioclavicular joint. Surgical exploration revealed massive rotator cuff tear

[17]. It is evident therefore that abnormalities of the rotator cuff may occur in a small percentage of Grade 2 shoulders, in about half of shoulders of Grades 3 and 4 and in the majority of end-stage shoulders.

Radiological Progression

In the rheumatoid shoulder the rate of progression of joint destruction, as in other joints, varies with the activity of the disease. To define patterns of progression, a retrospective radiological review of 20 painful shoulders was undertaken. The study was restricted to shoulders which presented initially with Grade 1 or 2 appearances. Serial radiographs had been performed because of recurring episodes of shoulder pain. Five shoulders showed no progression other than some increase in the size of erosions. The remaining 15 shoulders, however, showed significant deterioration to Grade 4 or 5. Two initial patterns of progression emerged; acute superior subluxation of the humeral head in 3 shoulders, and chronic superior subluxation of the humeral head in 12 shoulders. Subsequently, medial displacement of the humeral head occurred in 9 shoulders.

(i) Acute superior subluxation of the humeral head

In 3 shoulders an acute episode of disabling pain lasting for one to two weeks was associated with early and severe proximal subluxation of the humeral head, even in the absence of erosive disease (Figs. 7 and 8). In 2 instances arthrography confirmed the presence of a rotator cuff tear and surgical exploration of one shoulder revealed the presence of a massive tear. Similar observations have been noted by Weiss et al. [66].

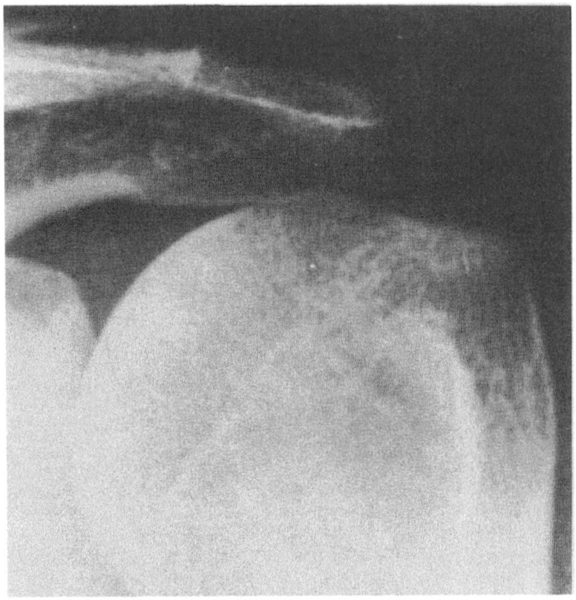

Fig. 9. Radiograph of rheumatoid patient with intermittent shoulder pain for one year. No evidence of erosive changes

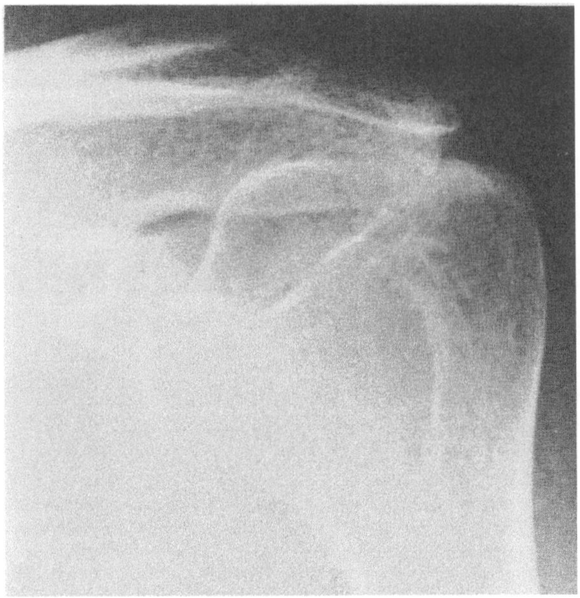

Fig. 11. The same shoulder four years after onset of symptoms showing Grade 5 appearances with segmental bone destruction in the upper part of the humeral head

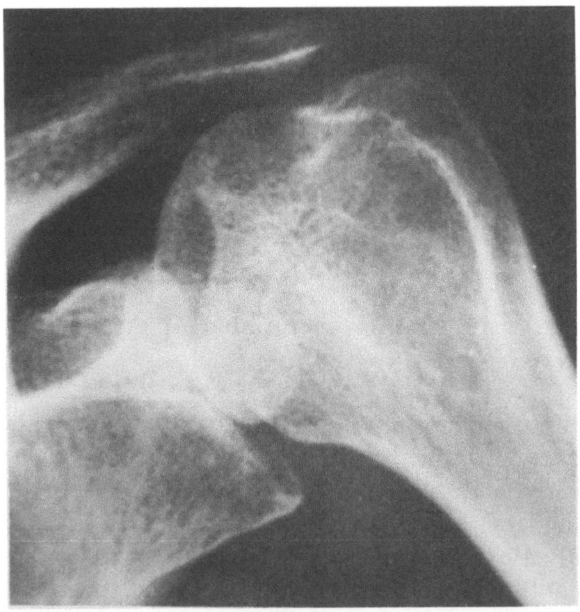

Fig. 10. The same shoulder two years later following recurring episodes of shoulder pain. Grade 4 appearances with proximal subluxation of the humeral head

(ii) Chronic proximal subluxation of the humeral head

In 2 shoulders a less dramatic and more insidious subluxation of the humeral head occurred over a period of between two and three years. This pattern of progression was associated with recurring episodes of shoulder pain. In 9 instances the end result was a Grade 5 shoulder (Figs. 9, 10, 11). Progressive reduction of the subacromial distance with time in these shoulders may indicate attenuation of the rotator cuff or cuff rupture. Changes in the humeral head consisted of bone loss either in a segmental fashion or as a generalised process involving the entire subchondral area. In the latter situation, medial displacement of the humeral head occurred.

(iii) Medial displacement of the humeral head

Nine shoulders eventually developed medial displacement of the humeral head beneath the acromion. This process was preceded by the appearance of sclerosis in the subchondral area of the humeral head, and subsequently rapid des-

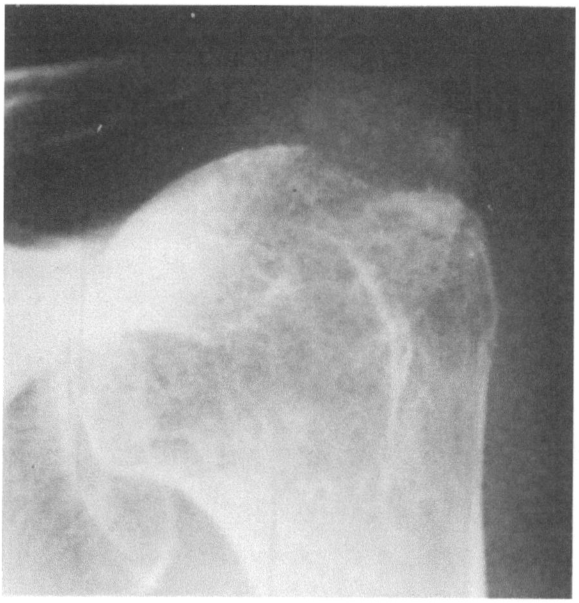

Fig. 12. Grade 4 shoulder with proximal subluxation of the humeral head. Note the early sclerotic changes in the subchondral area of the central part of the humeral head

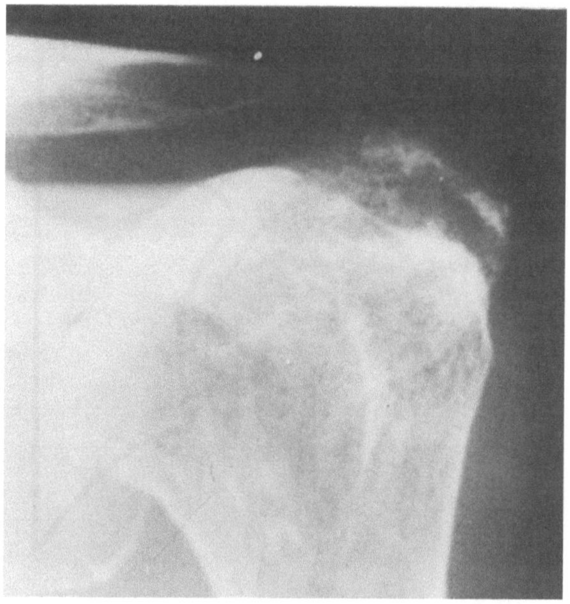

Fig. 13. The same shoulder two months later with central erosion in humeral head and extension of sclerosis

truction of bone on both sides of the glenohumeral joint resulting in a change from Grade 3 to Grade 5 in as little as six months or one year (Figs. 12, 13 and 14).

Forces Acting in the End-stage Shoulder

The line of action of the middle fibres of the deltoid muscle in the normal shoulder changes direction at the greater tuberosity of the humerus. When two surfaces are in contact and there is no friction between them, the force of reaction is at right angles to the surfaces at the point of contact. Thus the force R results from the change of direction of the deltoid muscle at the greater tuberosity and is transmitted through the subdeltoid bursa and humeral head in an inferomedial direction (Fig. 15). This is consistent with the static force analysis of the glenohumeral articulation described by Poppen and Walker [49]. Assuming isometric muscle conditions in a normal shoulder, the compressive force acting across the glenoid at the initiation of abduction acts in an inferomedial direction. From 30-60° of

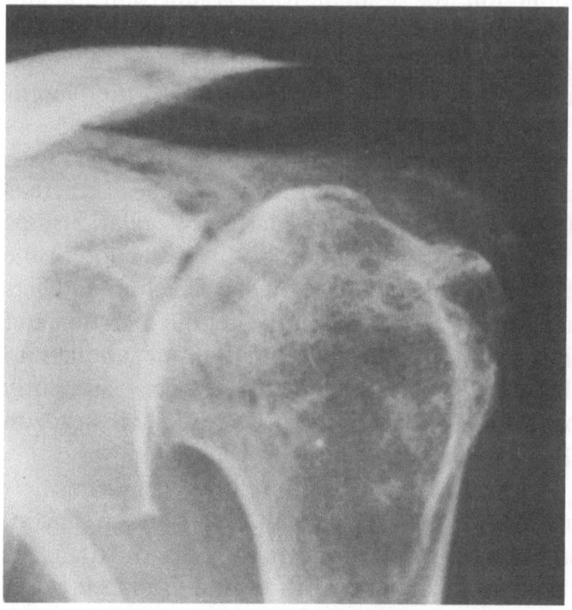

Fig. 14. The same shoulder two months later showing Grade 5 appearances with extensive subchondral bone resorption and pronounced osteoporosis

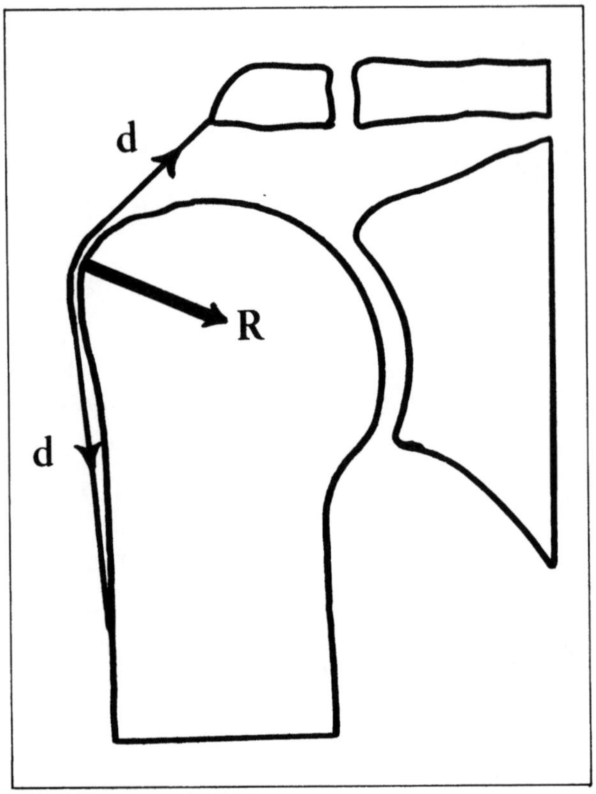

Fig. 15. In the normal shoulder, at the initiation of abduction, the deltoid exerts a resultant force *R* acting in an inferomedial direction

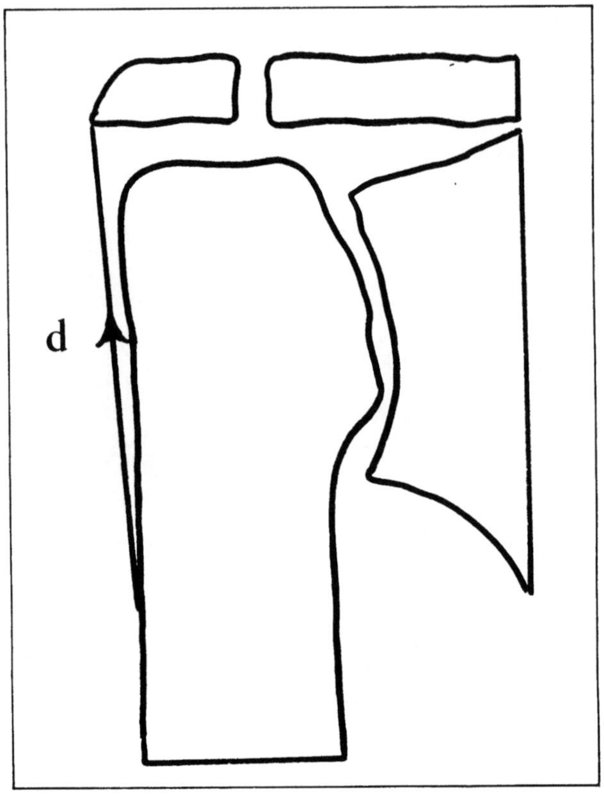

Fig. 16. End-stage shoulder with medial displacement of humeral head. At the initiation of abduction the deltoid exerts a force *d* acting in a superior direction

abduction, the resultant force is superomedial and passes through the superior surface of the glenoid fossa, but at no stage of abduction does the resultant force act superiorly through the supraspinatus tendon.

In the end-stage rheumatoid shoulder with medial displacement of the humeral head, there is a major alteration in anatomical relationships (Fig. 16). In this situation the line of action of the deltoid muscle does not change direction and acts in a straight line between the deltoid insertion and the acromion. At the initiation of abduction, therefore, the resultant force *d* acts superiorly producing impingement of the humeral head on the supraspinatus tendon.

These factors are of importance when considering prosthetic arthroplasty. Thus, if an unconstrained joint replacement is performed in the rheumatoid shoulder with medial displacement of the humeral head, it is important to establish normal anatomical relationships of the humeral prosthesis to the acromion and to establish a satisfactory repair of the rotator cuff. In the absence of such relationships it would be unrealistic to expect a good functional result. In addition, repeated compression of the supraspinatus tendon between the acromion and the prosthesis would occur each time abduction was initiated. Under these circumstances therefore, a fixed fulcrum type of total shoulder prosthesis would be more appropriate.

Summary

Involvement of the shoulder joint in rheumatoid arthritis is surprisingly common. In many instances the shoulder remains pain-free with satisfactory function even in the presence of significant joint destruction. However, a dramatic deterioration in function occurs in end-stage disease, and significant pain occurs in more than 50% of these shoulders.

Knowledge of the natural history of the rheumatoid shoulder may help to establish the role of prophylactic surgery, such as synovectomy, partial acromionectomy and double osteotomy. Total shoulder joint replacement, however, is likely to offer the patient with end-stage disease the most satisfactory result in forms of pain relief and function.

V.2. The Dynamic Study of Shoulder Movement

William Angus Wallace

Introduction

Studies of shoulder movement are essential in order to improve our understanding of how the shoulder complex functions when the arm is elevated. The knowledge gained will help both in detecting abnormal movement and in providing guidance to those designing shoulder replacement prostheses. A number of good studies have been reported, with the classic paper by Inman et al. in 1944 [30] and more recent work by Freedman and Munro [23], Doody et al. [19] and Poppen and Walker in 1976 [48]. These workers analysed shoulder movement using radiographs taken at a number of static phases during elevation of the arm. Thompson [61] used a different approach by measuring the position of the arm and scapula externally using bony points as markers and identifying the three-dimensional change in position of the bones, but again this was carried out during static phases of elevation of the arm. In practice when we examine a patient, we always study the shoulder while it is moving, observing as much as is possible the rotation of the scapula as the arm is raised in addition to the movement which occurs at the glenohumeral joint. Is it possible to study radiographically the shoulder as it moves?

The Dynamic Abduction Study

In Nottingham over the last three years I have developed a radiographic method of studying the shoulder during movement, the arm stopping only at full elevation. The study is carried out with the subject standing and positioned as shown in Figs. 1 and 2.

It is important that the blade of the scapula is aligned parallel with the calibration grid shown in Fig. 2, and the X-ray beam is directed at right angles to the grid. The grid was necessary to identify and correct any distortion which may occur between the image-intensifier tube used for the study and the final picture reproduced on a television monitor. In practice if the beam is centred on the glenohumeral joint, minimal distortion occurs in the area from which measurements are made. The glenoid normally lies almost perpendicular to the blade of the scapula, thus the outline given on radiographic views in this position is good, with clear views of the humeral head articulating on the glenoid. The shoulder region is screened using the image-intensifier and the arm elevated in the scapular plane (Freedman and Munro) [23] over a period of ten seconds. The arm is then returned to its dependent position over a further ten-second period. The image-intensifier

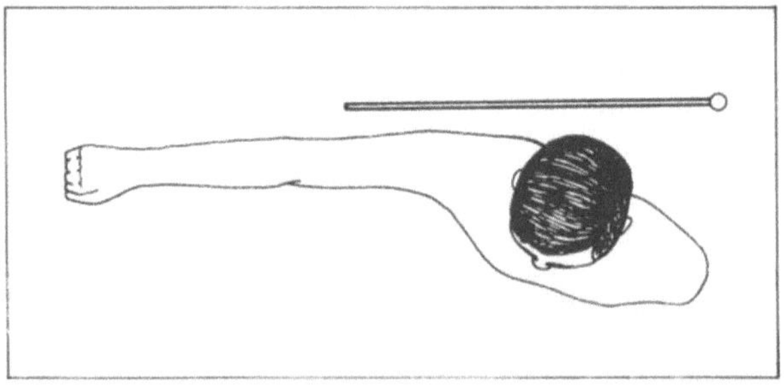

Fig. 1. Positioning of subject. The blade of the scapula should be parallel with the X-ray screen and grid. The X-ray beam is centred on the glenohumeral joint and directed onto the grid at right angles to it, so obtaining a true anteroposterior picture of the glenohumeral articulation

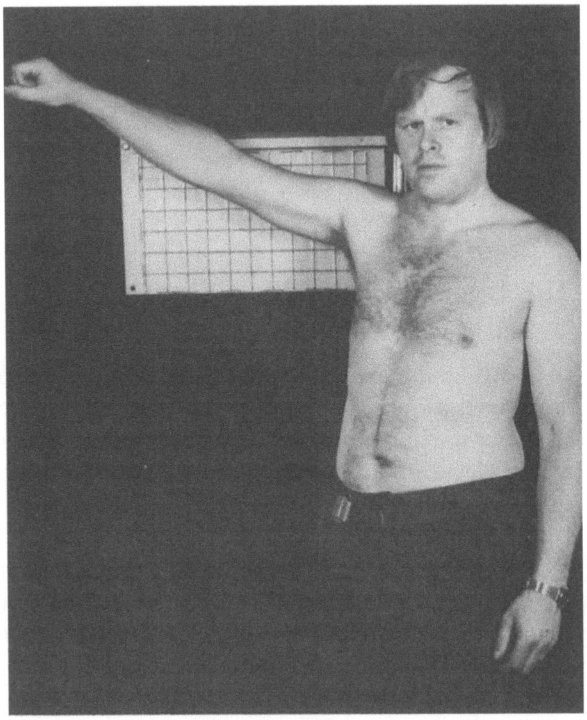

Fig. 2. Positioning of subject. Frontal view showing X-ray screen and calibration grid (*see text*)

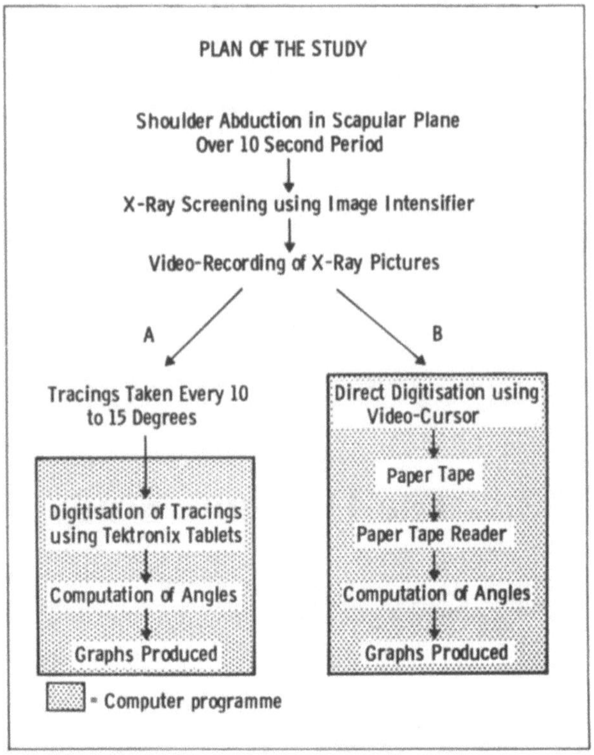

Fig. 3. Plan of study. The earlier method (A) of analysing radiographic film was time-consuming and was later replaced by a more automated method (B)

pictures are recorded on videotape for storage and later analysis. The study is repeated three times to ensure a good series with a total X-ray screening time of around two minutes. The analysis is carried out according to the plan shown in Fig. 3.

Initially I used Method A in Fig. 3, but accuracy has been markedly improved with Method B, using direct digitisation of the picture with a video-cursor designed in Nottingham by Trinder [62]. The computer program is written in FORTRAN for a Digital PDP-11 computer. Digitisation of the pictures is carried out every 10 to 15°, with a full analysis— both elevation and return to the dependent position— taking around one hour. Analysis of the pictures and production of a graph take under one minute.

Results

A total of 60 shoulder studies have been completed on fifty normal and abnormal shoulders. The computer graphs produced for one normal shoulder analysis are shown in Fig. 4.

There are four graphs— all show on the abscissa the *arm angle* measured as the angle between the long axis of the humeral shaft and the vertical. The first graph (upper left) shows the amount of scapular rotation which has taken place, measured by taking a line from the superior to the inferior pole of the glenoid and comparing this with the vertical. The second graph (upper right) identifies

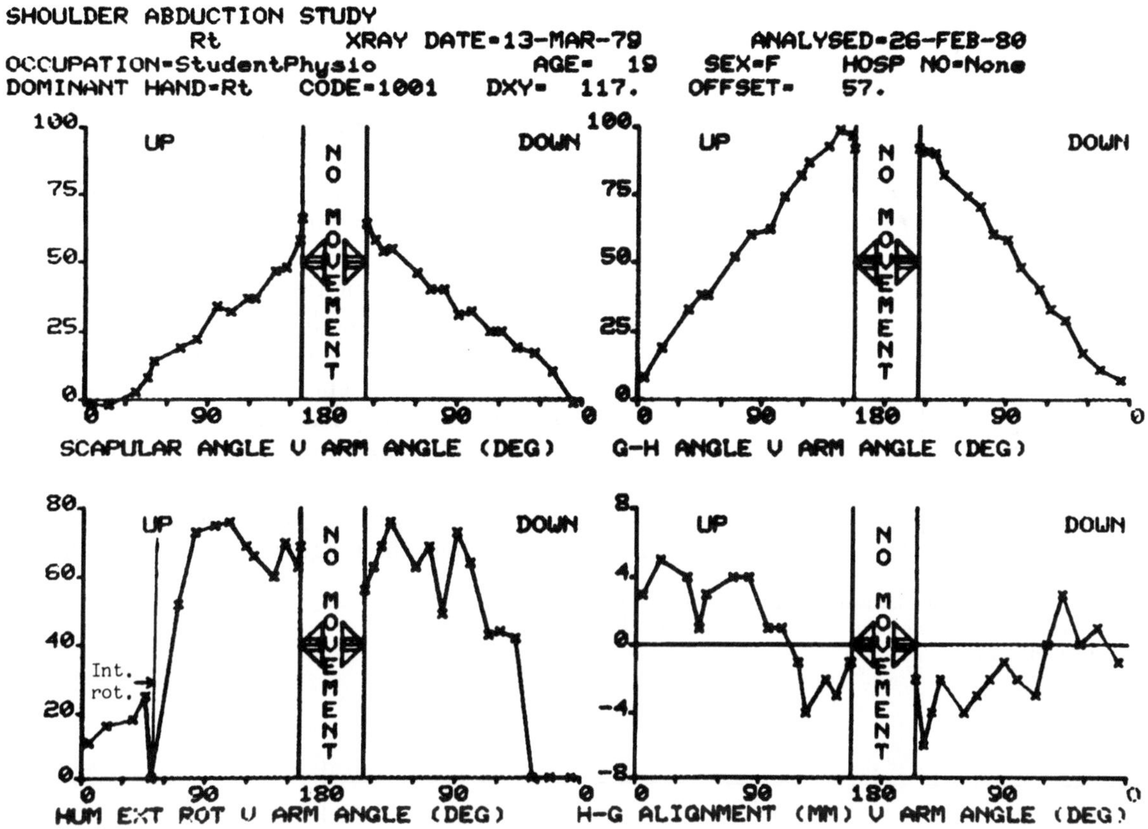

Fig. 4. Illustrative results from the shoulder abduction study: normal subject (*see text*)

the amount of glenohumeral movement by simple subtraction. These two graphs are accurate to within 5° at each point as shown by repeated analysis of the same shoulder movement. The lower two graphs provide information which has not previously been obtained. During abduction of the arm the humerus automatically externally rotates from an initial position of internal rotation. The pattern and range of external rotation are shown in the third graph (lower left). The method of recording this rotation is discussed below. Repeated analyses show this graph is less accurate with an error of ±20°, but the patterns of rotation are of value. The final graph (lower right) shows the alignment of the humeral head in relation to the glenoid, with the geometric centre of the articular surface used as a reference point. The results show the humeral head may slide up and down on the glenoid with an excursion of over 10 mm, but here again the accuracy of each point has an error of ±1.5 mm.

Humeral Rotation

Observation of the proximal humerus shows the articular surface of the humeral head forms part of a sphere [60]. This sphere does not sit centrally on the humeral shaft but is offset with its centre displaced up to 15 mm from the centre line or axis of the humeral shaft as shown in Fig. 5.

The perpendicular distance of the geometric centre of the humeral head from the axis of the humeral shaft is the true offset shown in Fig. 6.

Rotation of the humerus results in the offset distance being reduced to an apparent offset. The amount of humeral rotation can be calculated from the equation:

$$\cos \Theta = \frac{\text{Apparent offset}}{\text{True offset}},$$

where Θ = angle of rotation. The true offset is established from the *maximum* measured offset

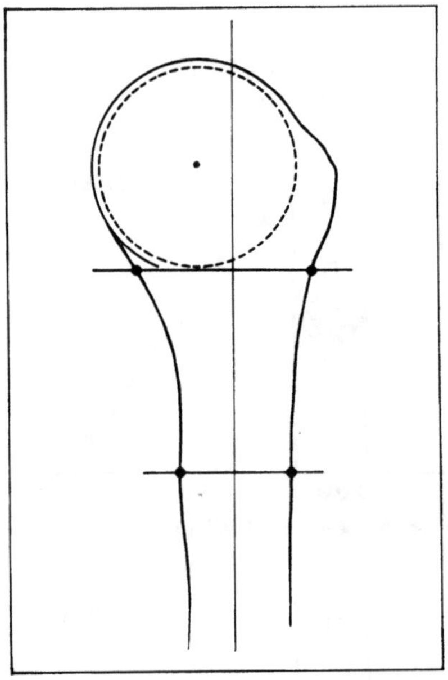

Fig. 5. Line drawing of humerus from medial aspect to show offset of humeral head anatomical centre from the centre line of the humeral shaft

where rotation = 0°. If the humeral head is damaged, rotation cannot be assessed.

Scapulohumeral Rhythm

In the normal shoulder when the arm is elevated, there is a smooth rotation of the scapula on the chest wall with scapular rotation contributing approximately one-third and the glenohumeral joint two-thirds to the total range of abduction. The definitions for normal, abnormal and reversed scapulohumeral rhythm are given below in order to clarify later discussion:

Normal scapulohumeral rhythm. Scapular rotation smooth throughout elevation of the arm *and* the range of glenohumeral movement is greater than the range of scapular rotation.

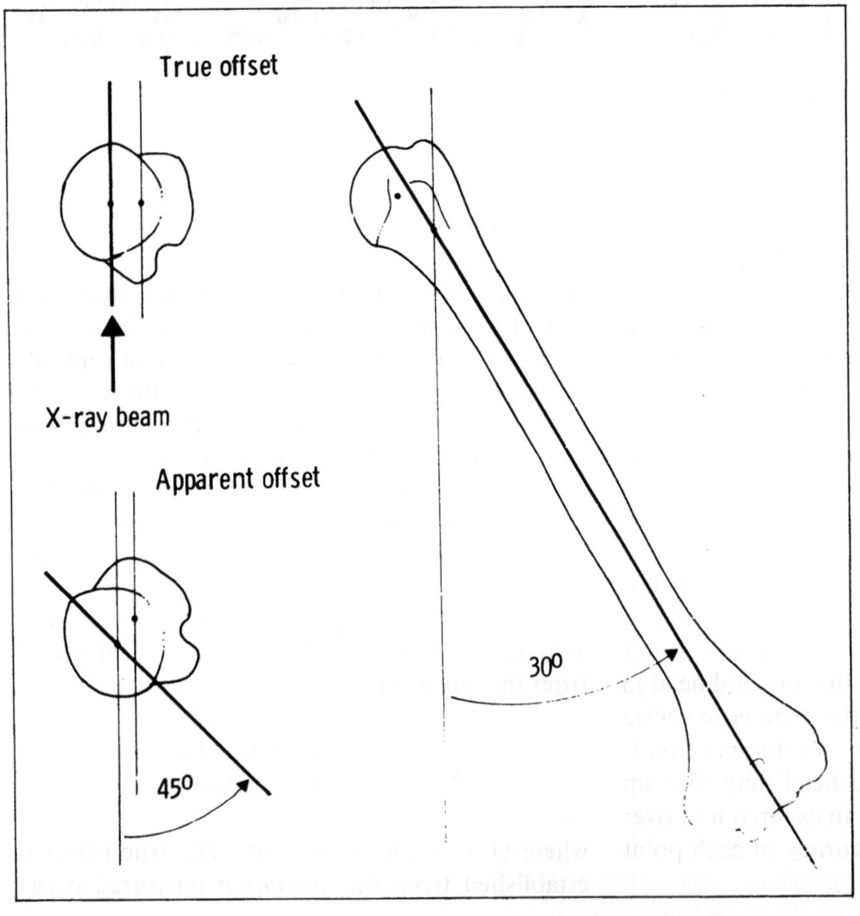

Fig. 6. The offset shown in Fig. 5 can be used to compute humeral rotation during abduction (*see text*)

Shoulders Studied

Studies have been completed on 12 normal shoulders, 14 with silastic cup interposition arthroplasty and 2 with total shoulder replacements. In addition patients with supraspinatus tendinitis, supraspinatus rupture, axillary nerve palsy, accessory nerve palsy and rheumatoid arthritis have been studied.

Summary of Findings from the Dynamic Abduction Studies

(1) The normal range of scapular rotation is 65°.

(2) The normal range of glenohumeral movement is 100°.

(3) There is a linear relation between scapular rotation and glenohumeral movement except at full elevation when the last 10° are almost pure scapular movement.

(4) The pattern of movement going up and coming down is similar.

(5) Abnormal scapulohumeral rhythm may be assessed using this study but only in one case was this not observed clinically prior to the study.

(6) Reversed scapulohumeral rhythm can be measured and was found valuable in assessing the progress of stiff shoulders.

(7) The humeral head excursion on the glenoid was large in young patients (< 30 years; 10+ mm) but much less in the middle-aged (6 mm).

(8) Following both silastic cup interposition arthroplasty and Stanmore total shoulder arthroplasty there is a slightly improved range of movement almost entirely due to increased *scapular* rotation.

(9) There is very obvious restriction of external rotation of the humerus following Stanmore total shoulder arthroplasty and this may be related to the poor range of glenohumeral movement (15°) recorded during abduction.

Discussion

The normal ranges of scapular rotation and glenohumeral movement recorded in the dynamic abduction studies are similar to those reported in previous studies [19,23,30,48].

Three reports— Inman et al. [30], Saha [60], and Poppen and Walker [48]— noted that at the beginning of abduction there was a setting phase during the first 30° to 60° of arm elevation, when scapular rotation was minimal. The dynamic abduction studies I have carried out show this setting phase is virtually absent when the moving shoulder is studied, which supports the views of Freedman and Munro [23].

The importance of humeral external rotation during abduction has been neglected in the past although Lucas [41] did emphasise this point. Limitation of abduction after supraspinatus rupture is common and may be a result of the loss of the external rotation force produced by this muscle as well as the abduction power. External rotation has also been ignored in the design of many constrained total shoulder prostheses— possibly one of the reasons for their poor function.

Conclusions

In all academic studies two criteria are important: the accuracy of the results and the clinical relevance of the findings. I have highlighted the inaccuracies and some of the problems which do occur in these shoulder studies. Using the initial results as a baseline, I hope to continue this work, concentrating on analyses of hemiarthroplasty and total shoulder replacement.

Acknowledgements

I should like to thank Dr Frank Johnson and Professor W Waugh for their continuous encouragement and help, the Medical Research Council for the support they gave me as a Research Fellow, and the Special trustees for the Nottingham University Hospitals who provided a grant for materials. Finally, my thanks to all the orthopaedic consultants in Nottingham for allowing me the opportunity to examine their patients, and to Mr Geoff Lythe for help with the illustrations.

V.3. Biomechanical Considerations in the Design of a Semi-constrained Total Shoulder Replacement

Reinhard Kölbel, Antonius Rohlmann and Georg Bergmann

Anatomy and Biomechanics of the Shoulder

The shoulder joint is, as an approximation, a spherical joint with incongruent surfaces. The shallower one, the glenoid, covers only one-half of the humeral head in the scapular plane and one-third in the anteroposterior plane. In consequence the joint depends upon muscle forces for stability. In the healthy articulation the resultant force must act normal (at right angles) to the instantaneous area of contact. Their possible spatial angle with respect to the glenoid can only vary between around 50° in the AP plane and 75° in the scapular plane. That proportion which the glenohumeral joint contributes to the overall range of active motion of the arm relative to the trunk and through which the joint is stable appears to be smaller than the extreme of passive glenohumeral mobility. There is gliding and some element of rolling in the relative motions, but the vertical movement of the centre of the head is negligible for practical purposes [48]. At the extremes of the passive range of motion the glenohumeral joint is secured by the capsule and its ligamentous reinforcements. The tensile strength of this complex was determined to be in the range of 30-60 kg, or 300-600 N. This is equivalent to a moment of 9-18 Nm applied to the humerus in order to cause dislocation [54].

Forces acting across the joint have been determined to be in the range of 0.9 times body weight in 90° of abduction of the stretched arm [30]. The upward component of the resultant force amounts to 0.42 times body weight at 60° of abduction [49]. When the arm hangs down by the side the humeral head sags. When active abduction starts it rises again to a position stabilised by muscular forces and joint geometry.

Indications for a Constrained or Semi-constrained Joint Replacement

A constrained or semi-constrained implant for replacement of the glenohumeral joint is indicated when the structures providing muscular stabilisation are absent or non-functional (irreparable rotator cuff tears, bone loss or resection inclusive of the rotator attachments).

Reconstruction with a constrained joint is clearly a salvage procedure for severely involved shoulders for which simple joint resurfacing will do nothing and in which reconstruction of the stabilising soft tissues is not feasible. By implication it will be seen that we believe the indications for non-constrained or resurfacing implants to be distinct from those for constrained or semi-constrained devices.

Design Considerations

When a joint implant provides stability, its anchorage to bone will be subjected to moments transmitted through the joint. Shear components of the resultant (i.e. transverse forces acting on the scapular part of the implant) will be prevalent in all modes of loading. This is more pronounced the more the scapular part projects from its point of fixation to the bone.

Early studies with the Stanmore shoulder have drawn attention to the smallness of the space enclosed by the glenoid vault, and even if the prosthetic centre of rotation is shifted medially from its natural locus, the glenoid vault will not wholly accommodate a prosthetic socket.

Ingenious use of fixating pins cemented into separate drill holes in the cancellous bone of the glenoid [55] and the use of cement injection in the liquid state [51] achieve the maximum possible mechanical bonding in an intact glenoid vault, but

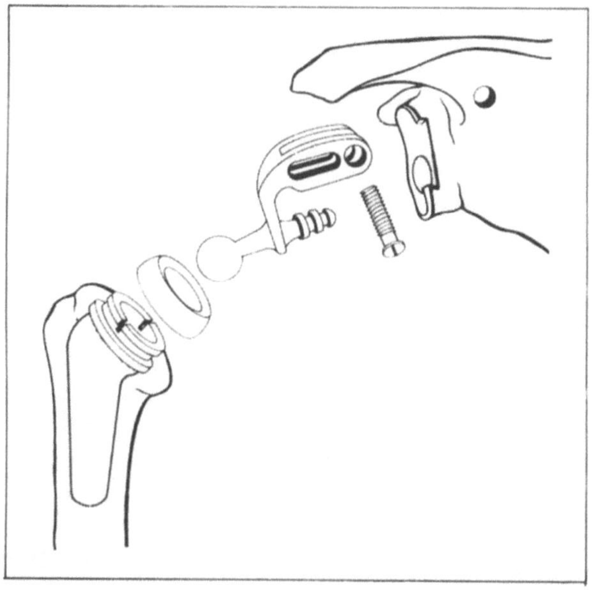

Fig. 1. Exploded diagram of implant (*see text*)

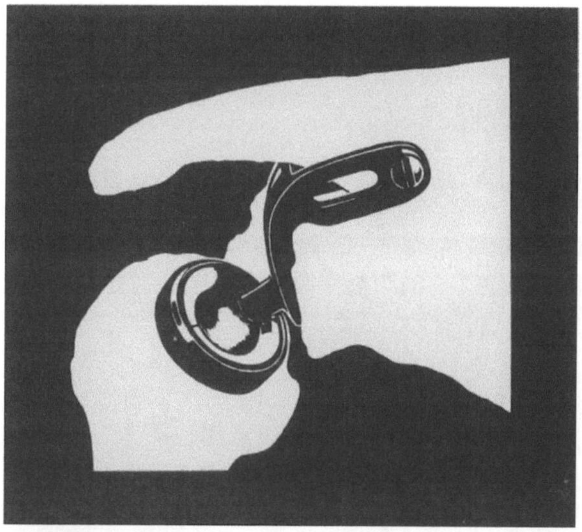

Fig. 2. Detail showing fixation of outrigger to base of scapular spine

in the diseased shoulder loss of bone stock may render such fixation inadequate. Maximum mechanical fixation is therefore an important design consideration in the preclinical stages of implant development.

In the design of our implant two ways of protecting the anchorage in the scapula were chosen: limitation of the transmission of moments by allowing dislocation of the implant joint at a certain moment and extension of the basis of fixation to a cortical structure [38]. This would eliminate peak moments acting on the fixation and also reduce the stresses occurring under each load.

Implant Design

The scapular part of the implant carried the ball and neck on a serrated bolt which is cemented into the glenoid (Fig. 1). The forked outrigger goes to both sides of the base of the scapular spine where it is clamped tightly to the bone by a transfixing screw which goes through a drill hole in the cortical bone of the base of the spine (Fig. 2). The humeral part is made of polyethylene and is cemented into the humerus. After fixation of both components to bone a retaining ring is slipped over the ball. Then the joint is reduced and the ring is snapped on to the rim of the socket.

The joint subtends 90° of angular motion— allowing rotation of the humerus around its long axis and angular motion in the scapular and coronal planes— and rotation around the axis of the prosthetic neck— allowing angular elevation of the humerus in the plane of the glenoid (flexion/extension).

Clinical Experience

This implant has been used in twenty patients with some modifications of the humeral part. A posterior approach was used. At the time of writing the follow-up is between six years and one month

Table 1. Shoulder joint replacement: complications related to implant

1. Wear of retaining ring, dislocation after 5 years 6 months	*Revision*: Replacement of humeral component
2. Loosening of screw, breakage of cement after 10 months	*Revision*: Tightening of screw
3. Dislocation after 8 months	*Revision*: Open reduction
4. Dislocation; scapular component fixed upside down	*No revision*

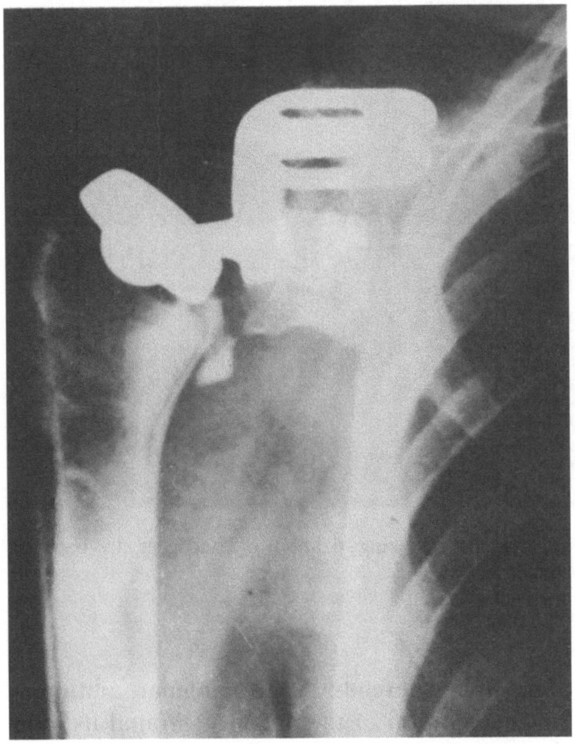

Fig. 3. Postoperative radiograph showing implant in situ

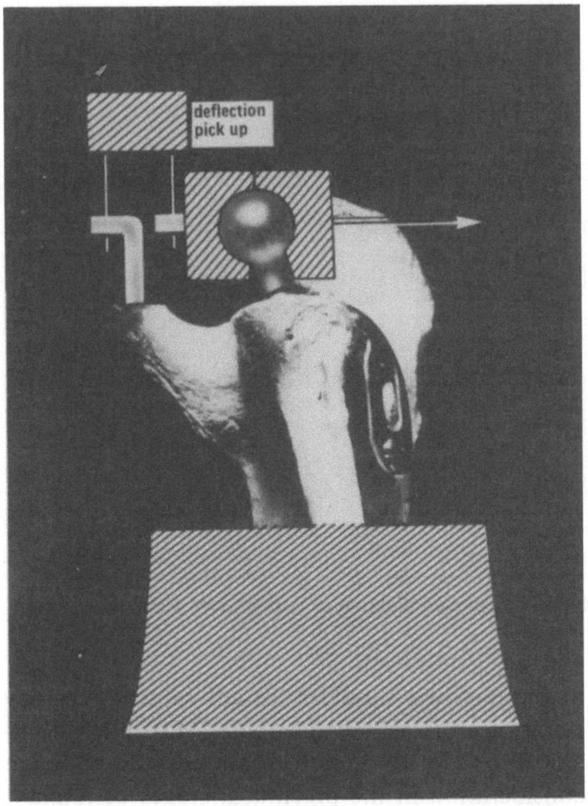

Fig. 4. Implant mounted in cadaveric scapula for fixation tests

(Fig. 3). It has been shown that a normal active range of motion can be achieved.

Complications related to the implant or its fixation are listed in Table 1. Problems are anticipated in some patients in whom impingement occurs in adduction. There were no infections. There were no clinical manifestations of long-term loosening, although radiolucent lines were frequently seen.

Laboratory Tests of Fixation to the Scapula

Prior to clinical use an early prototype of the scapular part was fixed to fresh cadaveric scapulae and loaded transversely, i.e. at right angles to the neck. Loads of up to 400 N were supported without failure of the fixation [36].

After modification and improvement resulting in the present design [37] loading tests were again performed using 20 fresh frozen cadaveric scapulae [39]. The specimens were potted in plaster of Paris (Fig. 4) and transverse loads of 200 N were applied in several directions. The deflection of the implant relative to the bone was least in the plane of the spine, i.e. the outrigger (Fig. 5). When we tested the specimens to failure (Fig. 6), the first sign of loosening was a gap which appeared between the cement and the cancellous bone of the glenoid. This was regarded as a failure. When the load was then redirected, e.g. the direction reversed, it was found, that an even higher load might be applied before failure in the new direction. Failures of the bone never occurred near the transfixing screw.

The majority of loads were between 500 N and 1000 N. Pull-out loads, applied along the axis of the neck were above 2000 N. The implant joint itself pulls apart at 700 N. Torque applied to the neck led to failure of the fixation beyond 20 Nm. The implant joint dislocates at 9 Nm and the neck bends at 23 Nm (Fig. 7).

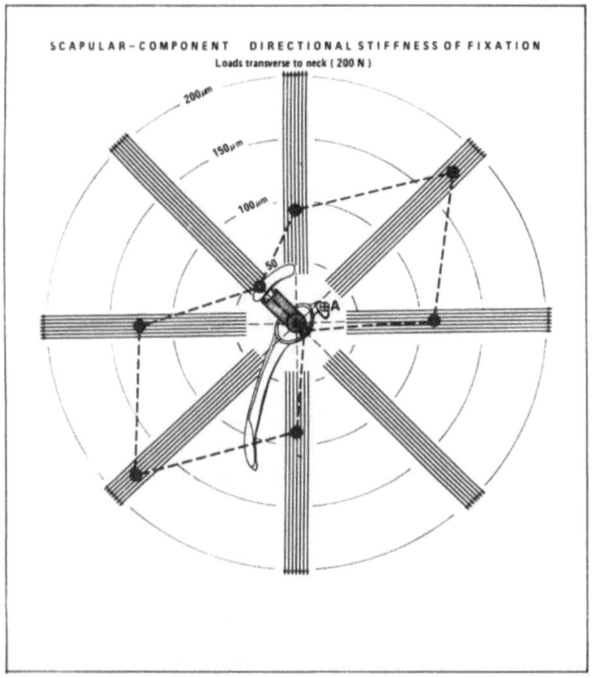

Fig. 5. Fixation studies: deflection response in several directions to a standard 200 N load. Note the least deflection occurs in the plane of the implant outrigger

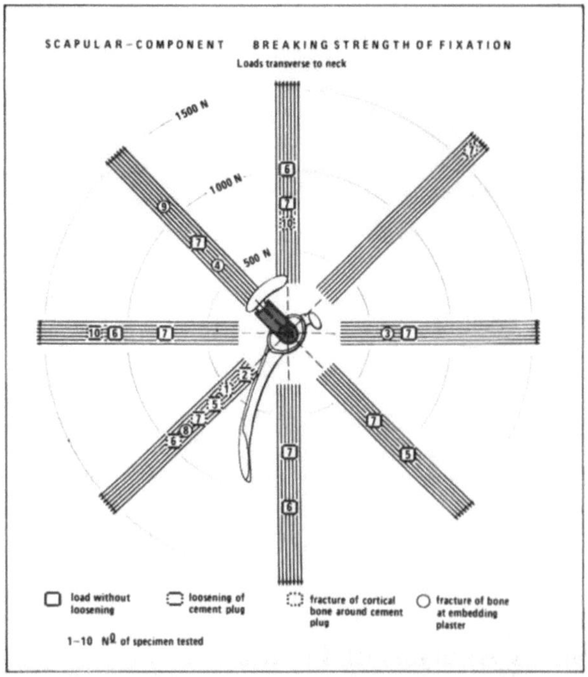

Fig. 6. Fixation studies: load applied to failure of bone, implant or fixation. Results are shown for loading in several directions

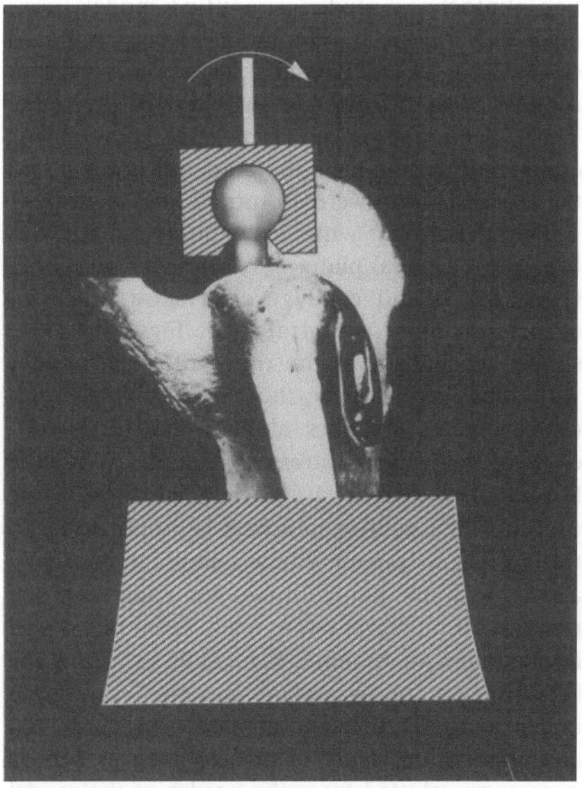

Fig. 7. Fixation studies: loads were also applied to test implant resistance to dislocation (*see text*)

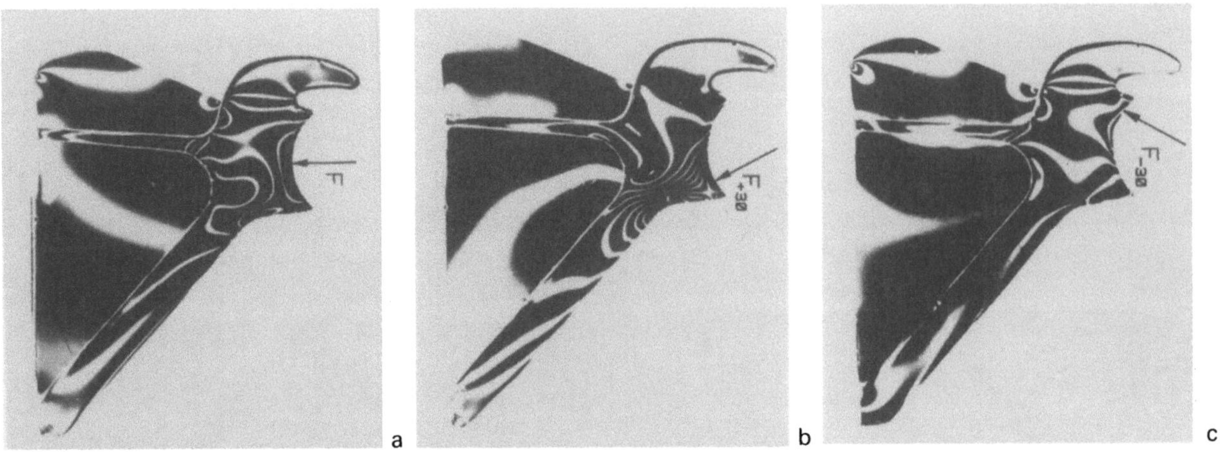

Fig. 8 a-c. Photoelastic studies to assess stress within a scapular model under load from three directions (*arrow*)

Stress Analysis of Fixation to the Scapula

Photoelastic Studies

For photoelastic studies simplified models were made of Araldite B. The models were composed of plates of 2 and 10 mm thickness to represent roughly areas of different thickness of the bone. The scapular spine, an appendage representing either the acromion or the coracoid process and the lateral margin were all turned into one plane.

The glenoid of a model without implant was loaded by a metal plunger over a layer of rubber (Figs. 8a, b and c). Figure 8a shows the isochromates under a central load, Figs. 8b and c show the changes in the order of isochromates with loads acting near the rim of the glenoid. (Isochromates are lines along which the differences of the principal stresses are equal. When the borders of the model are not loaded directly, the order of the isochromates there is proportional to the surface stresses.) Various implant configurations, with one pin, with two pins, and with one pin and an outrigger, were made from metal and bonded on with Araldite. Figures 9a to c show the isochromates for an implant with one fixating pin under loads in different directions. Figures 10a and c show the calculated surface stresses. Tensile stresses are plotted from the border of the model to the outside, compressive stresses to the inside. A load acting from above would occur when the patient lifts a bag, a load acting from below when the patient uses a cane (Figs. 10a and c).

The surface stresses are clearly related to the direction of loading. They are reversed as the direction of loading is reversed. Near the implant only compressive stresses are shown. Tensile stresses did not occur under the collar, as this was not bonded to the surface of the glenoid.

Figures 11a to c show the isochromates, and Figs. 12a to c show the surface stresses for different types of fixation under identical loads. In Figs. 11a and b (two bonded pins plus a wide area of bonding to the glenoid surface versus one bonded pin with an unbonded collar) there are marked differences in the order of the isochromates near the fixating pins. As far as the stresses near the borders are concerned, the effects of the different fixations appear to be irrelevant.

In Figs. 11c and 12c (fixation as in Fig. 12b plus an outrigger with a transfixing screw through the appendage) the order of the isochromates and the surface stresses show that the appendage takes part in carrying the load. It follows that the distribution of the load is improved.

The results of our photoelastic studies must be viewed with caution and with a knowledge of photoelasticity in general and our simplified models in particular: stresses which occur in the appendage (at its base), when no load is introduced there, raise doubts about the configuration of this model. The acrylic is quite stiff around the

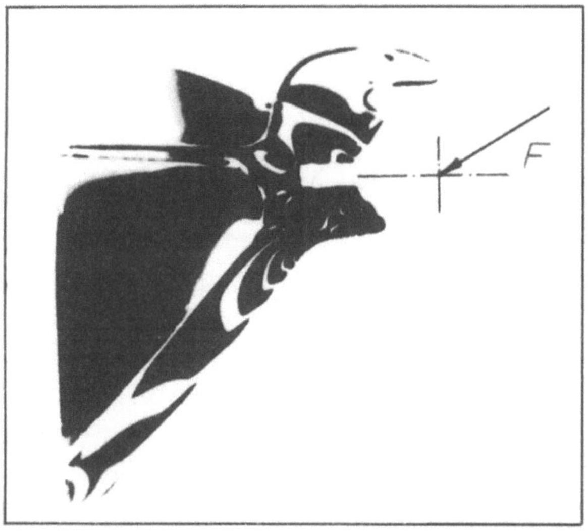

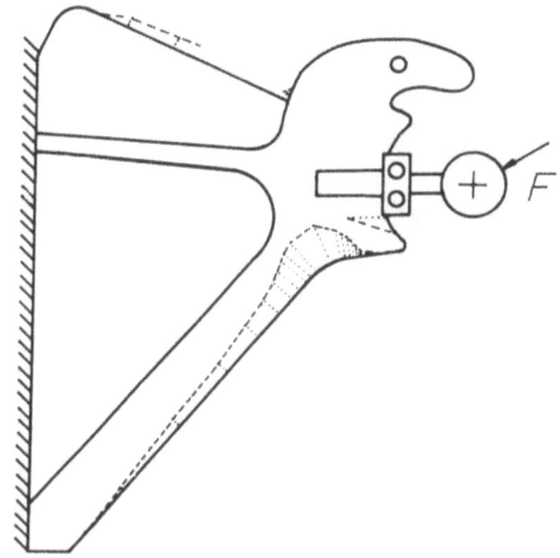

a

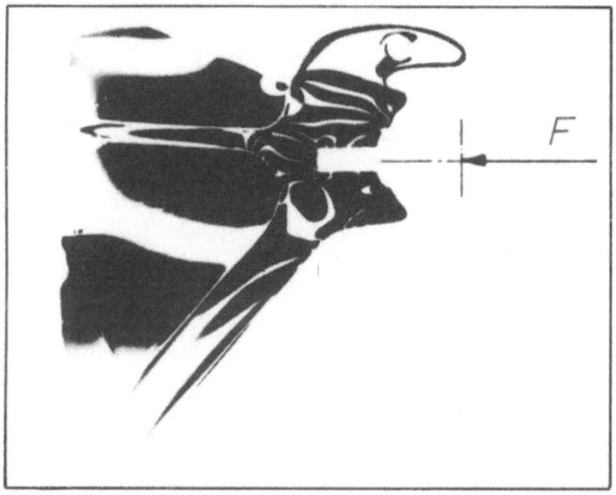

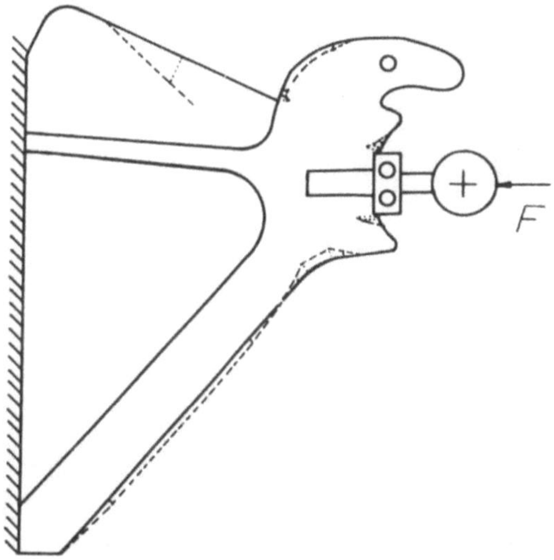

b

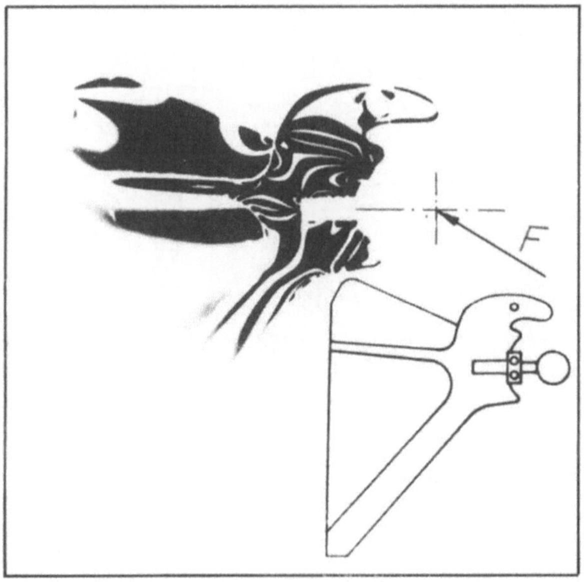

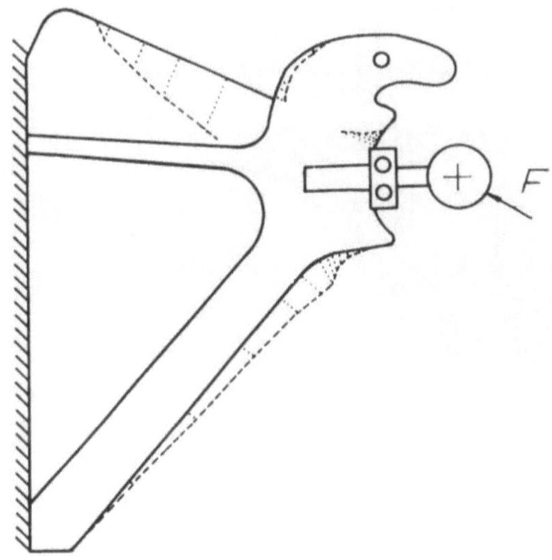

c

Figs. 9 and 10 a-c. Photoelastic studies to show stresses within a scapular model when load is applied to a single pin implant from one of these directions (*arrows*). Compressive stress is plotted within the model and tensile stress outside its margins

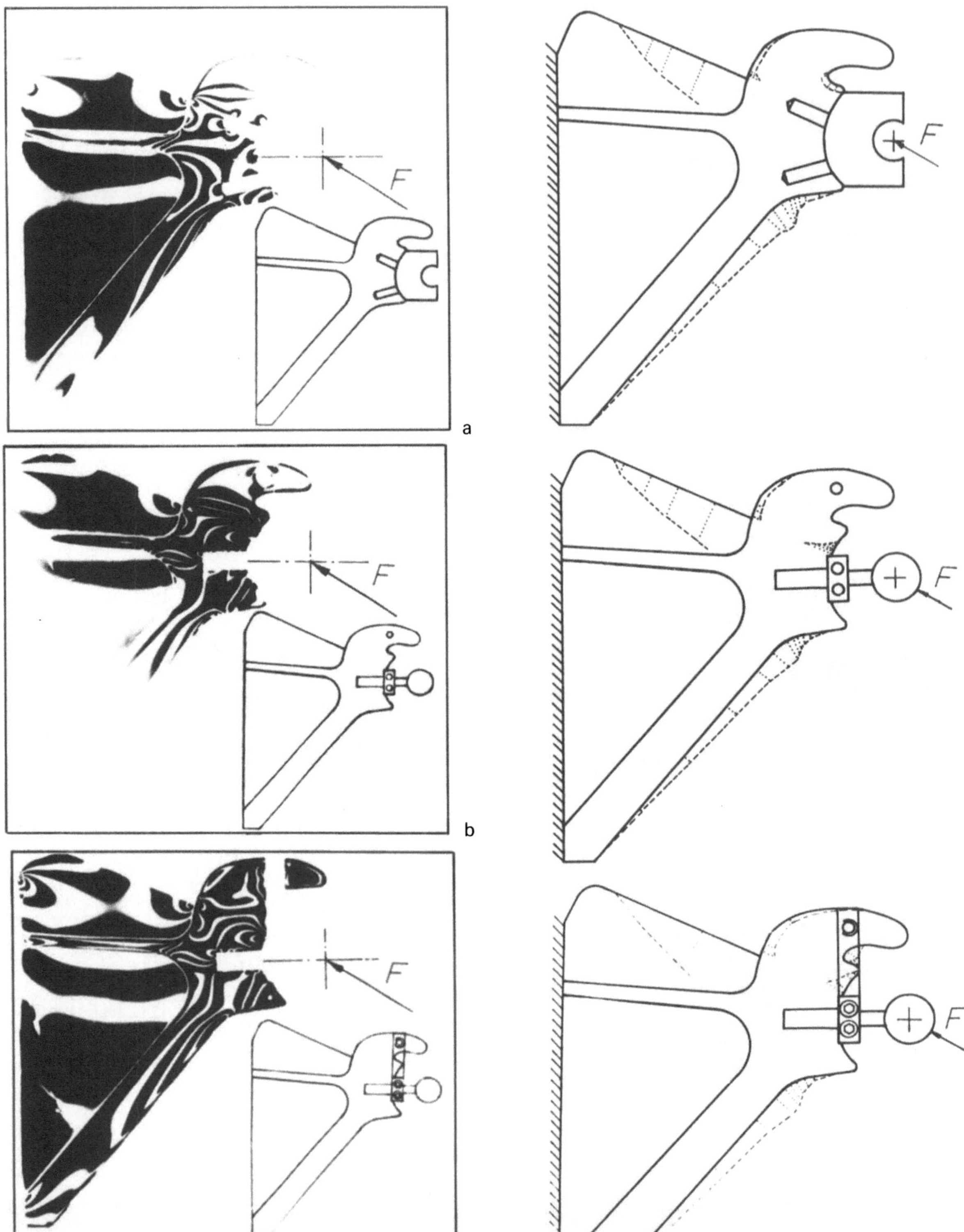

Figs. 11 and 12 a-c Photoelastic studies for three methods of fixation (a) double pin with collar bonded to face of glenoid (b) single pin with unbonded collar (c) single pin with unbonded collar plus outrigger fixating pins as compared to the real situation and under load deformation of the model there is less than in reality. This prevents loading of the scapular appendage to the extent which occurs when the pins are fixed in the cancellous bone of the glenoid. (The stiffness of the scapular fixation with the outrigger has been well demonstrated in our loading tests.) The state of stress around the fixating pins in the model is three-dimensional. Evaluation of the isoclines which would be required for determination of stresses within the model is irrelevant in our plane model. Consequently the stresses within the borders were not determined. We would expect a more detailed picture of the state of stress in the scapula from a three-dimensional finite element study.

Finite Element Model

The three-dimensional finite element (FE) model is composed of nearly 1200 volume elements with more than 3000 nodal points (Figs. 13a and b).

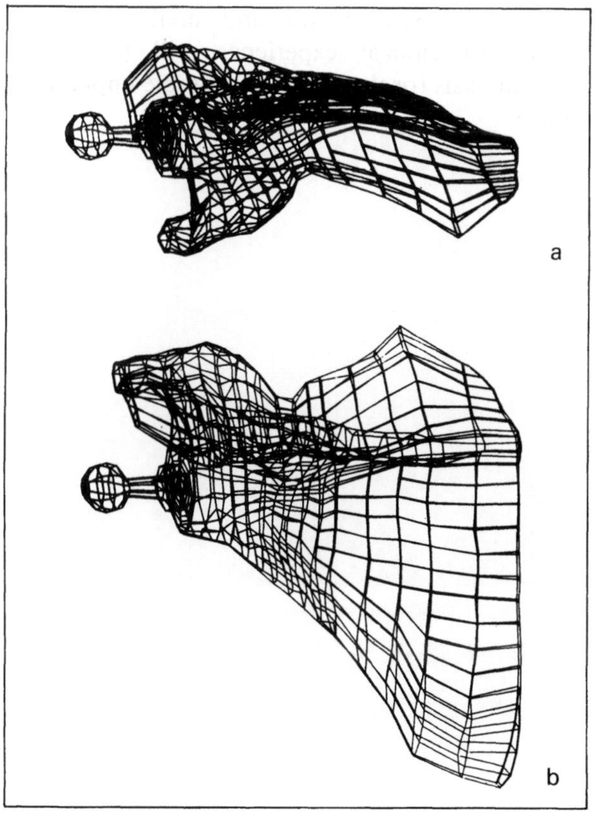

Fig. 13 a, b. Finite element model of scapula and implant in two planes (*see text*)

The figures show the outer net of elements as seen in the scapular plane and roughly at right angles to it. With this type of model the geometry and the distribution of the material properties of the bone can be simulated in a realistic fashion. For the scapula the assumptions of the mode of clamping of the model could present considerable problems because this bone is surrounded by muscles almost completely. However, we feel that simplification is justified as long as we are interested only in the state of stress around the fixation of the implant. A modified FE program SAP and a CYBER 175 computer were used for the computations. Evaluation of a whole volume of results is in progress.

Discussion

Our good intentions to optimise shoulder joint replacement in the biomechanics laboratory are somewhat frustrated when it comes to relating our results to what is known of the biomechanics of the shoulder. Biomechanical data on fixation of non-constrained resurfacing implants might be compared to what is known about normal joints. For implant joints which require changes from the normal anatomy, geometry, centre of rotation, etc., nothing is known quantitatively about loads occurring in clinical use.

Range of Motion

Near normal range of motion can be achieved with a constrained or semi-constrained joint which is positioned correctly in a patient with functional musculature. When a patient lacks muscle power to stabilise the artificial joint for abduction, this movement can only be performed with the joint in impingement and by rotation of the scapula. The implant then acts as an arthrodesis. If the patient has an implant with two centres of rotation, he cannot abduct unless his implant joints both impinge to act as an arthrodesis. With two centres of rotation the passive range of motion can of course be increased.

Joint Stability

The stability of the joint to dislocation irrespective of active muscular stabilisation is the great advantage of the constrained and the semi-constrained implant joint. This is indeed appreciated by patients with previously unstable shoulders in whom any muscular effort leads to painful subluxation or useless motion of a floating humerus. Traumatic dislocation of our semi-constrained joint occurs at dislocating moments which are very similar in magnitude to those which would rupture the anterior capsular structures in a normal joint.

Fixation

Limitation of the dislocating moment to 9 Nm protects the scapular fixation against moments which would disrupt it (15 Nm).

In a joint with functional musculature the shear (tangential) component of the resultant force is 0.42 times the body weight. The stability of the fixation under static loads of 500 to 1000 N applied transversely to the neck of the scapular part is difficult to relate to that figure. Such loads could occur when a patient pushes herself up from a seat. There appears to be a margin of safety of the fixation for that group of patients who are candidates for total shoulder joint replacement. Sudden, accidental (dynamic) loads to the shoulder may easily be much higher. They have not been reported to be responsible for accidental loosening of a properly fixed implant. It appears that the muscular suspension of the scapula absorbs dynamic loads effectively.

Conclusions

Our work concerned with a semi-constrained shoulder joint which includes some clinical experience has convinced us that "inherent stability" [55] and lasting fixation can be achieved with this type of implant. Proper load tests in the laboratory are the closest possible in vitro simulation of actual use and they should be used to improve fixation. Photoelastic studies are useful to demonstrate the state of stress for different implant configurations and fixations with simple models. For a detailed stress analysis of the implant-bone composite the three-dimensional FE model can be used. As in all such projects involving complicated bony structures, analytical approaches must be supplemented by experimentation with the real thing, bone. It is hoped that the data resulting from such experimental and analytical work related to clinical experience will provide a rational basis for the choice of suitable implants in future.

V.4. The Trispherical Total Shoulder Replacement

Anthony G. Gristina and Lawrence X. Webb

In fulfilling its function of positioning the arm in space, the shoulder joint is unique in its requirements for motion. Osseous congruity of the articular surfaces of humeral head in the glenoid is minimal and so motion is maximal. Soft fibrous tissue, in the form of a lax capsule with its reinforcing ligaments, keeps the humeral head in the vicinity of the glenoid. Fine-tuning of this association is brought about by the proprioceptor-rotator cuff (feedback-effector) mechanism.

Disruption of the glenohumeral joint architecture, whether by disease or trauma, may result in pain and restricted motion. Reconstruction of the glenohumeral joint is still in its infancy. The advances made in aseptic operative techniques and the development of antibiotics provided the right background for Neer's ingenious development of a humeral head prosthesis in the late 1950s [44]. That prosthesis was a much needed addition to the available alternatives of arthrodesis [9,52,64] or humeral head resection and advancement of the rotator cuff insertion to the proximal shaft, as had been described by Jones in 1933 [31,32]. For patients with severe fractures of the humeral head where avascular necrosis is anticipated or for patients with severe degenerative arthritis and an intact rotator cuff, the Neer prosthesis serves well [44,46].

However, the Neer prosthesis, being an unconstrained device designed to replace the articular surface of the humeral head, depends, once it is implanted, on the integrity of surrounding soft-tissue structures including the rotator cuff, for support. When the destruction of the glenohumeral joint is extensive with disruption of the soft tissues and the rotator cuff mechanism, a prosthesis of the constrained variety is advocated, because it must act as a fulcrum for the shoulder in the absence of a rotator cuff.

A constrained prosthesis may be defined as a prosthesis whose components are related to one another in such a way that they provide a mechanical block to subluxation or dislocation. We acknowledge that constraint is not an absolute concept, i.e. there are breakdown points for all interconnected materials. Our framework for the use of the term constrained is within what we would consider the normal kinetics of the joint concerned. With reference to the glenohumeral joint, a constrained prosthesis fixes the humeral head portion to the glenoid portion and maintains that relationship within certain parameters. By so doing, it establishes a fulcrum which does what cannot be done by an extensively torn, scarred, or paralysed rotator cuff.

In the normal shoulder [18], 50% of the scapulohumeral muscle mass is rotator cuff. Hence, nature has invested one-half the scapulohumeral muscle mass in rotator cuff alone. Calculation of the significant shear forces at the glenohumeral interface indicates the wisdom of Nature's investment. It also shows up the magnitude of the problem of restoring the extensively disrupted glenohumeral joint to painless function.

A variety of constrained prostheses have been reported in recent years [7,22,27,40,50,57,59,67]. It is fair to say that their development has presented difficult challenges to the bioengineer and has spurred new interest in basic research on the shoulder as well as in new requirements of design and biomaterials.

The *trispherical total shoulder* prosthesis consists of a vitallium glenoid component, a vitallium humeral component, and an interposed high-density polyethlylene sphere reinforced by a vitallium shell (Figs. 1, 2 and 3). It is a variable-fulcrum three-bar linkage system that allows a greater than anatomical range of motion. Those features of the prosthesis were demanded by its design, which allows the surrounding soft tissues rather than the prosthesis or its bony anchorage to be the check-reins at the extremes of movement. That is, the more physiological situation of soft-tissue stretch-proprioceptor stimulation is preserved and called into play before the prosthesis and its bony anchorage are stressed at the extremes of glenohumeral motion. The variable ful-

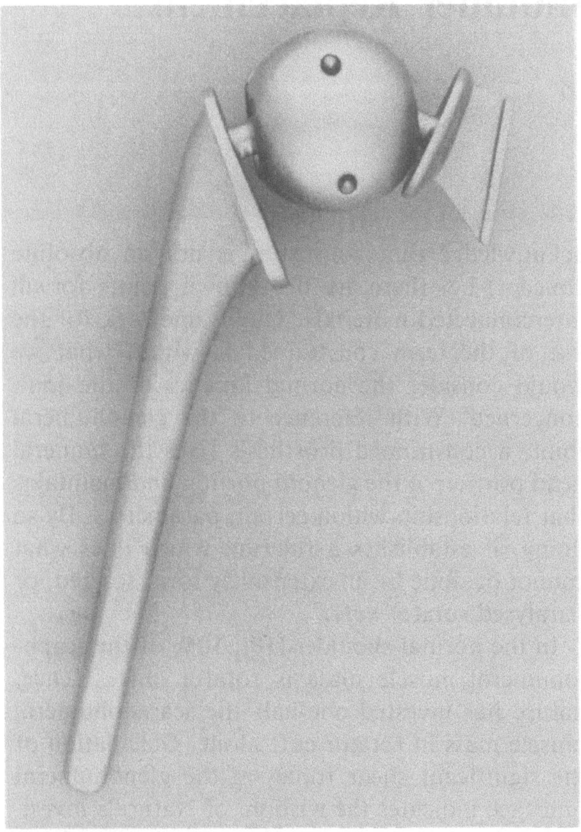

Fig. 1. Trispherical total shoulder prosthesis

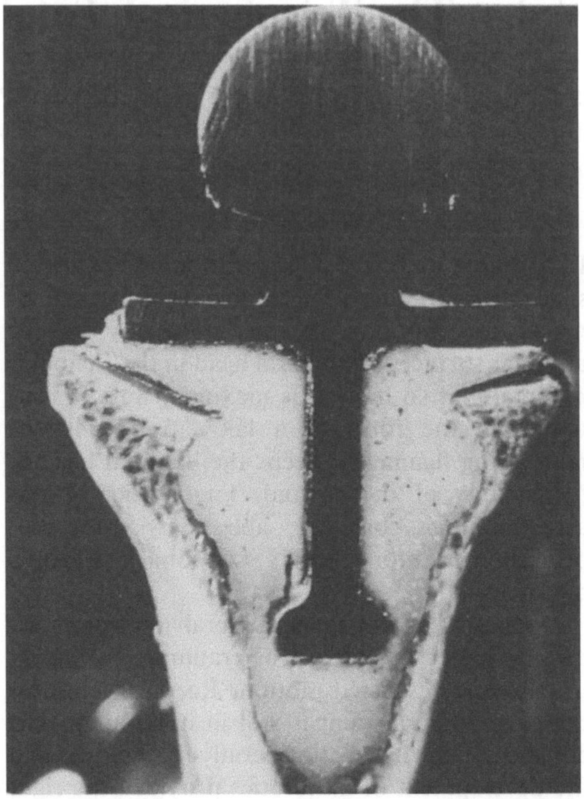

Fig. 3. Cross-section of cadaver scapula and glenoid component of trispherical total shoulder prosthesis showing firm anchorage of keel behind cortical bone on glenoid surface

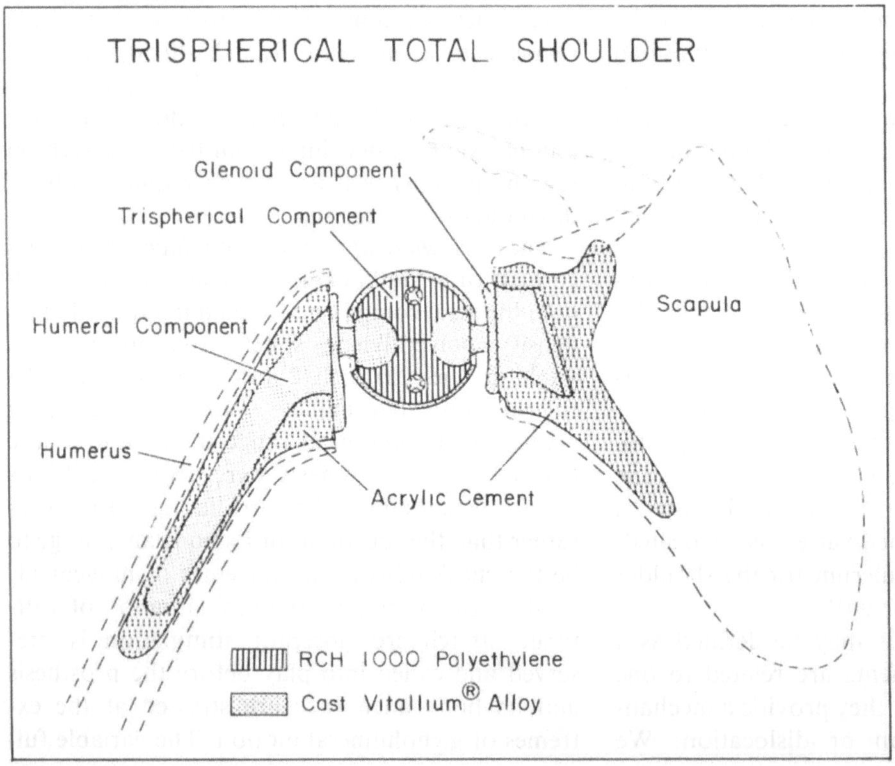

Fig. 2. Schematic drawing of trispherical total shoulder prosthesis showing physical relationship to humerus and scapula

crum is similar to the anatomical fulcrum in that it allows for abduction by the anterior and middle deltoid musculature, even though the rotator is absent.

We have developed a great respect for the forces acting on the prosthesis and its bony anchorage. The prototype of the polyethylene sphere was devoid of a vitallium shell. Two of those prostheses were implanted, but dislocation of one of them in the postoperative period spurred the redesign of the prosthesis to its current form. Addition of the vitallium shell to the retaining polyethylene sphere increased the dislocation tolerance of the prosthesis from 150 inch-pounds to 500 inch-pounds.

There are theoretical problems with a design that calls for absolute resistance to dislocation. Absolute resistance may result in fracture when maximal shoulder forces are applied, for example in a fall or when the patient is using crutches over the long lever arm of the upper extremity, especially when the prosthesis is invested by weak musculature. The ideal resistance to dislocation or degree of constraint remains to be determined by clinical experience.

Insertion of a constrained prosthesis is probably indicated for:

(1) Patients who have severe shoulder pain that has not responded to the usual conservative measures and who lack a functional rotator cuff. Patients with rheumatoid arthritis affecting multiple joints and severe involvement of the shoulder with fibrous scarring of what once was a capsule and rotator cuff are typical candidates in that category.

(2) Patients who have severe end-stage post-traumatic arthritis or osteoarthritis that has disrupted joint architecture and surrounding soft tissues (rotator cuff) to the extent that a resurfacing procedure or a hemiarthroplasty would not result in resumption of function.

(3) Patients who have an erosive tumour with involvement of the humeral head and soft tissues, provided some glenoidal bone stock remains intact.

A constrained prosthesis is relatively contra-indicated for (1) patients with inadequacy of the glenoidal bone stock (as might result from earlier failure of another constrained total shoulder prosthesis), (2) patients with active or recent infection or neurotrophic arthritis, and (3) patients whose rotator cuffs can be reconstructed with restoration of function. The last group of patients are probably best served by an unconstrained prosthesis of the Neer variety.

Operative Technique

On the night before operation, the shoulder is shaved and scrubbed with betadine and detergent. Just before operation, 1 g cephalothin is administered intravenously, and if the patient has severe rheumatoid arthritis, a stress dose of steroid is also started and continued postoperatively in a tapering dose. The patient is placed in the supine position on the operating table with the shoulder propped up at 45° to the horizontal. The shoulder area is scrubbed with betadine solution, and all but the upper extremity is draped. Steridrape™ is used to cover the area of prepared skin. Through an elongated deltopectoral incision, the deltopectoral groove is developed and the anterior 1 to 3 cm of the origin of the deltoid is removed with some attached periosteum and bone flecks. Next, the tendinous origins of the short head of the biceps brachialis and the coracobrachialis are detached from the tip of the coracoid.

In patients with severe rheumatoid arthritis, the humeral head has usually become fixed in maximal internal rotation and in a posterior position. For those patients, a longitudinal incision is made in the joint capsule (usually a scarred mass of what was once rotator cuff and capsule, adherent to the humeral head), and the joint space (or what was once the joint space) is developed, exposing the humeral head and glenoid. The humeral head is removed with a power saw. Next, the glenoid is exposed, a step that usually requires removal of adherent fibrohaemorrhagic tissue, and a dental burr is used to excavate a fenestration large enough to admit the fin of the glenoid component (Fig. 1). A curette is used to finish the excavation, and care is taken to preserve the subchondral bone. After a trial seating of the glenoid component, it is cemented with methyl methacrylate under pressure. The proximal humerus is reamed in standard fashion, a trial seating of the humeral component is done, and the humeral component is cemented in place in an appropriate amount of retroversion (usually 35°).

Next, the prosthetic components are assembled to complete the 3-bar linkage. The limb is then put through a range of motion, and contractures of the rotator cuff and capsule are released as required. The tissues are then irrigated copiously with bacitracin/sterile saline solution (50 000 units of bacitracin in 1.5 l saline), the muscles are reapproximated at their origins, and the wound is closed in a standard fashion over a Haemovac drain, which has been brought out through a separate stab wound in the skin.

Postoperatively, cephalothin prophylaxis is continued for a short while and the shoulder is placed in a soft, bulky immobiliser for three weeks. Motion of the elbow, wrist and fingers is encouraged during that period.

Results

Twenty trispherical total shoulder prostheses have so far been implanted in 18 patients. Fourteen were done at our medical centre; 6 were done elsewhere. Eighteen were implanted in patients with severe rheumatoid arthritis; 2 in patients with severe degenerative arthritis. All patients had severe shoulder disease that had required heavy doses of analgesics for control of pain. All had severe limitation of motion; 9 had had internal rotation contractures. The follow-up period has been from 12 to 42 months. Pain relief has been most dramatic (Table 1). The gain in overall shoulder movement has been uniform; the average gain at one year after operation is shown in Table 2.

Table 1. Pain relief

	Average preoperative pain rating: 4.9	
	Average 1 year postoperative: 1.8	
	Pain rating scale	
1.	None	
2.	Slight	– no compromise in activity
3.	Mild	– after unusual activity
4.	Moderate	– interfering with activity requiring analgesics occasionally
5.	Severe	– with serious limitations of activity

Table 2. Average range of motion (active scapulothoracic and glenohumeral)

	Preoperative (degrees)	1 year postoperative (degrees)	Average gain (degrees)
Flexion	36	54	18
Extension	25	41	16
Internal rotation	45	71	26
External rotation	1	43	42
Abduction	22	58	36

Discussion

For patients for whom a trispherical total shoulder is indicated, the therapeutic goals are relief of pain, stability, and increased function, in that order. The results to date are excellent as far as relief of pain is concerned, postoperative pain being either low-grade or non-existent.

As regards stability, as has been reported previously [28], two of the earlier, minimally constrained prostheses malfunctioned, the first dislocating in the postoperative period, the other fracturing at the anterior glenoid lip 42 months after operation while the patient was doing some heavy house cleaning. Up to the time of the fracture, this patient had had excellent use of her operated shoulder. The radiographs of the patient, who had severe rheumatoid arthritis and who had had other joints replaced as well, indicated extensive generalised osteoporosis including the glenoid.

Two of the current prostheses with a vitallium shell reinforcement of the middle sphere have undergone subluxation/dislocation at the humeral ball-middle sphere junction within three months of insertion. The two affected patients remain pain-free, and the glenoidal and humeral components appear to be intact with solid anchoring. Reoperation to replace the middle sphere is scheduled for both patients.

Retrospectively, we believe that the passive motion rehabilitation which these patients underwent may have been a factor in exceeding the design specifications of the prosthesis. In passive motion exercises, the movement of the arm can generate tremendous force on the shoulder. Thus, passive motion exercises may lead to high-molecular-weight polyethylene creep and generation of forces in excess of prosthesis design, instead of loosening soft tissue and overcoming muscle spasticity. Of all the patients who were rehabilitated with active motion exercises, begun only after a suitable healing period of six to twelve weeks, none has had the problems of the two patients mentioned above.

We believe that once muscle spasm has abated and a pseudocapsule has formed, the patient will learn the limits of shoulder movement. Over a period of time, with appropriate exercises, the soft tissues will adjust and accommodate the movement of the sphere and its armatures, so that a gain in active shoulder motion will be obtained.

Conclusions

A variable-fulcrum, or three-bar linkage, shoulder prosthesis affords a much greater range of motion than could be achieved in the same space by a simple ball and socket prosthesis [26]. Indeed, Nature uses the three-bar concept in the normal shoulder, the three bars being the thoracic wall, the scapula, and the humerus, and the links being the scapulothoracic and glenohumeral joints.

The development of the trispherical total shoulder is still in the clinical trial stage. It has been used only in the most severely affected shoulders that are not suitable for a Neer-type prosthesis, and all of the patients in whom it has been inserted have had multiple joint involvement.

Considering the severity of disease in these patients and the diminished shoulder muscle mass in many of them, one should choose relief of pain as the primary goal, and should expect only modest gains in stability and function. Pain relief has indeed been uniformly good in all of these patients; stability and increased function have been surprisingly good in the 16 of the 18 replacements with the current constrained prosthesis which were subjected postoperatively to the currently advocated rehabilitation programme of active motion exercises.

V.5. Neer Total Shoulder Arthroplasty

Charles S. Neer III and R. Peter Welsh

Total shoulder arthroplasty is not merely the replacement of a destroyed shoulder articulation. Rather, it is an essential adjunct to soft-tissue reconstruction and rehabilitation of the shoulder when disease has destroyed bone and/or the joint surfaces such that salvage by soft-tissue surgery alone is impossible.

The Neer total shoulder emphasises three vital principles:

(1) The resurfacing of destroyed joint surfaces. A low-friction arthroplasty of stainless steel articulating with high-density polyethylene aims at minimal bone resection.

(2) Non-constraint by mechanical stops. Any device with mechanical restriction imposes what must ultimately become intolerable loads on the fixation of the glenoid component predisposing such device to failure. The Neer device is restricted like the normal shoulder only by soft-tissue forces.

(3) The reconstruction and rehabilitation of

supporting soft-tissue elements. The objective throughout being to provide a painless fulcrum for soft-tissue rehabilitation and function.

Total shoulder arthroplasty therefore demands a careful rebuilding of soft tissue-support if normal function, i.e. normal range and strength of movement, is to be achieved. This may require multiple associated procedures in addition to the implantation of the prosthetic device and includes:

Clearing of the subacromial space by acromioplasty

Freeing of the rotator cuff and obliterated muscle planes

Release of contractures

Reconstruction of the rotator cuff

Acromioclavicular joint excision arthroplasty

Careful preservation of deltoid function

Above all, a carefully structured rehabilitation programme must be pursued if restoration of normal function is to be achieved.

Indications

Simply stated, the indications for arthroplasty embrace those conditions unsalvagable by soft-tissue surgery alone and include:

Osteoarthritis: primary, post-traumatic and cuff arthropathy

Rheumatoid arthritis

Trauma: acute and late

Congenital dysplasia

Tumour

Previous failed surgery: fusion or prosthesis

Because the objective is restoration of normal anatomy and soft-tissue function, there are really only two contra-indications to shoulder salvage by arthroplasty:

Too few muscles, i.e. no rotator cuff or deltoid function.

Active sepsis.

Under these circumstances fusion remains the only possible alternative following poliomyelitis or septic arthritis.

The Neer Total Shoulder

The stainless steel humeral component has been modified from the original design and now offers two different head diameters, three different stem diameters, and two different stem lengths. This versatility enables full restoration of the soft-tissue advantage and the rebuilding of the cuff envelope around the humeral head. An extra long stem prosthesis is available for situations where there has been major bone loss or resection for tumour. In such instances an associated fibular graft may be employed to aid stability.

Methyl methacrylate cement fixation of the humeral component is optional but recommended with osteoporosis or where there is poor bone stock.

The high-density polyethylene glenoid component presents a concave surface to reface the glenoid and reciprocate with the opposing humeral head. Two component sizes are available, one of polyethylene alone, the other metal backed. Both types must be cemented in the glenoid where it is emphasised that minimal bone need be removed to mount the component. If necessary, the glenoid can be reconstructed with bone graft, utilising the resected portion of humeral head to provide adequate bone stock.

A special semi-constrained glenoid component has been devised for situations where there is a gross cuff deficiency as in severe rheumatoid arthritis or rotator cuff arthropathy. With a subacromial extension this modification prevents ascent of the head yet allows 90° elevation at the glenohumeral joint and has the advantage over fusion of preserving rotation in the shoulder.

Technique

A brief description of the surgical technique is presented to emphasise the importance of the soft-tissue reconstruction of the shoulder which is facilitated by the use of the prosthetic device.

A deltopectoral incision is employed with complete preservation of deltoid and careful protection of the circumflex nerve during retraction. Subscapularis is released with a Z plasty lengthening to facilitate later reconstruction. An anterior acromioplasty allows clearance of the subacromial space and coupled with an acromioclavicular resection arthroplasty affords even further visualisation and mobilisation of the rotator cuff. The humeral head is resected removing only the destroyed joint surface: the angle of the head being cut parallel to the undersurface of the prosthesis.

Soft tissues are now fully mobilised, the capsule released, and the cuff mobilised before the glenoid is prepared. The glenoid can now be prepared carefully preserving its strong cortical rim for support. The glenoid component is implanted with cement fixation followed by the humeral component which is positioned in 35° of retroversion. Rotator cuff reconstruction around the head must then be complete and the soft-tissue envelope totally restored.

The rehabilitation phase is vital. Following rest in an abduction wedge pillow for five days a programme of active assisted exercises is instituted. For four weeks emphasis is on regaining active assisted flexion, extension and rotation. Then a programme of strengthening exercises is added and from the eighth week the programme is further supplemented with flexibility routines. Although rehabilitation must initially be under physiotherapy guidance, the ongoing programme must be continued five to six times daily by the patient himself and maintained for at least six months.

Results

The results achieved depend on the nature of the primary pathology, the quality of soft-tissue repair and the cooperation of the patient in the rehabilitation programme. In terms of the original stated objectives of a full soft-tissue reconstruction and complete rehabilitation of the shoulder this can be the expected goal in primary osteoarthritis. In rheumatoid arthritis or cuff arthropathy however, our goals must be tempered. That is, one seeks complete pain relief, improved range of motion to 110°, and greatly improved function. However, to expect a full range of motion and function in such instances is unrealistic. None the less, such a result in these individuals constitutes an excellent response to surgery and can be defined as such.

Overall, in 250 total shoulder replacements 75% have achieved excellent pain relief, a range of flexion greater than 110°, approaching within 25° of the opposite normal side, all measurements being recorded in the supine position. Dislocation of the prosthesis has not been a problem, because the soft-tissue envelope has been completely reconstructed.

Summary

The present policy regarding the use of the Neer Shoulder Arthroplasty may be summarised as follows:

(1) Preservation of rotator cuff and glenoid as for example, following acute trauma or avascular necrosis.	Replace head of humerus only.
(2) Inadequate glenoid as in advanced osteoarthritis or rheumatoid arthritis.	Resurface both humerus and glenoid.
(3) Inadequate rotator cuff or deltoid as in severe rheumatoid arthritis or old trauma.	Humeral replacement plus semi-constrained glenoid component.
(4) Deficient bone stock following trauma or excision of a tumour.	Long-stemmed humeral component with bone graft plus glenoid resurfacing ± bone graft as necessary.

Conclusions

The Neer total shoulder arthroplasty aims to resurface a joint so destroyed by disease that reconstruction by soft-tissue repair alone would be impossible. The prosthesis itself is considered adjunctive to the soft-tissue rehabilitation of the shoulder, and emphasis is placed on the reconstruction of soft-tissue support at surgery followed by a carefully structured postoperative programme of rehabilitation. The prosthesis is completely non-constrained, but because of the soft-tissue repair, no problems with dislocation are encountered and a constrained shoulder prosthesis is unnecessary. It is this careful soft-tissue reconstruction which is the key to successful total shoulder replacement, not the device itself.

V.6. The Kessel Total Shoulder Replacement

J.I.L. Bayley and Lipmann Kessel

Prosthetic replacement of the shoulder is not a new procedure (Péan 1894) [47], but only in recent years has it become a practical therapeutic device. That the pace of advance in this joint has lagged behind the hip is hardly surprising when one considers the complexity of shoulder biomechanics. Global mobility is controlled by such a powerful yet delicately balanced series of muscle couples that function would be difficult enough to reproduce in health, quite apart from its restoration in diseases which themselves weaken the controlling muscles. Nor does the bone stock available for implant fixation in the least resemble the comparatively welcoming environment of the hip; the glenoid has so diminished in size during evolution (to liberate shoulder movement) as to be incapable of enclosing a prosthetic cup.

In practice, current shoulder joint replacements represent a compromise in design whose roots are to be found in three basic considerations: first, most shoulders coming to replacement are affected by end-stage rheumatoid arthritis in which the rotator cuff is likely to be deficient [16]; secondly, in the present state of knowledge it is advisable to adopt a metal-to-plastic type of bearing; thirdly, adequate fixation of the scapular component is difficult to achieve using acrylic cement.

To compensate, somewhat inefficiently, for rotator cuff deficiency most implants are of the constrained or semi-constrained type and most are of a metal-to-plastic ball and socket design. Thereafter the similarities end, and the great variation between methods of scapular component fixation bears witness to the central role played by this factor in prosthetic replacement of the shoulder.

Eschewing the use of acrylic cement on the scapular side and opting for a metal-to-plastic bearing, one arrives at the type of replacement which has been used virtually unaltered in our service since 1973 (Fig. 1). Of simple reversed design, it consists of a strong ball carrying self-tapping lag screw, which is fixed to the scapula without recourse to cement and which articulates with a semi-captive high-density polyethylene cup whose stem is cemented into the proximal humeral shaft. Thirty-six of these devices have been used in 35 patients.

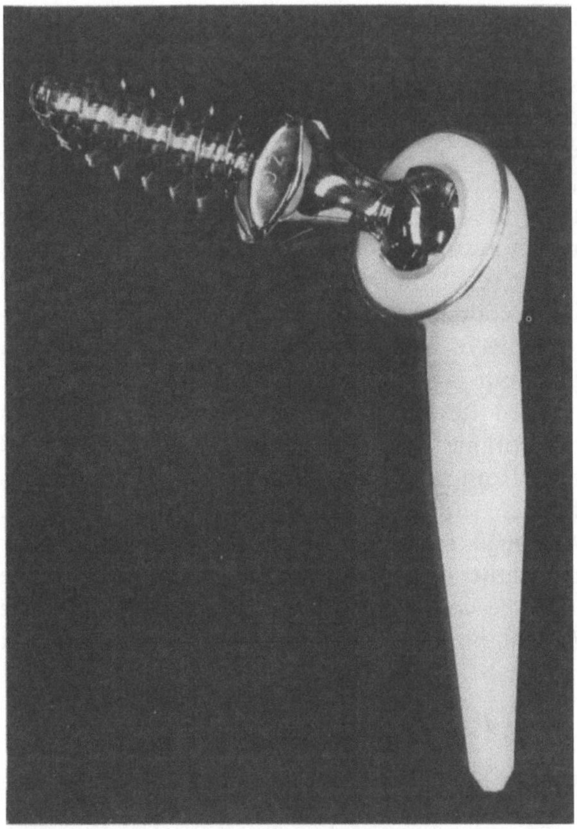

Fig. 1. Reversed ball and socket design. The scapular component is screwed into the glenoid vault and the humeral stem is cemented into bone. The components "clip" together

Operative Technique

The operative technique is straightforward, requiring few instruments (Fig. 2); it has been described elsewhere [35]. Briefly, the shoulder joint having been displayed via a standard delto-

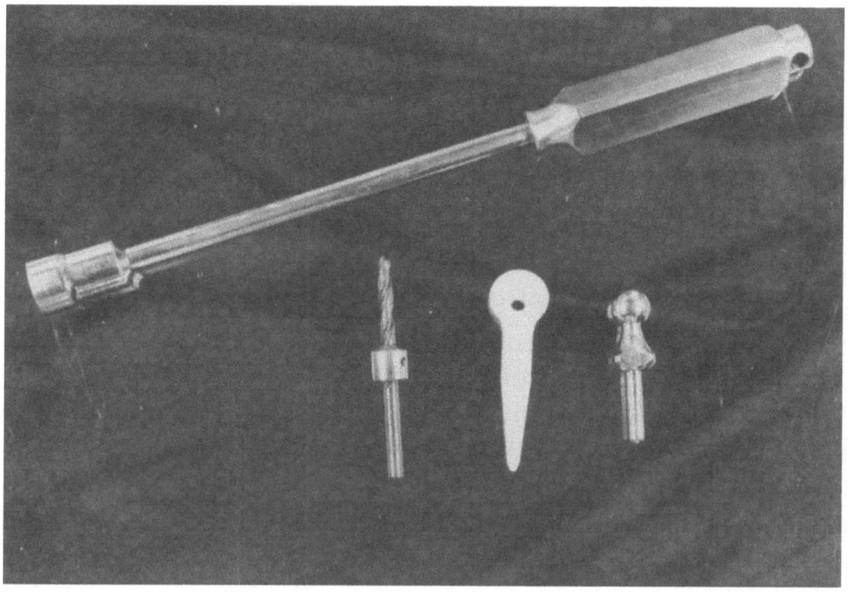

Fig. 2. Instrumentation: a guarded drill is used to pre-drill the glenoid vault. A trial reduction is achieved using the test components. The scapular component is inserted using the introducer

pectoral approach, the humeral head is resected in 60° of retroversion. The line of humeral neck transection is dictated by the degree of anteversion occupied by the scapular component. The insertion track for the lag screw is directed into the cancellous bone of the glenoid at an angle 20° anteverted to the plane of the scapula. This is to make full use of the limited space and length of the glenoid vault. Bearing in mind the normal forward inclination of the scapula on the chest wall, the resultant anteversion of the glenoid component is of the order of 50°. Failure to neutralise this on the humeral side would limit the postoperative range of external rotation. After a trial reduction using the test prosthesis (Fig. 2), the components are fixed into their respective bones and articulated with a snap fit. Postoperatively the arm is supported on an abduction wedge, bandaged to the trunk, for two to three weeks prior to commencing a graded programme of mobilising and strengthening exercises.

Clinical Material

Thirty-six shoulders have been replaced in 35 patients. Follow-up in the last 3 shoulders has been less than 6 months, and although they are all satisfactory to date they have been excluded from this review. In the remaining 33 shoulders (32 patients) rheumatoid arthritis accounted for the majority of conditions treated (21 patients) whilst 11 patients suffered from a variety of disorders (Table 1). The 28 women and 4 men had an average age of 64 years and 6 months (range 38 to 84 years), and follow-up ranged from 6 months to 7 years (average 3 years and 6 months). Two patients died from unrelated causes and have therefore been excluded from analysis of the up-to-date results: one had achieved a very good result, but the other had been less than satisfactory in that continuing pain had led to removal of the prosthesis. There were therefore 31 shoulders in 30 patients left for analysis.

Table 1. Conditions treated

Condition	Patients
Rheumatoid arthritis	21
Post-traumatic destruction	4
Synovial chondromatosis	2
Occupational osteoarthritis	1
Failed rotator cuff repair	2
Syringomyelia	1
Spastic monoplegia	1
Total	32

Results

Prosthetic fate

Of 31 shoulders 26 remain in situ and functioning. Four replacements required removal for the reasons given in Table 2, and in one patient the prosthesis remains in situ but dislocated. This lady, being 87 years of age, is rather frail, and prone to frequent falls. Having initially enjoyed a good result she then dislocated her shoulder in a fall, but she is unfit for further surgery and when recently reviewed she reported herself to be essentially free of pain.

Table 2. Prosthetic fate (31 shoulders)

Fate	Shoulders
A. In situ	26
B. Removed	
1. Wrenched shoulder	1
2. Recurrent early dislocation failing to respond to revision	1
3. Late dislocation – cause unknown	1
4. Failure to relieve pain after total shoulder replacement for multiple failed rotator cuff repair	1
C. Late dislocation – in situ	1
Total	31

Assessment of Results

Whilst the prime indication for shoulder replacement is the relief of pain, results have been assessed according to four criteria: pain relief, enhancement of function, restoration of mobility, and patient's response. Summation of performance in these parameters allows an overall grading to be given to each shoulder. We cannot yet achieve normal function and we have avoided the use of an "excellent" grade. To be regarded as "very good" a shoulder must have been improved in all aspects and the patient must be enthusiastic. Failure to achieve significant pain relief dictates inclusion in the "poor" category regardless of performance in other parameters.

Pain Relief

Pain was a major feature in all shoulders prior to surgery. It was abolished in 28 shoulders, unchanged in 4 and worse in 1.

Enhancement of Function

In 19 shoulders (18 patients) function was improved and in 12 it was unchanged. Failure to improve function was often due to involvement of other joints in the same limb or to prosthetic complications of the type mentioned above, but removal of the components did not necessarily lead to vitiation of function as compared with the preoperative rating.

Restoration of Mobility

The main gains occurred in the arcs of flexion and rotation in which 19 shoulders achieved enhanced active mobility. Eight shoulders were unchanged and 4 lost movement.

Patient Response

On the whole, patients rated their results with greater optimism than we were prepared to on the basis of the stated parameters (Table 3). Of 25 patients (26 shoulders) who were satisfied and would have the operation again, no less than 22 were unreserved in their enthusiasm.

Overall Results

In terms of composite grading (Table 3) 25 shoulders (24 patients) were classified as "good" or "very good", and 6 were rated as "fair" or "poor". When all factors are considered there was therefore an overall success rate of 80 per cent.

Complications

The shoulder region, possibly by virtue of its generous blood supply, seems to enjoy a relative immunity to infection similar to that of the scalp,

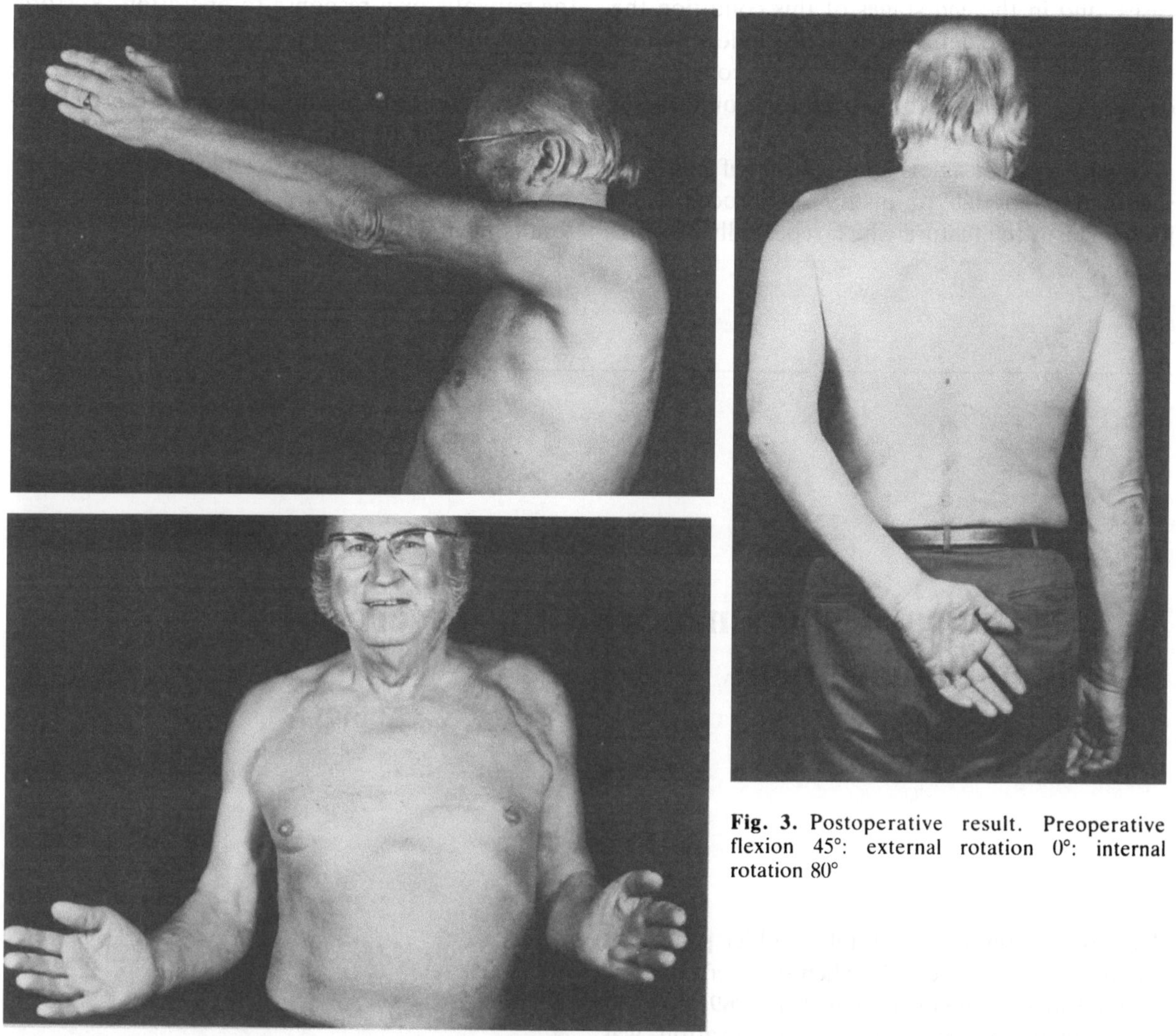

Fig. 3. Postoperative result. Preoperative flexion 45°: external rotation 0°: internal rotation 80°

and we have been fortunate in avoiding any complications of sepsis. Apart from the cases previously discussed which came to secondary excision arthroplasty or suffering prosthetic dislocation, the only other complication has been a traction lesion of the medial cord of the brachial plexus. This occurred in two cases and was diagnosed by nerve conduction studies. For some reason the medial cord therefore appears to be particularly at risk, possibly from traction, and great care should be exercised during operation to avoid excessive retraction of the humerus.

Conclusions

Prosthetic shoulder replacement is in its infancy and in the majority of cases it is not possible to re-establish normal function. This is due to a combination of related factors, including constraints on prosthetic design and severity of shoulder joint destruction, because only those shoulders causing major problems of pain and disability are considered for replacement. It is no accident that rheumatoid arthritis accounted for most of our cases, and in the end stages of this condition the soft tissues are so deficient as to preclude anything other than a constrained or semi-constrained device. The results of the procedure should therefore be judged accordingly.

By any scale of assessment pain relief has been satisfactory enough to justify the procedure in itself. This is the feature which repeatedly governs the patient's own response to operation. Restoration of mobility and function can be encouraging (Fig. 3), but gains are more usually due to the patient's ability to use his movement more effectively by virtue of pain relief. Given strict indications for selection, worthwhile results can be achieved in 80% of cases. In our experience these results have not deteriorated with time.

V.7. Clinical Experience with the Liverpool Shoulder Replacement

F.H. Beddow and M.A. Elloy

The present low-friction total shoulder prosthesis has been in use since 1975 when it superseded the original metal implant designed in 1969. A semi-constrained ball and socket configuration was used to prevent upward humeral subluxation to which an unconstrained prosthesis is prone, particularly in rheumatoid shoulders in which the superior rotator cuff is extensively damaged.

The Prosthesis

The prosthesis is of reversed ball and socket type. Placing the ball on the scapula and the socket on the humerus [56] enables the anatomical centre of articulation to be preserved and prevents impingement between the greater tuberosity and the acromion during abduction. The stainless steel or cobalt chrome scapular component (Fig. 1) has a stem which is inserted into the medullary cavity of the axillary border of the scapula to a depth of approximately 50 mm. A short stem variety was

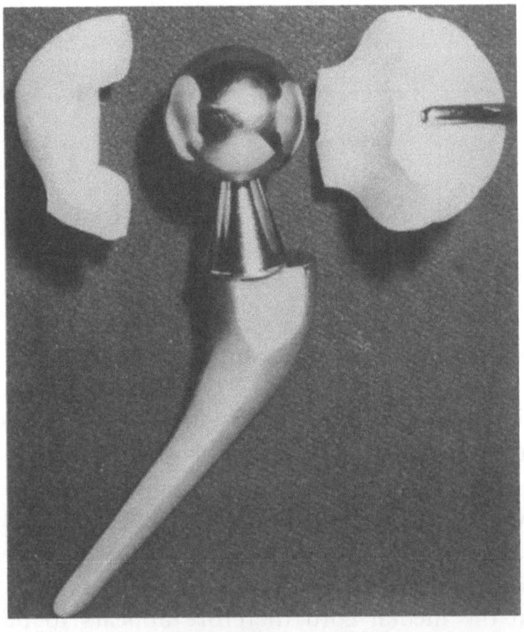

Fig. 1. The prosthesis: the scapular stem carries the ball and the humeral component consists of a polyethylene socket with external metal support. Note the projecting polyethylene lugs (see text). The removable protective cap is also shown

later introduced where excavation to the required depth was not possible. It has a 20 mm diameter head which articulates with an ultra-high-molecular-weight polyethylene humeral socket. The humeral component has no stem, but its external surface is deeply grooved to key into the acrylic cement, a material which is used to enhance the fixation of both components.

Dislocation in the first few postoperative weeks before the formation of a new capsule is prevented by two diametrically opposed lugs on the cup, extending just beyond the equator of the ball and reinforced by an external metal support that also serves as a radiological marker (Fig. 1). A removable protective cap serves to position the lugs during insertion that they do not subsequently impinge on the neck of the prosthesis during normal movements of the shoulder. Radiographs of the implants in situ are shown in Figs. 2 and 3.

Clinical Material

A total of 19 shoulder replacements have been performed using this prosthesis; 14 patients were female and 5 male; the average age was 52 years.

Indications

The main indication has been pain from a joint that has suffered severe mechanical damage: 16 patients had rheumatoid arthritis; 2 suffered old fracture dislocations; there was 1 case of osteoarthritis.

Technique

All the operations were performed in a Charnley Howarth sterile air enclosure or laminar air flow theatre. The operation has been carried out via an anterior approach through the deltopectoral groove. Originally, the anterior third of the deltoid muscle was divided close to its origin and retracted to give additional exposure. In the last twelve patients the anterior third of the lateral end of the clavicle was removed and retracted with the deltoid origin intact, thus avoiding any denervation of deltoid muscle fibres and providing a firm base for the reattachment of the deltoid using strong sutures passed through holes in the bone.

The humeral head is removed through its anatomical neck, and a synovectomy is carried out if there is significant synovial proliferation. The glenoid and axillary border of the scapula are excavated using gouge, curette and small reamers whilst a finger is passed down the axillary border as a guide. The cancellous bone of the humeral head is then excavated with a curette and a trial prosthesis is inserted. Although the prosthesis was designed to be implanted pre-articulated using one

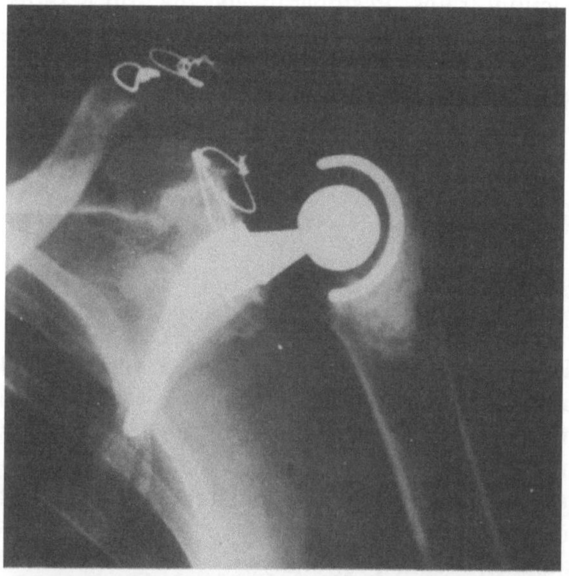

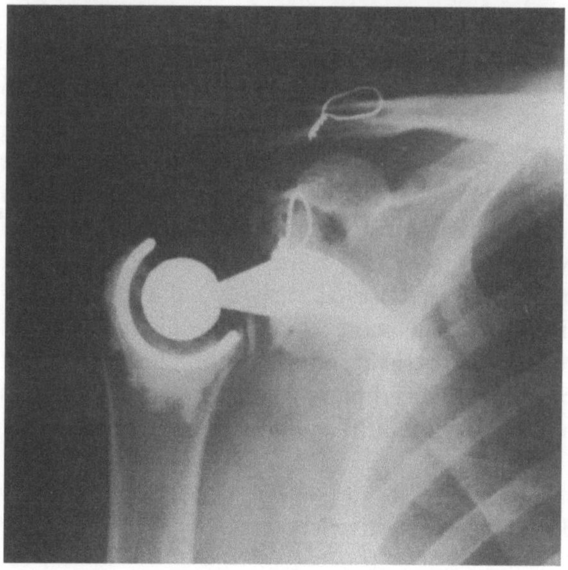

Figs. 2 and 3. Postoperative radiographs of the standard and short stemmed prostheses respectively

mix of acrylic cement [2,3] some difficulty was experienced in complete removal of excess cement from behind the prosthetic neck. Therefore, after the first few cases, the prosthetic components have been implanted separately. The position to be occupied by the lugs of the humeral cup is marked on the humerus, and the trial scapular prosthesis is withdrawn.

The humeral component is first cemented in position flush with the anatomical neck. The scapular component is then cemented in place with its neck at right angles to the glenoid. The components are articulated by gentle pressure. The wound is closed in layers over two closed suction drains. Postoperatively, the arm is rested in a collar and cuff for two weeks. The drains are removed at 48 hours, and active assisted exercises performed from five days.

Results

1. Follow-up

The longest follow-up has been 5 years and 4 months and the average about 2 years and 6 months. Two shoulders done in the last 6 months have been excluded because of inadequate follow-up (these are satisfactory to date) and one patient aged 74 years has been lost to follow-up, so 16 shoulders remain for analysis.

2. Pain Relief

Preoperatively, all patients had severe pain on movement and 12 were wakened at night by the pain. Pain relief following the operation has been rapid, most patients reporting such marked relief within two days that it has been possible to begin mobilising exercises as early as 5 days postoperatively without more than mild discomfort. At review, 11 patients reported complete or almost complete relief of pain; 2 said that their shoulders had become painful again after early relief.

3. Range of Active Movement

Improvement in the range of active movement was less satisfactory than pain relief: 9 patients obtained an increased range of movement and 2 of these achieved an almost full range (Fig. 4). In 1 case the range was unchanged and in 6 the range was reduced.

4. Function

Although pain relief is the most important parameter, improvement in function was also examined: 10 patients reported improvement in

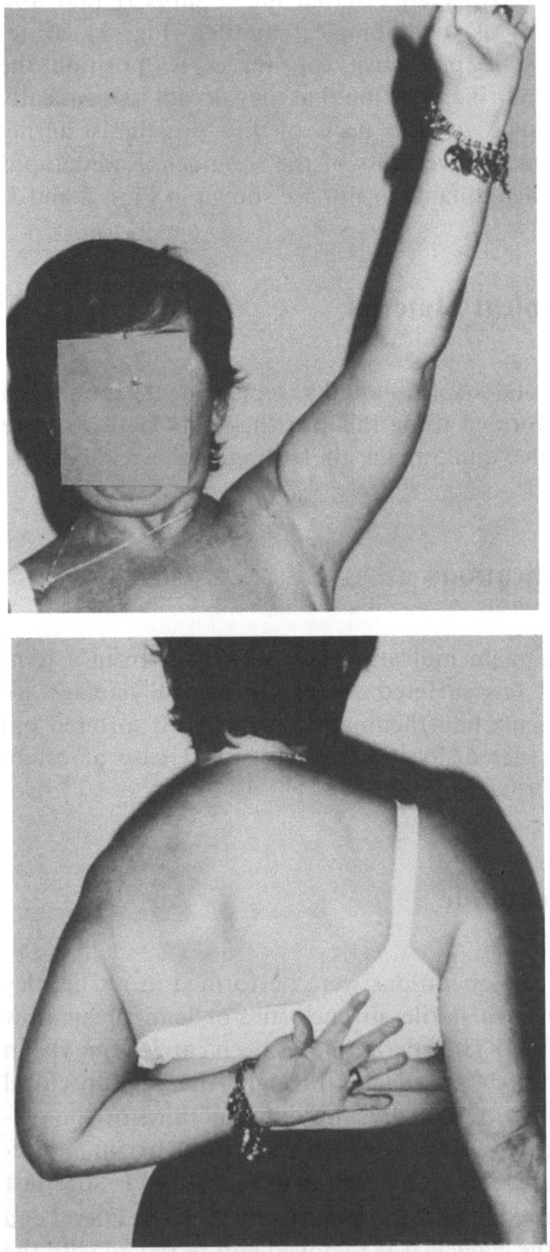

Fig. 4. Postoperative movement (*see text*)

function, being able to comb the hair and dress more easily and also able to undertake more household duties; 6 patients reported unchanged function.

5. Patient Response

Patient response was generous: 13 patients expressed themselves pleased, 1 was undecided, and 2 felt they had not been helped.

6. Complications

There have been no cases of infection or dislocation.

Loosening has occurred in 4 shoulders, 1 of which followed a fracture of the scapula as a result of a fall. The loosening has been confined to the scapular component, but none of these was of the short stem type. One patient has very limited movement but little pain, and because of her other extensive rheumatoid problems the position has been accepted. Another patient had her prosthesis removed and replaced with an unconstrained prosthesis of new design which is being separately evaluated. In this prosthesis the upward subluxation to which an unconstrained prosthesis is liable is controlled by a shaped block of ultra-high-molecular-weight polyethylene fixed to the undersurface of the acromion and articulating with the head of the metal humeral component. The glenoid is resurfaced with a separate ultra-high-molecular-weight polyethylene component. This patient has been relieved of her pain and has regained a good range of movement. The remaining two patients currently await re-exploration.

One patient developed ossification in the lower part of the capsule and this has restricted the range of movement to half the preoperative range.

One patient sustained a stress fracture of the clavicle at the anterior end of the osteotomy during exercise. This did not unite but was successfully treated by excision of the outer end of the clavicle.

Conclusions

The Liverpool shoulder replacement has been performed for just over five years, but as with many series of shoulder replacement the numbers are small [35].

The main difficulty has been finding the medullary cavity of the scapula when the bony architecture has been more than usually badly damaged. This technical difficulty assumes increased importance when a semi-constrained prosthesis of reversed ball and socket design is used, because both reversal and constraint add to the strains to which the scapular fixation is subjected. For these reasons the results with this prosthesis are being carefully compared with the results of a parallel series, in which an unconstrained prosthesis is used but the upward subluxation to which it is subject is controlled by a component on the undersurface of the acromion.

V.8. Taking Stock — Ten Years Experience of Shoulder Arthroplasty

Alan Lettin

The introduction of the Stanmore Total Shoulder Replacement into clinical practice in 1969 was a direct consequence of early experience in prosthetic replacement of the proximal part of the humerus for resectable tumours. The muscles attaching the upper humerus to the scapula and chest wall were inevitably divided, leaving the deltoid as the only muscle spanning the shoulder joint. It is perhaps, therefore, not surprising that the prosthetic humeral head invariably subluxed upwards and forwards on the glenoid (Fig. 1). This was assumed to be due to the loss of the stabilising influence of the rotator cuff leaving the deltoid without a stable fulcrum on which to exert its force. A similar situation follows primary excision arthroplasty of the head of the humerus for severe fracture dislocation. Although the rotator cuff in this instance is present, the bony fulcrum is missing and once more the deltoid is unable to elevate the arm, although passive movement may be full.

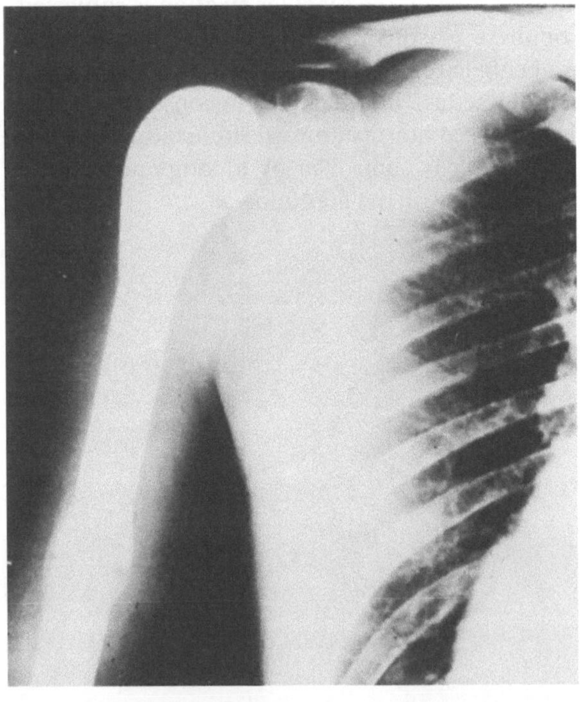

Fig. 1. Upward subluxation of Prosthesis used in replacement of Upper Humerus for giant cell tumour

The unsatisfactory results of the Neer prosthesis in patients suffering from rheumatoid arthritis may also be due to the lack of a rotator cuff or the trapping of the cuff under the acromion by the upward subluxation of the arm. A ball and socket total replacement for the glenohumeral joint (Fig. 2) was designed to provide a stable fulcrum after resection of the head of the humerus and in the absence of the rotator cuff, and with minor modifications has been used in more than fifty patients over the last ten years. The prosthesis itself allows a full anatomical range of internal and external rotation and flexion, and 90° of abduction, and so with the addition of scapulothoracic movement a full range of shoulder movement is theoretically possible. In the event, abduction and flexion above shoulder level is rarely achieved and then only by a matter of 10° or 20°, although full rotation, especially internal rotation, is commonplace (Table 1).

From a functional point of view this proved to be no serious disadvantage, for most everyday activities are carried out below shoulder level, and in fact internal rotation proved to be the most important functional movement and pure abduction (the commonly used index of shoulder function) the least important (Table 2). The relief of

Table 1. Average range of movement (40 patients)

Movement	Average range (degrees)	
	Preoperative	Postoperative
Abduction	50	70
Internal rotation	45	85
External rotation	10	20
Extension	10	30
Flexion	55	75

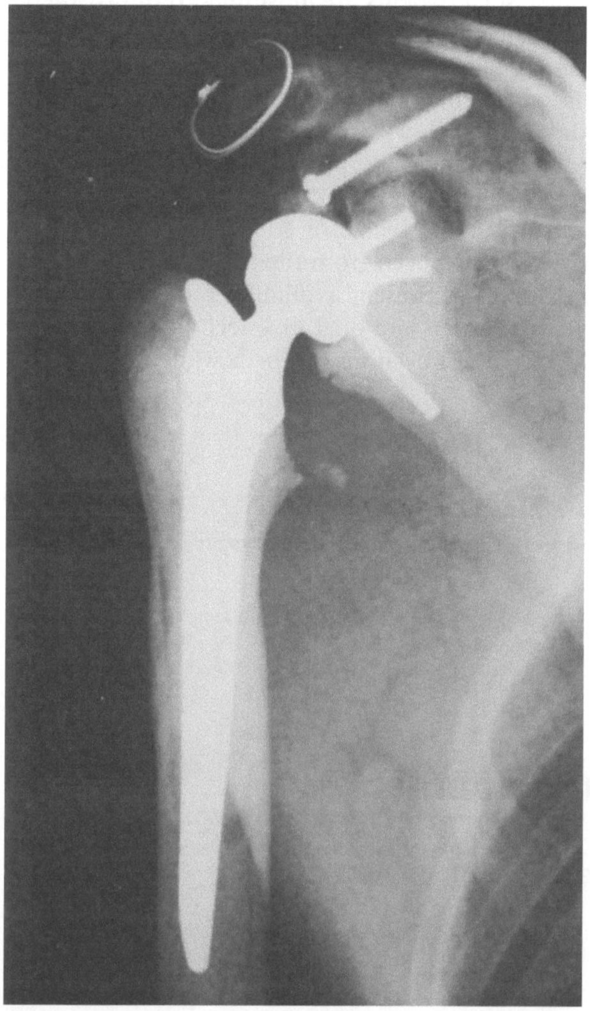

Fig. 2. Radiograph of Stanmore Total Shoulder Replacement (The upper screws is re-attaching the Coracoid Process)

pain, as well as such improvement in the range of movement that did occur, greatly facilitated many everyday tasks and enabled them to be carried out much more quickly, a hitherto unrecognised measure of improved function.

Impingement, either of the greater tuberosity against the acromion or of one component of the prosthesis against the other, did not seem to be the cause of the limited movement. Undoubtedly weakness and wasting of the deltoid, especially after multiple operations, may have been a contributing factor limiting active movement. The detachment of the lateral portion of the deltoid from the clavicle during the anterior approach may also have devitalised this part of the muscle, and recently prosthetic replacement has been performed through a transacromial approach.

Table 2. Assessment of function

	Number of patients	
	Preoperative	Postoperative
Able to get hand to mouth	18	33
Able to comb hair	4	31
Able to dress and to attend to personal toilet with aids	22	32
Able to carry out normal occupation	12	21

The presence or absence of the rotator cuff appeared to make little difference to the range of movement. Some of the best results were achieved in patients in whom the cuff was irreparably damaged, but conversely deliberate sacrifice of the cuff did not ensure a good result.

The studies of Poppen and Walker [48] suggest that the instant centre of movement of the normal shoulder lies within 6 mm of the centre of the humeral head. The instant centre of the Stanmore prosthesis lies 12.5 mm medially, and perhaps even this small difference is critical to the efficient working of the deltoid, the better results occurring when the prosthetic instant centre lay close to the true instant centre for that particular shoulder.

It seems more likely, however, that the head of the humerus glides as well as rotates on the humerus (Wallace) [63] and the contraint inherent in the Stanmore prosthesis prevents this; perhaps the semi-constrained joints now under trial will prove to be more satisfactory. It may of course be unrealistic to expect an artificial shoulder joint to reproduce the very wide range of movement of the normal shoulder and at the same time remain stable.

Finally, perhaps the limited range of movement is the result of the well-known propensity of the shoulder to stiffen after injury or operation.

The prosthesis was removed from nine of the first fifty patients treated: Once for infection, once for recurrent dislocation and in seven patients for loosening of the glenoid component. Removal of the prosthesis left a surprisingly stable and, in the main, pain-free, useful excision arthroplasty. No patient was worse off than before the original operation, no doubt due to the severity of the preoperative pain and disability, and secondary excision arthroplasty of the shoulder certainly seems to be less disabling than excision arthroplasty carried out as a primary procedure.

The fixation of the glenoid component of a total shoulder replacement presents problems by virtue of the very flimsy nature of the scapula. Excavation of the subglenoid bone leaves a cavity which is rarely large enough to contain even a small cup and is often smaller than might be expected from preoperative radiographs. The glenoid often proves to be no more than a ring of osteophytes, and after their removal the residual bone affords poor fixation for a prosthesis. What is more, the quality of the bone in patients suffering from rheumatoid arthritis, especially after prolonged steroid treatment, is often poor, but of course such patients are most in need of prosthetic replacement.

Although the need for prosthetic shoulder replacement may be infrequent, there are undoubtedly patients with resectable tumours, post-traumatic arthritis, primary osteoarthritis, and particularly rheumatoid arthritis of the glenohumeral joint, who are sufficiently disabled to derive benefit even from the far from satisfactory prostheses at present available. Further improvement in design and operative technique will make the operation even more worth while.

V.9. Double Osteotomy of the Shoulder

A. Benjamin, D. Hirschowitz, G.P. Arden and N. Blackburn

Severe pain with loss of sleep and profound incapacity can arise from an arthritic shoulder. The success of double osteotomy at the knee for the relief of pain of both rheumatoid arthritis and osteoarthritis [4] prompted the development of double osteotomy of the shoulder [6]. Early results [5] showed this simple procedure to be effective for the relief of pain and incapacity and to be free of serious complications. We have therefore continued to develop and evaluate double osteotomy at the shoulder, and this report records our extended experience and follow-up.

Method and Material

Between 1967 and 1979 double osteotomy at the shoulder has been performed on 29 shoulders in 28 patients. The indication in every case was severe incapacitating shoulder pain, unresponsive to conservative measures, in an arthritic joint with advanced radiological changes (Fig. 1). The pathology was rheumatoid arthritis in 15 shoulders, juvenile rheumatoid arthritis in 4 and osteoarthritis in 10. The age range was 14-74 years (average 54.2 years). Five patients were men (Tables 1 and 2). The combined glenohumeral and scapulothoracic range of abduction was measured pre- and postoperatively. Pain was recorded in four grades: 0 representing no pain; 1, mild occasional ache; 2, moderate pain requiring analgesics; and 3, severe pain. Follow-up has been from 1 to 13 years (average 30 months).

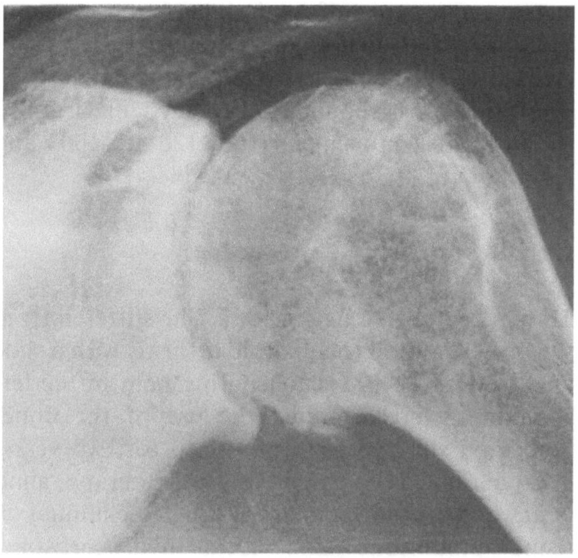

Fig. 1. Case No. 2. Degenerative arthritis

Table 1. Clinical material

Patients	28
Shoulders	29
Age range (years)	14–74 (average 54.2)
Men	5
Women	23

Table 2. Conditions treated

Osteoarthritis	10
Rheumatoid arthritis	15
Juvenile rheumatoid arthritis	4

Operative Technique

The operation is performed under general anaesthetic. Through an anterior shoulder-strap incision the fibres of the deltoid muscle are separated parallel to and half an inch lateral to the medial border of the muscle, preserving the cephalic vein. The coracoid process is detached. The subscapularis muscle is divided in its tendinous portion. The anterior aspect of the neck of the scapula is exposed, and retractors are placed above and below. The anterior shoulder capsule is opened and the glenoid fossa visualised. An osteotomy is performed 5 mm medial to the glenoid fossa, the osteotome being directed posteriorly and slightly laterally in a plane parallel to that of the articular surface of the glenoid. By opening up the osteotomy, the posterior cortex is cracked and hinged on the posterior periosteum but not displaced. The humerus is now approached just distal to the subscapularis and an osteotomy, without displacement, is performed at the surgical neck (Fig. 2). The coracoid process is replaced with sutures, and the capsule and muscle layers are repaired.

Once the surgeon is conversant with this technique, it is possible to perform the operation without detaching the coracoid process. The conjoint tendon can be retracted medially and the subscapularis split in the line of its fibres instead of transecting its tendon. This more limited exposure may be sufficient.

Table 3. Effect of operation on pain

Grade*	0	1	2	3
Preoperative	0	0	0	29
Postoperative	12	13	1	3

*For details of grade see text.

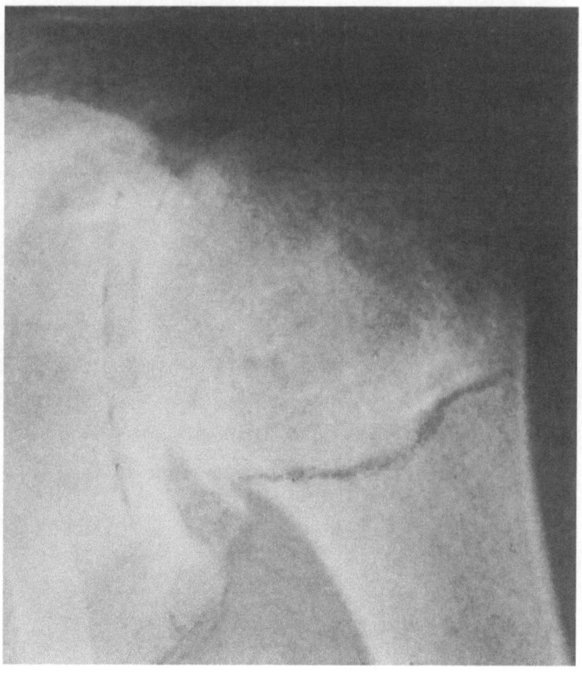

Fig. 2. Case No. 2. After osteotomy

Results

The effect of the operation on pain is shown in Table 3. Pre-operatively all patients had severe pain (Grade 3). Every patient experienced good early pain relief (Grade 0 or 1) within a month of surgery. Often the arthritic pain was completely relieved the day after the procedure. Pain relief was maintained to the latest follow-up in 25 shoulders (86%). The remaining 3 shoulders had deteriorated, 1 to Grade 2 and 3 to Grade 3. One of the latter has subsequently had, and another is awaiting, total shoulder replacement.

The active range of total abduction (i.e. scapulothoracic and glenohumeral combined) was increased in 19 shoulders by 20°-30° (average 46°). The range in 8 shoulders was unchanged and 2 shoulders lost movement from 120° to 100° and from 80° to 70° respectively (Table 4).

Case Report 1

JB was 25 years of age in 1967. She suffered from severe generalised rheumatoid arthritis with a slide latex test of 1246. Incapacitating pain in the left shoulder severely limited the use of the upper limb, and she had disturbed sleep for two years. The pain failed to respond to physiotherapy, analgesics and anti-inflammatory drugs including systemic prednisone and local hydrocortisone.

Table 4. Effect of operation on abduction

Increased abduction (degrees)	19 (average 46)
Decreased abduction (degrees)	2 (average 15)
Unchanged	8
Average abduction (degrees)	
Preoperative	52 (range 0–120)
Postoperative	81 (range 15–175)

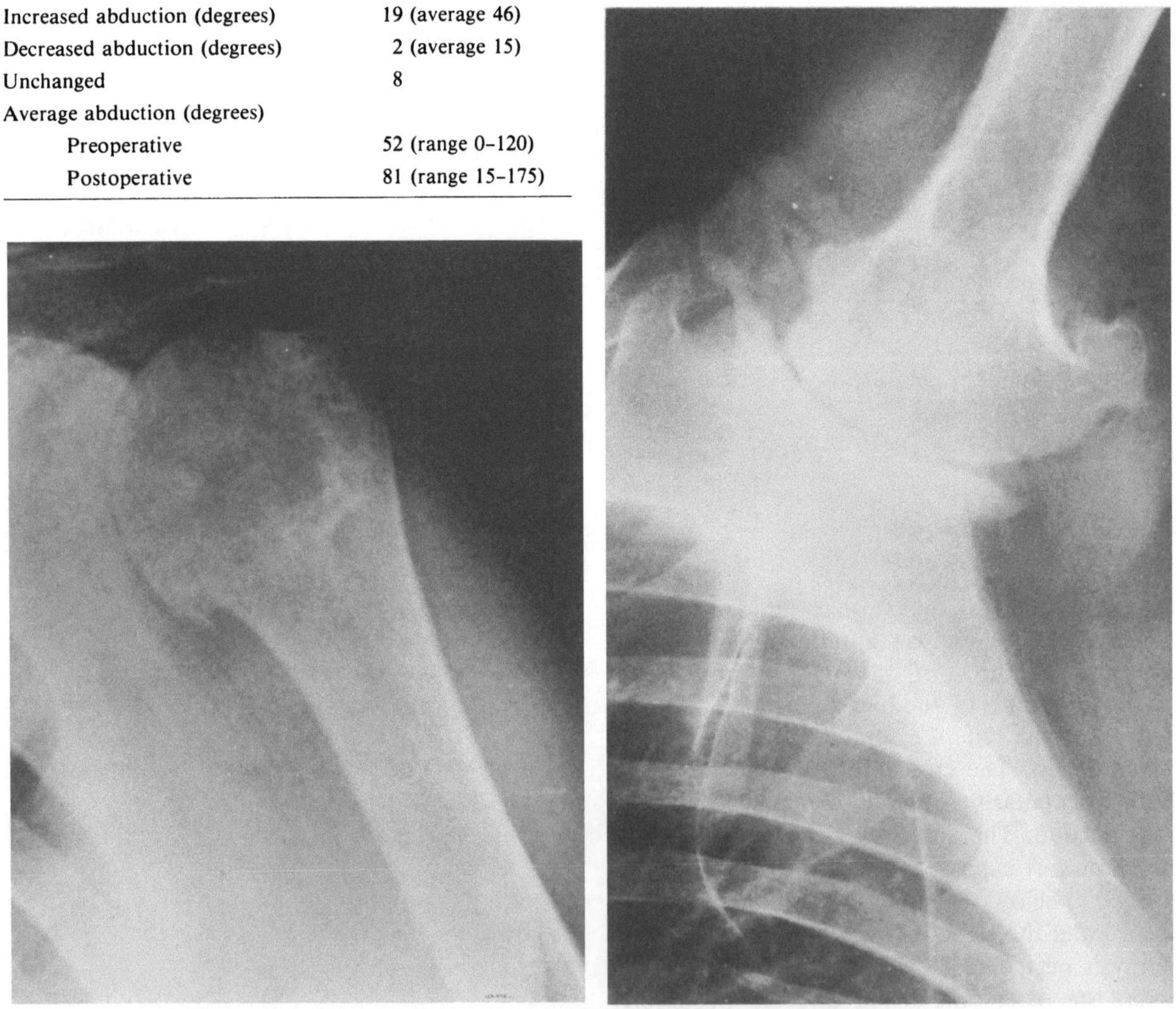

a b

Fig. 3. Case No. 2. **a** One year after operation **b** in full abduction

Radiographs revealed severe rheumatoid arthritis in the shoulder. She was referred from the Rheumatology Department for arthrodesis. It was decided to perform a double osteotomy and she became the first patient to have this operation. Two weeks after the operation her pain was entirely relieved and she could abduct to 90°. She remains pain-free with an excellent range of movement 13 years later.

Case Report 2

DK was 55 years of age in 1979. In 1948 he had sustained an injury at rugby following which there was increasing left shoulder pain. He became unable to play golf and was kept awake at night. Radiographs revealed loss of joint space, irregularity of the joint and subchondral sclerosis (Fig. 1). In 1979 a double osteotomy of the left shoulder was carried out (Fig. 2) and now one year later he is entirely free from pain and has regained a remarkable range of movement (Figs. 3 to 6).

Complications (Table 5)

There was one non-union of the humerus in a patient who preoperatively had a glenohumeral ankylosis. The shoulder remained fused, but she lost all her pain and has 90° useful abduction at the pseudo-arthrosis. There was one delayed union of the humeral osteotomy. Two patients lost some active abduction, as described above.

Table 5. Complications of operation

Non-union of humerus	1
Delayed union of humerus	1
Loss of movement	2
Postoperative sepsis	2

Discussion

Double osteotomy of the shoulder has achieved good or excellent pain relief in 86% of our patients. The pain is often relieved within twenty-four hours. This analgesic effect may be related to the reduction of intra-osseous hypertension which has been shown to exist in the subchondral bone in arthritic conditions [1,29]. The results of double osteotomy at the shoulder are more satisfactory than at the knee, because the shoulder does not have the problems of weight-bearing.

We have recorded clinically the total active range of abduction in the glenohumeral and scapulothoracic articulations. In those we measured with radiographs glenohumeral movement was not increased by double osteotomy.

The increase in total movement reflects the ability of the patient to utilise all potential abduction at both joints once pain has been reduced. The ability of the joint to sustain load is similarly increased as demonstrated by two rheumatoid patients who were able to weight-bear through crutches after the operation, whereas preoperatively they had been chair-bound because of shoulder pain.

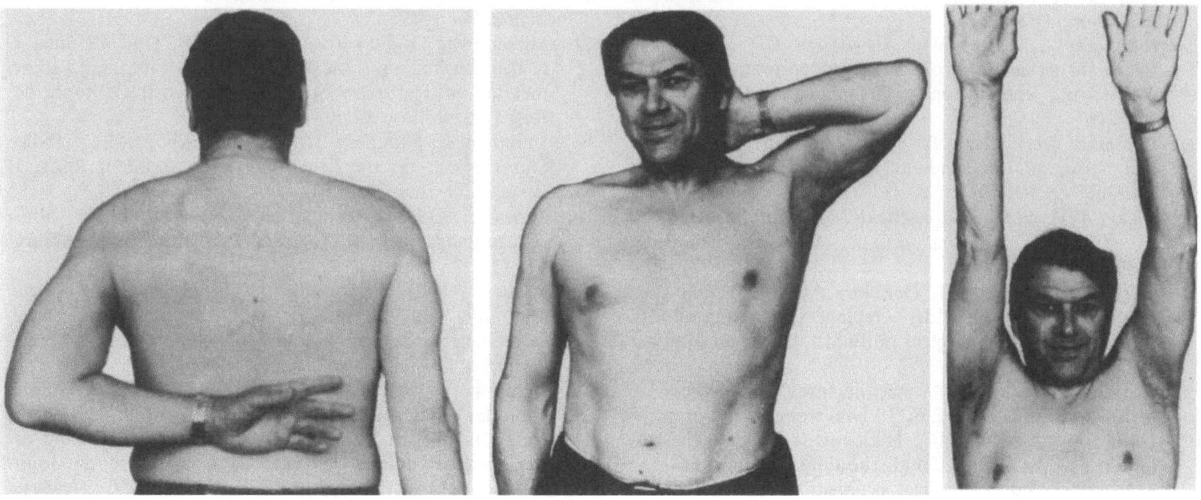

Figs. 4-6. Case No. 2. Postoperative range of movement

During the last decade, many authors have advocated total shoulder replacement for the painful arthritic shoulder [3,8,10,11,12,13,14,20, 22,25,33,34,40,43,46,53,56]. It is clear, however, that fixation of the glenoid component and restoration of stability following attenuation of the rotator cuff in the rheumatoid patient remain major problems. Destruction of bone stock and complications such as infection and loosening, with no satisfactory salvage procedure, make total shoulder replacement a less than ideal procedure. Complications following double osteotomy, however, are few and none is serious. Bone stock is improved as a result of the reversal of disuse atrophy with pain relief.

Total shoulder replacement is a salvage procedure for failed double osteotomy but is rarely indicated. We believe that double osteotomy of the shoulder should be considered before total replacement.

References

1 Arnoldi CC, Lemperg RK, Linderholm H (1971) Immediate effect of osteotomy on the intramedullary pressure of the femoral head and neck in patients with degenerative osteoarthritis. Acta Orthop Scand 42: 454-455
2 Beddow FH, Elloy MA (1975) An improved shoulder prosthesis. The Proceedings of the 15th International Conference of the Biological Engineering Society London
3 Beddow FH, Elloy MA (1977) The Liverpool total replacement for the gleno-humeral joint. Joint replacement in the upper limb. I Mech E Conference Publications 1977-5: 21-25
4 Benjamin A (1969) Double osteotomy for the painful knee in rheumatoid arthritis and osteoarthritis. J Bone Joint Surg 51-B: 3
5 Benjamin A, Hirschowitz D, Arden GP (1979) The treatment of arthritis of the shoulder joint by double osteotomy. International Orthopaedics (SICOT) 3: 211-216
6 Benjamin A, Helal B (1980) Surgical repair and reconstruction in rheumatoid disease. Macmillan, London: pp 101-103
7 Bickel WH cited by Linscheid, RL, Cofield R (1976) Total shoulder arthroplasty: Experimental but promising. Geriatrics, 31: 64-69
8 Buechel F, Pappas MJ, DePalma AF (1978) "Floating Socket" total shoulder replacement; anatomical, biomechanical and surgical rationale. J Biomed Mat Res 12: 89-114
9 Brittain HA (1952) Architectural principles in arthrodesis. 2nd Edit. E & S Livingstone, Edinburgh
10 Clarke IC, Amstutz HC, Hirschowitz D, Sen Hoy A, Gruen TAW (1979) Total shoulder replacement—an anatomical and mechanical problem. Proc Amer Acad Orthop Surg Paper 156 San Francisco
11 Clarke IC, Gruen TAW, Sen Hoy A, Hirschowitz D, Maki S, Amstutz HC (1979) Problems in gleno-humeral surface replacements—real or imagined? Mech E Vol 8: 161-175
12 Clayton ML, Ferlic DC (1974) Surgery of the shoulder in rheumatoid arthritis. Clin Orthop 106: 166-174
13 Corfield RH (1977) Total shoulder arthroplasty; the current state of development. "Total Joint Replacement" Proceedings of a Workshop Sponsored by RSA, Northwestern University Chicago
14 Corfield RH, Stauffer RN (1977) The Bickel gleno-humeral arthroplasty. Joint replacement in the upper limb. I Mech E Conference publications 1977-5: 15-19
15 Cotton RE, Rideout DF (1964) Tears of the humeral rotator cuff. J Bone Joint Surg 46-B: 314-328
16 Crossan JF, Vallance R (1980) Clinical and radiological features of the shoulder joint in rheumatoid arthritis. Journal of Bone and Joint Surgery 62B, 1-116
17 Cruess RL (1980) Rheumatoid arthritis of the shoulder. Orth Clin N Amer 11: 333-342
18 Data extrapolated from Inman V, Saunders JBdeCM, Abbott IC (1944) Observations on the function of the shoulder joint. J Bone Joint Surg 26: 1-30
19 Doody SG, Freedman L, Waterland JC (1970) Shoulder movement during abduction in the scapular plane. Arch Phys Med & Rehab 51: 595-604
20 Englebrecht E, Stellbrink G (1976) Totale schulterendoprothese modell "St George". Chirurg 47: 515-530
21 Ennevaara K (1967) Painful shoulder joint in rheumatoid arthritis. Acta Rheum Scand (Suppl 11) 1-116
22 Fenlin JM (1975) Total gleno-humeral joint replacement. Orthop Clin N Amer 6: 565-583
23 Freedman L, Munro RR (1966) Abduction of the arm in the scapular plane: Scapular and gleno-humeral movements. J Bone Joint Surg 48-A: 1503-1510
24 Golding FC (1962) The shoulder—the forgotten joint. Brit J Radiol 35: 149
25 Gristina AG, Forte MR (1977) The trispherical total shoulder prosthesis—biomechanical, anatomical and surgical considerations. Symposium in Trans Soc for Biomaterials. Paper 121. New Orleans
26 Gristina AG (1978) Presentation to AAOS New York. Sept 1978
27 Gristina AG, Forte MR, Rovere GD, Poehling GG, Nicastro JF (1978) The trispherical total shoulder prosthesis—Biomechanical, anatomical, and surgical considerations. Trans 24th Ann Meeting ORS 3: 302
28 Gristina AG (1979) Presentation to AAOS New York. September 1979
29 Hirschowitz D, Edwards J, Arden GP, Hart G, Shea J (1978) Intraosseous hypertension and knee pain. Joint meeting of Heberden Society and British Orthopaedic Research Section, London, March 1978
30 Inman VT, Saunders JB de CM, Abbott LC (1944) Observations on the function of the shoulder joint. J Bone Joint Surg 26: 1-30
31 Jones L (1933) Reconstructive operation for non-reducable fractures of the head of the humerus. Ann Surg 97: 217-225
32 Jones L (1942) The shoulder joint—observations on the anatomy and physiology with an analysis of a reconstructive operation following extensive injury. Surg Gynaecol Obstet 75: 443
33 Kenmore PI, MacCartee C, Vitek B (1974) A simple shoulder replacement. J Biomed Res Symp 8: 329-330
34 Kessel L, Wright KJW (1977) Prosthetic replacement of the shoulder joint. Delivered at Conference on Joint Replacement in the Upper Limb. I Mech E Conference Publications. (unpublished data).

35 Kessel L, Bayley I (1979) Prosthetic replacement of the shoulder joint– a preliminary communication. J Roy Soc Med Vol 72: 748-752

36 Kölbel R (1972) Total shoulder joint replacement. M Sc Thesis, University of Surrey, Guildford, Surrey

37 Kölbel R, Friedebold G (1975) Schultergelenkersatz. Z Orthop 113: 452-454

38 Kölbel R, Rohlmann A, Bergmann G, Friedebold G (1977) Shoulder joint replacement. In: Endoprostheses and alternatives for the arm shoulder joint. Editors C Burri, Coldeway J, Rüter A. Hans Huber Publishers, Bern, Stuttgart, Vienna, pp 47-60

39 Kölbel R, Rohlmann A, Bergmann G (1980) Experimentalle Untersuchungen der verankerung einer schultergelenkendoprothese. In: Osteosynthese, Endoprothetik und Biomechanik der Gelenke. Editors Jager M, Hackenbroch MH, Refior HJ. Georg Thieme, Verlag-Stuttgart, pp 54-61

40 Lettin AWF, Scales JT (1972) Total replacement of the shoulder joint. Proc Roy Soc Med 65: 373-74

41 Lucas DB (1973) Biomechanics of the shoulder joint. Arch Surg 107: 425-432

42 Macnab I (1979) Rotator cuff tendinitis. In: Recent advances in orthopaedics. McKibbin (Ed) Vol 3. Churchill Livingstone, p 95

43 Maki S, Gruen T (1976) Anthropometric studies of the glenohumeral joint. Trans Orthop Res Soc Paper 162, New Orleans

44 Neer CS (1955) Articular replacement for the humeral head. J Bone Joint Surg 37-A: 215-228

45 Neer CS (1970) Displaced proximal humeral fractures Part I. Classification and evaluation. J Bone Joint Surg 52-A: 1077-1089

46 Neer CS (1974) Replacement athroplasty for gleno-humeral osteoarthritis. J Bone Joint Surg 56-A: 1-13

47 Péan JE (1894) Gazette des hôpitaux civils et militaires (Paris) 67: 291

48 Poppen NK, Walker PS (1976) Normal and abnormal motion of the shoulder. J Bone Joint Surg 58-A: 195-201

49 Poppen NK, Walker PS (1978) Forces at the gleno-humeral joint in abduction. Clin Orthop 135: 165-170

50 Post M, Haskell S, Finder J (1975) Total shoulder replacement. J Bone Joint Surg 57-A: 1171

51 Post M, Jablon M, Miller H, Singh M (1979) Constrained total shoulder joint replacement: a critical review. Clin Orthop 144: 135-150

52 Putti V (1933) Arthrodesis for tuberculosis of the knee and of the shoulder. Clin Org Morimento 18: 217

53 Ranawat CS, Poppen NK (1977) Total shoulder arthroplasty– Hospital for Special Surgery Design. Read at Conference on Joint Replacement in the Upper Linb. I Mech E London (unpublished data)

54 Reeves B (1968) Experiments on the tensile strength of the anterior structures of the shoulder joint in man. J Bone Joint Surg. 50-B: 858-865

55 Reeves B, Jobbins B, Dowson D, Wright V (1971) The development of a total shoulder joint endo-prosthesis. In: Conference on human locomotor engineering. I Mech E pp 108-122

56 Reeves B, Jobbins B, Dowson D, Wright V (1972) A total shoulder endo-prosthesis. Engineering in Medicine. Vol 1 No 3: 64-67

57 Reeves B, Jobbins B, Flowers M (1972) Biomechanical problems in the development of a total shoulder endoprosthesis, abstracted. J Bone Joint Surg 54-B: 193

58 Rohlmann A, Bergmann G, Kölbel R (1980) The relevance of stress computations in the femur with and without endoprosthesis. In: International conference on finite elements in biomechanics. Simon BR (Edit) University of Arizona Tucson pp 549-566

59 Romano RL, Burgess EM (1975) Total shoulder replacement abstract. J Bone Joint Surg 57-A: 1033

60 Saha AK (1961) Theory of shoulder mechanism: description and applied. Charles C Thomas, Springfield, Illinois

61 Thompson G (1974) Measurement of glenohumeral articulation. M Sc Thesis, Victoria University of Manchester

62 Trinder JR (1980) Digital video-cursor for computer logging the co-ordinates of features displayed on a video-monitor (in press)

63 Wallace WA (1980) The dynamic study of shoulder movement. Proceedings of inaugural international conference on surgery of the shoulder: Institute of Orthopaedics, University of London. Ed Kessel L & Bayley JIL Publishers: Springer-Verlag (in press)

64 Watson-Jones R (1933) Extra-articular arthrodesis of the shoulder. J Bone Joint Surg 15: 862

65 Weiner DS, Macnab I (1970) Superior migration of the humeral head. J Bone Joint Surg 52-B: 524-527

66 Weiss JJ, Thompson GR, Doust V (1975) Rotator cuff tears in rheumatoid arthritis. Arch Int Med 135: 521-525

67 Zippel J (1975) Luxationssichere Schulterendoprothese Modell BME. J Orthop 113: 454-57

Section VI. Fractures and Dislocations

Moderator—Bo J. Lundberg

VI.1. A Biomechanical Appraisal of the Acromioclavicular Joint

William Angus Wallace and Frank Johnson

The acromioclavicular (AC) joint has two main functions: to allow movement to occur between the clavicle and the scapula and to act as a load-bearing joint for the clavicle which acts as a strut between the chest wall and the scapula. Movement at the AC joint is essential in allowing full movement of the shoulder complex during elevation of the arm. This has been confirmed personally when observations were made on the shoulder movement of a patient who inadvisedly had an AC joint dislocation treated by rigid screw fixation. The patient was unable to raise the arm in abduction or flexion higher than shoulder level. Full movement returned on removal of the screw.

Confirmation that the AC joint acts as a load-bearing joint is provided by the relatively common occurrence of osteoarthritis in the AC joint in later life, as highlighted by Kessel and Watson [14] and Watson [28]. Unfortunately no studies have shown the magnitude of the forces transmitted across the AC joint, and because of the complexity of this articulation the only way this is likely to be possible is by implantation of pressure transducers into the joint—a method unikely to be adopted.

Anatomy of the Acromioclavicular Joint

Movement of the AC joint can only be appreciated if the anatomy of the normal joint is fully understood. Figure 1 shows the appearance of the shoulder as viewed obliquely from above. The clavicle articulates with the sternum at the sterno-clavicular joint. Although there are ligaments between the sternum and clavicle, the main stabilising ligament of this joint is the costoclavicular ligament passing from the first rib up to the medial end of the clavicle. The clavicle articulates at its lateral end with the acromion process of the scapula. Again although there are ligaments joining the clavicle to the acromion, the main stabilising ligament lies some distance from the joint; the coracoclavicular ligament, divided into two parts the medial conoid part and the lateral trapezoid part. Because of the sigmoid shape of the clavicle and the attachment of its ligaments, the inter-relation of movements of the clavicle and the scapula may be described with reference to an anatomical model.

Movement of the Scapula and Clavicle in the Anatomical Model

All previous work on the AC joint has concentrated on the two-dimensional changes in position of the clavicle and scapula as seen on a radiograph, with three-dimensional movements ignored. By using a three-dimensional model of the shoulder girdle the importance of correlating movements of the clavicle with the movements of the scapula will be demonstrated. Thus rotation of the clavicle around its long axis should be compared with angulation of the scapula as seen in the scapular anteroposterior view; upward angulation

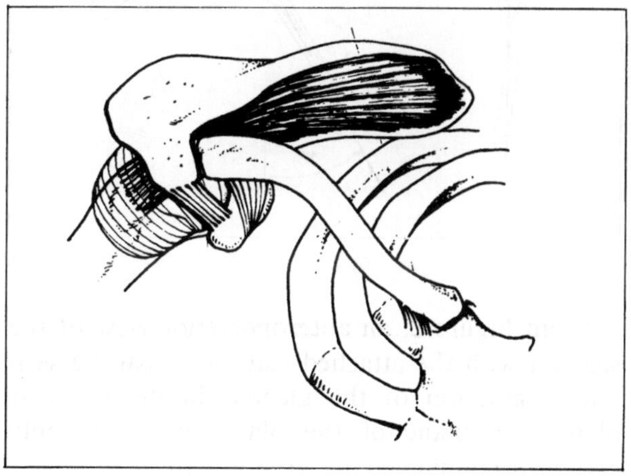

Fig. 1.

of the clavicle should be matched with forward tilting of the scapula as seen in the lateral scapular view; and backward angulation of the clavicle should be matched with posterior angulation of the glenoid and scapular blade as seen in the lateral scapular view. Figures 2, 3 and 4 illustrate the relation of clavicle to scapula during movements.

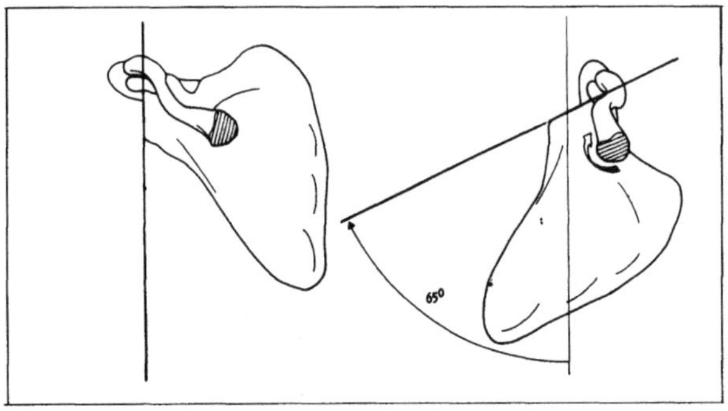

Fig. 2.

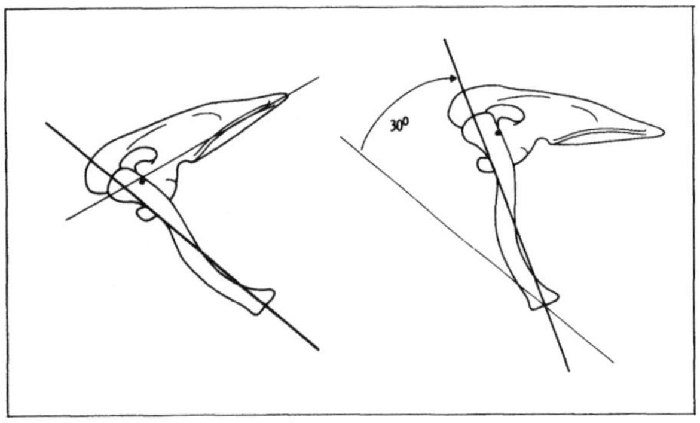

Fig. 3.

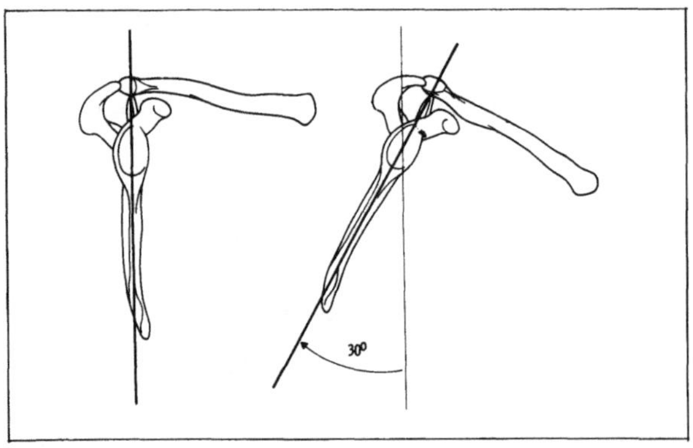

Fig. 4.

From Figure 2, an anteroposterior view of the scapula with the attached clavicle, it can be seen that angulation of the glenoid in the scapular plane— the plane of the blade of the scapula [9]— is accompanied by rotation of the clavicle around its longitudinal axis.

Figure 3 shows the plan view of the scapula and explains the direct relation between rotation of the scapula about the axis from the superior to the inferior pole of the glenoid and posterior angulation of the clavicle.

The lateral view of the scapula (Fig. 4) clearly identifies the scapular angle as seen in this lateral view of the scapula and its direct relation to upward angulation of the clavicle.

Failure to appreciate these relations of scapular to clavicle movement has been obvious in diagrams and movement studies of the acromioclavicular joint after surgery published in the past [11,12].

Dynamic Bi-planar Radiographic Study of the Acromioclavicular Joint

In Nottingham we have developed a bi-planar study of the shoulder which was designed to show the movements which occur at the AC joint. The study has been completed on two normal shoulders with a further twelve radiological studies recorded but not yet analysed.

The study is carried out using two image-intensifiers placed perpendicular to one another at rest. The subject stands erect with the blade of the scapula in the same plane as one of the image-intensifiers as shown in Fig. 5. Because of the restriction imposed by the radiological equipment the study is carried out with the arm elevated in flexion— at right angles to the scapular plane. The plan of the study is shown in Fig. 6 and has been reported previously [25,26].

Distortion of the image-intensifier pictures has been the subject of a separate study [27], and must be corrected prior to a full three-dimensional analysis of the results using a computer programme developed in Nottingham, run on a Digital PDP-11 computer.

Results

This complex study produces as a final result three graphs showing the relation of the clavicle movements to the scapular movements described earlier. The computer graphs of one of our studies is shown in Fig. 7.

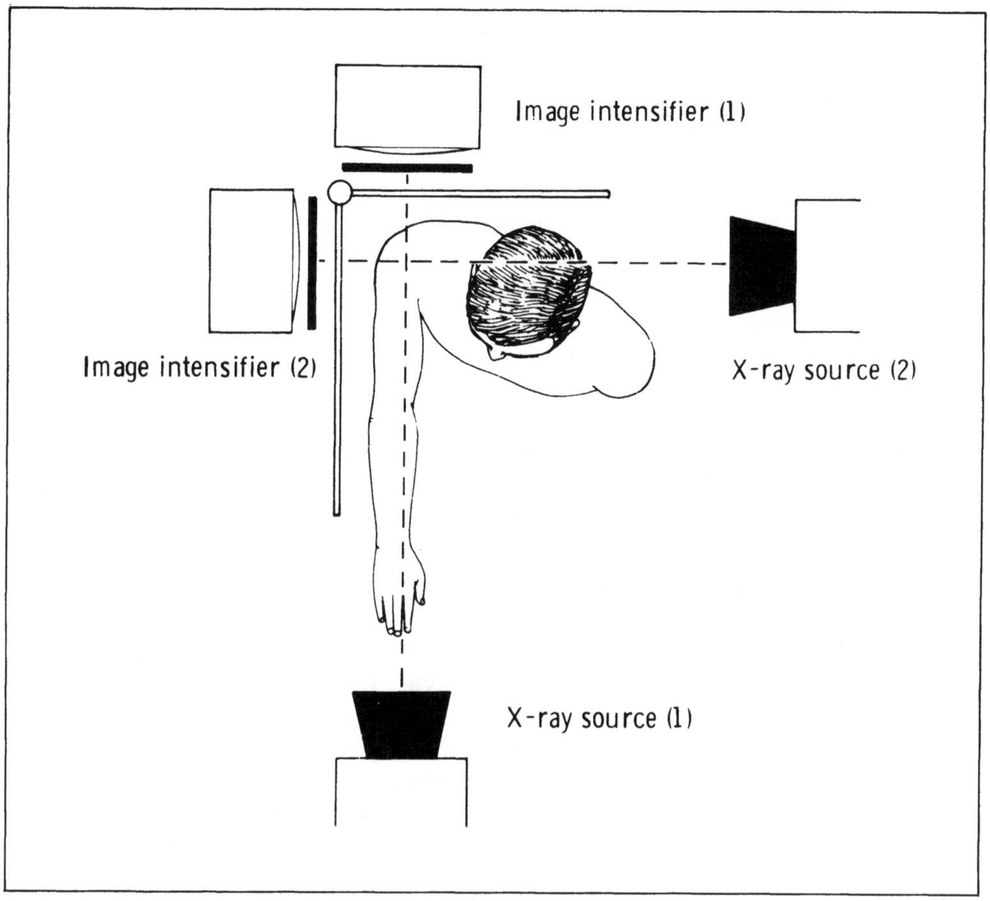
Image intensifier (1)
Image intensifier (2)
X-ray source (2)
X-ray source (1)

Fig. 5.

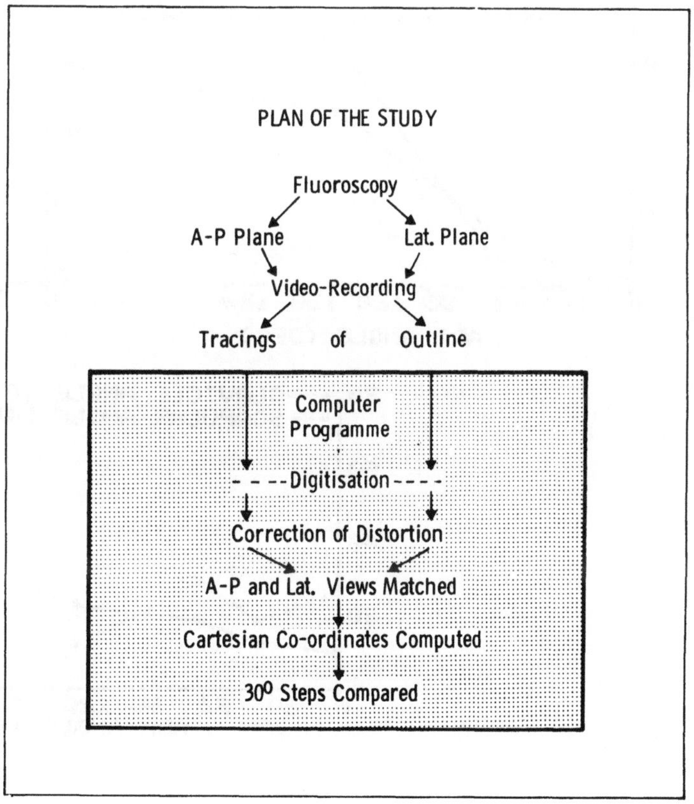
PLAN OF THE STUDY
Fluoroscopy
A-P Plane
Lat. Plane
Video-Recording
Tracings
of
Outline
Computer
Programme
Digitisation
Correction of Distortion
A-P and Lat. Views Matched
Cartesian Co-ordinates Computed
30° Steps Compared

Fig. 6.

In all three graphs the arm angle, measured against the vertical as the arm was elevated is recorded on the abscissa. If no movement were to occur at the acromioclavicular joint, all three graphs should show parallel lines. This is obviously not the case. In the first graph (Fig. 7, *upper left*) clavicular rotation around its longitudinal axis is compared with scapular angle recorded in the anteroposterior view. Clavicular rotation was difficult to measure above 120° of arm elevation and may be inaccurate, but the results indicate that at 90° of elevation very little movement has taken place at the joint and at full elevation 30° to 40° of clavicular rotation has been "taken up" at the AC joint. The accuracy of the data in the other two graphs is considered to be good. In the second graph (Fig. 7, *upper right*) the clavicle angle and scapular rotation as seen in the plan view are compared. At 90° of arm elevation little relative movement has occurred, but at full elevation up to 50° of angulation has been "taken up" at the AC joint. In the final graph (Fig. 7, *bottom*) the clavicle angle to the horizontal is compared with the scapular angle recorded on the lateral view. Here again little movement occurs at the joint during the first 90° of arm elevation, but at full elevation almost 40° of angulation has been "taken up" at the AC joint.

These results show movement at the acromioclavicular joint does take place and occurs increasingly from 90° of arm elevation to full elevation, with maximal movement occurring during the last 30°.

Discussion

Knowledge of the movement which occurs at the AC joint has been limited in the past because of inability to palpate or visualise the joint as the arm is elevated. Simple deduction of the movements were made by Poirier and Charpy [22]. Only recently has more accurate work been carried out by Dvir and Berme [8] using sequential radiographs, but no allowance was made for errors due to perspective. Our work, although complex, is able to establish that movement of the AC joint is an important component of shoulder movement.

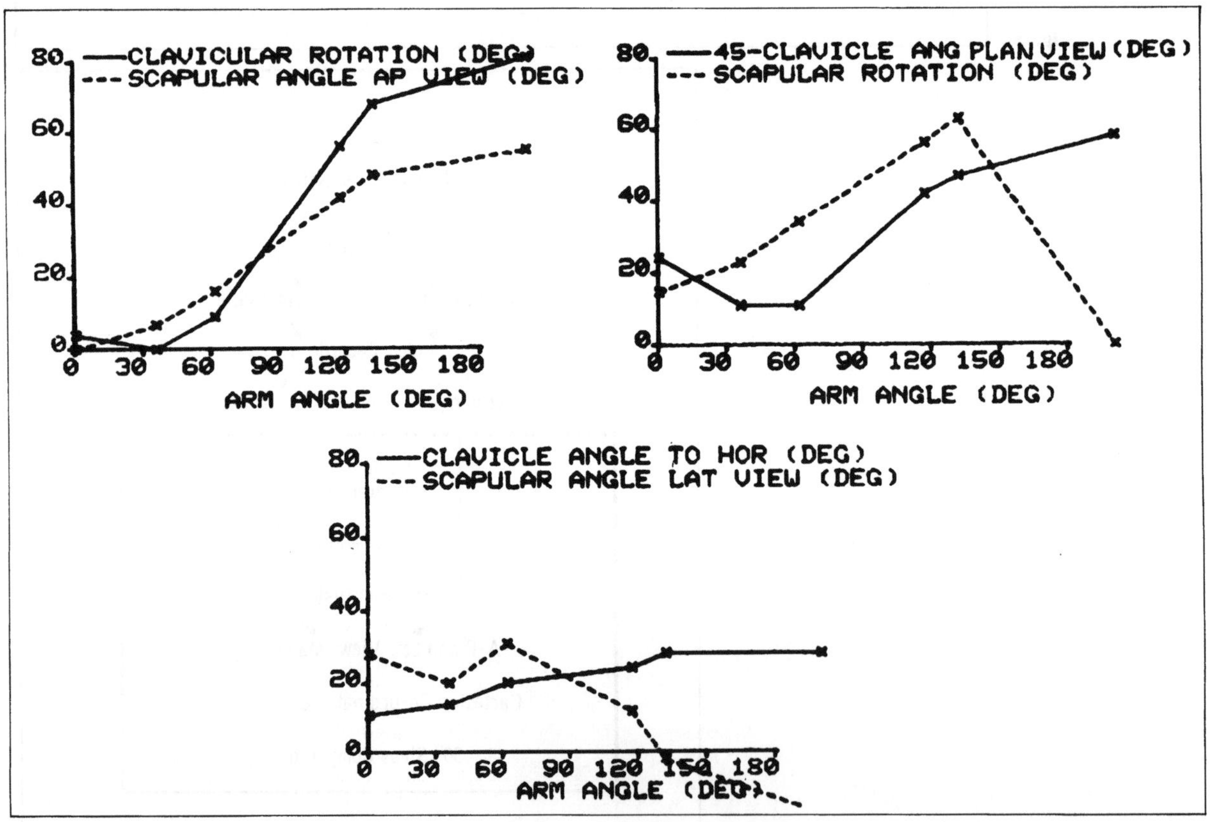

Fig. 7.

VI.2. Post-traumatic Osteolysis of the Distal Clavicle

Anthony Leyshon and Lipmann Kessel

The acromioclavicular joint is a more frequent site of shoulder pain than is commonly realised [31]. Certainly degenerative change in this joint is common after the third and fourth decade [6], the radiological and histological changes being similar to those seen in other synovial joints.

Less frequently, the acromioclavicular joint is the site of an unusual pathological process— distal clavicular osteolysis. The condition has been described in rheumatoid arthritis [3], hyperparathyroidism [23], and scleroderma [17], when it is usually bilateral, and unilaterally in disappearing bone disease [10]. Infrequently, osteolysis of the distal clavicle may occur following trauma [16,18,30].

The physical signs and radiological changes are subtle and easily overlooked. The condition differs from degenerative arthritis of the joint by the absence of subchondral sclerosis and osteophyte formation and the presence of a normal acromial articulation.

Material

Ten patients referred to the Shoulder Unit at the Royal National Orthopaedic Hospital, London form the basis for this study. There were 9 men and 1 woman, aged from 26 to 71 years (mean 43 years).

The dominant limb was involved in all cases. Five patients gave a definite history of trauma, usually involving a fall on to the point of the shoulder some 3 to 6 weeks prior to the onset of symptoms. Two other patients were "one-handed", due respectively to an Erb's palsy and to a persistent posterior dislocation of the shoulder on the other side, and had pain in their useful shoulder. One patient was a competitive freestyle swimmer practicing 6 hours a day with repeated rotatory movements of the shoulder. No patient showed any evidence of generalised arthropathy.

All patients complained of severe pain in the shoulder usually well localised to the epaulette region without radiation proximally or distally. Night pain occurred in 5 patients and a single patient noted restriction of shoulder movements.

Clinical Features

Clinical examination revealed a number of useful physical signs. Well-defined local joint tenderness was seen in 7 cases. A high painful arc of abduction (140°-180°) (Fig. 1) was observed in 7

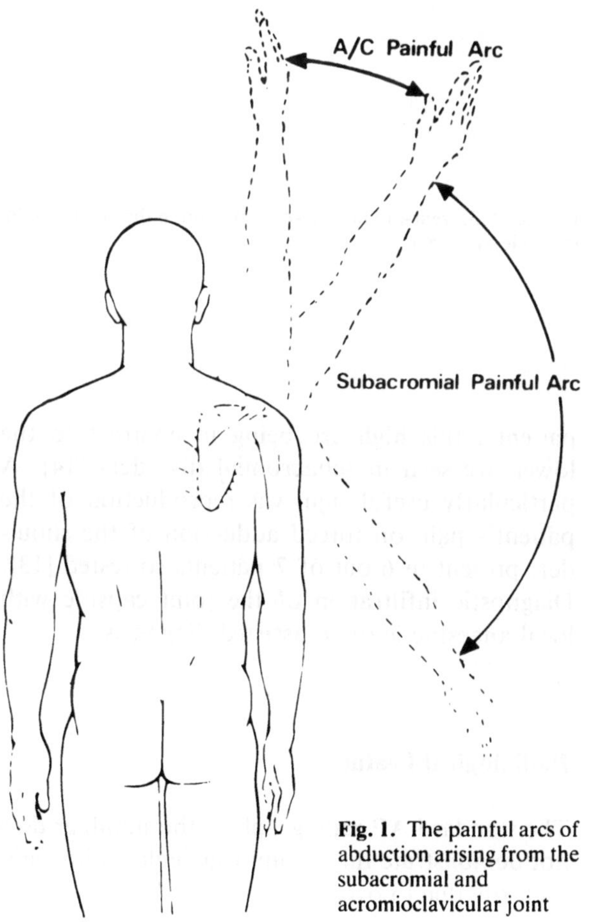

Fig. 1. The painful arcs of abduction arising from the subacromial and acromioclavicular joint

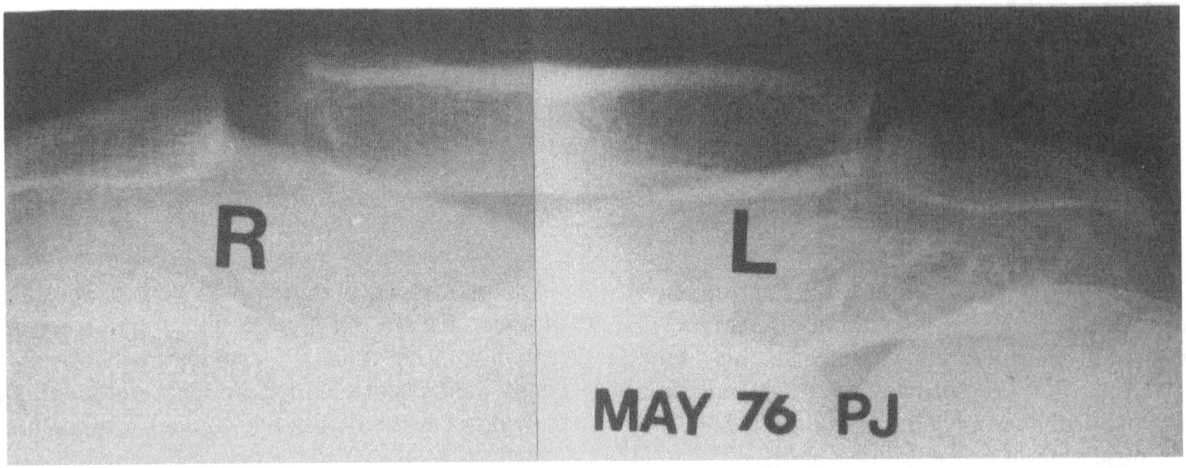

Fig. 2. **Radiographs of the acromioclavicular joints of a 27-year-old male, with pain in the right shoulder of 11 months duration, after a fall**

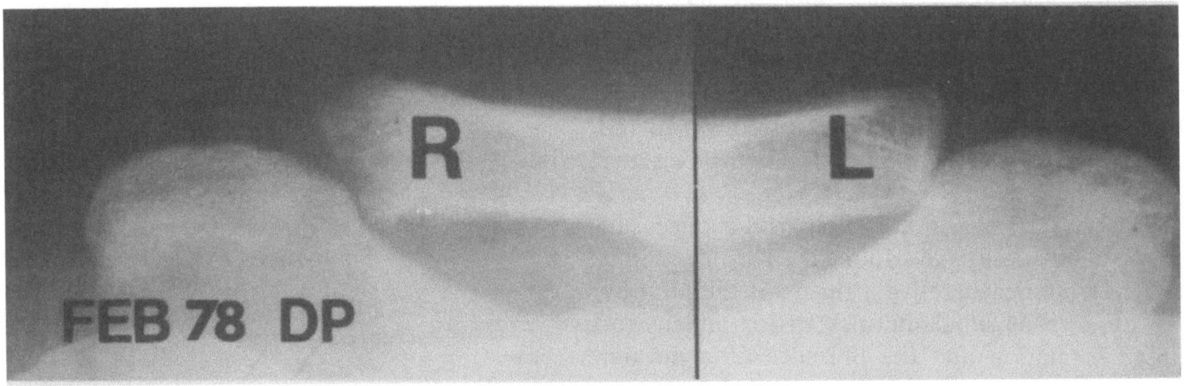

Fig. 3. **A 37-year-old taxi driver with pain in the right shoulder for 7 months. There was no history of injury but he was a keen freestyle swimmer**

patients, this high arc being in contrast to the lower arc seen in subacromial disorders [14]. A particularly useful sign was reproduction of the patient's pain on forced adduction of the shoulder, present in 6 out of 7 patients so tested [13]. Diagnostic infiltration of the joint capsule with local anaesthetic often assisted diagnosis.

Radiological Features

The standard AP radiograph of the shoulder does not demonstrate the acromioclavicular joint satisfactorily due to overlapping bony shadows. If the radiograph tube is tilted upwards some 20°-30° the joint is seen clearly and subtle changes are more readily noted [24]. Radiographs of both joints are compared.

In post-traumatic osteolysis the radiographic changes are confined to the clavicular surface of the joint and are always unilateral. The earliest change is widening of the joint space from its normal 2-3 mm (Fig. 2). Irregularity of the clavicular articulation follows, and there is loss of definition of the subchondral bone plate (Fig. 3). Progression may result in subchondral cyst formation (Fig. 4).

Abnormalities may not be present in the early stages of the condition. The earliest reported changes have been seen one month following injury [2].

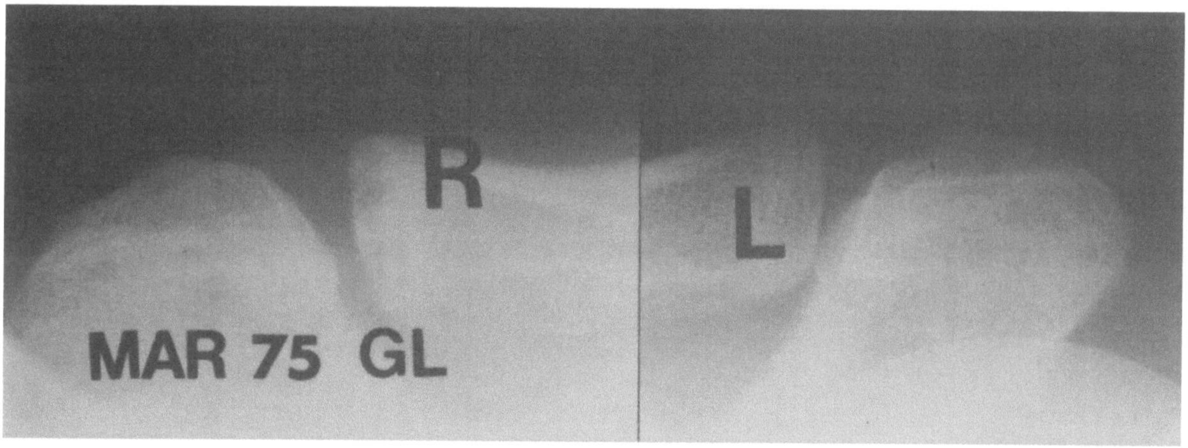

Fig. 4. Subchondral cysts in the right clavicle of a 45-year-old caretaker with a 5-month history of shoulder pain after lifting a sack of potatoes

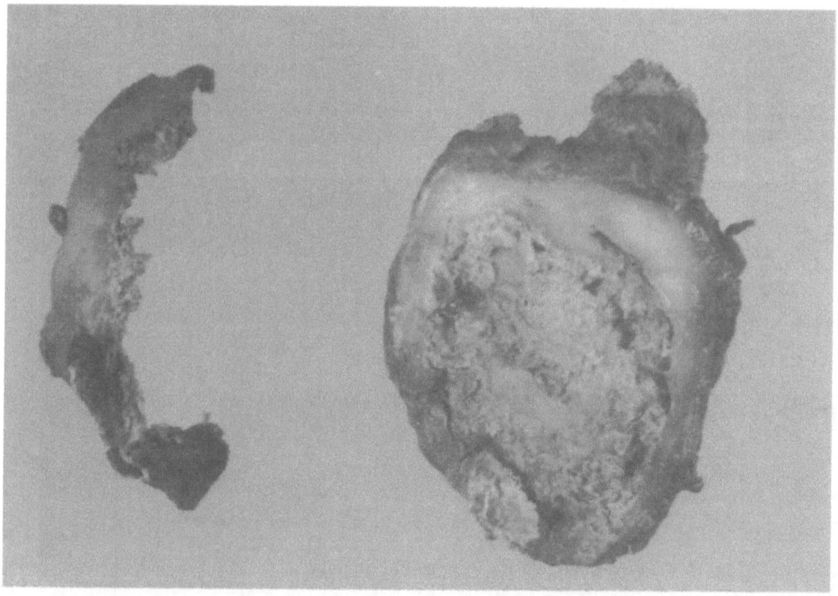

Fig. 5. The clavicular articulation of a 37-year-old engineer, excised for pain, present for 6 months following a fall on to the point of the shoulder. Note the grossly degenerate intra-articular disc

Treatment and Results

Conservative measures such as rest, physiotherapy and local injections of steroid have not been of value.

All patients responded well to excision of the outer centimetre of the clavicle. This is carried out easily with a reciprocating saw through a small coronal incision. Provided the line of section is lateral to the insertion of the coracoclavicular ligaments, no instability results. The cut surface of the clavicle is thoroughly covered with bone wax to discourage bleeding and new bone formation.

The operative findings have been constant. The intra-articular disc is very degenerate and frequently adherent to the acromial side of the joint. The acromial joint cartilage is normal. The articular surface of the clavicle exhibits pitting, roughening and areas of exposed eburnated bone (Figs. 5 and 6). Osteophytes are not seen.

All specimens of excised clavicle have been examined by slab radiographs and histology. These show that the pathological changes are no

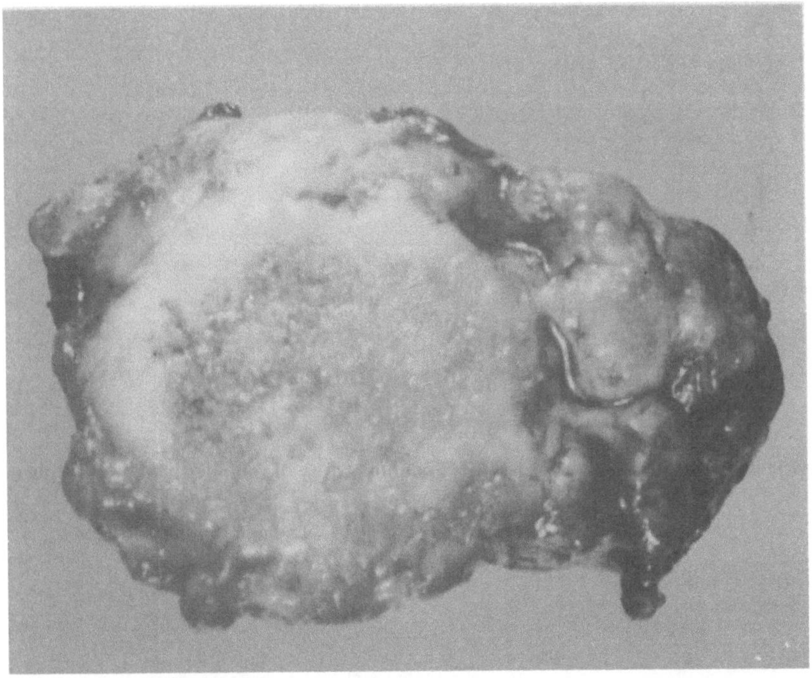

Fig. 6. The articular surface of the clavicle shows pitting and eburnation. It was excised from a 58-year-old driver with pain dating from a fall 10 months before

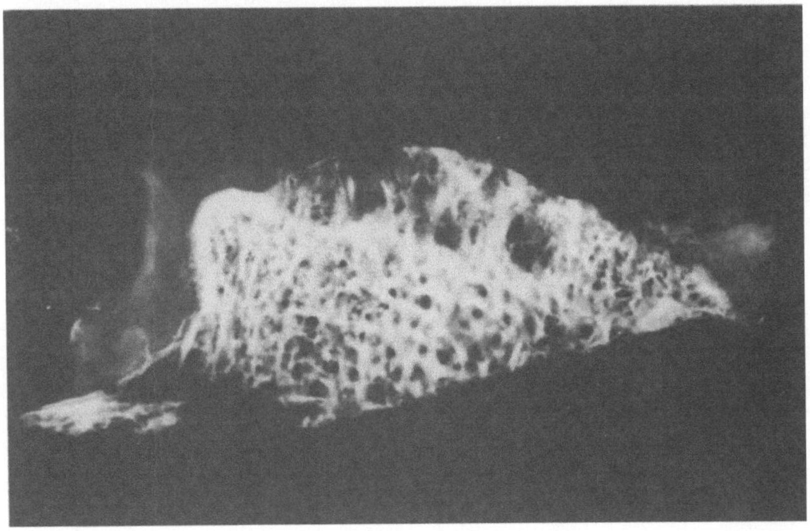

Fig. 7. A fine-detail slab radiograph of the specimen obtained from the case described in Fig. 5. The thinning of the subchondral bone plate and the cyst formation are well demonstrated

more and no less than those seen in degenerative arthritis. Cartilage fibrillation and thinning and loss of the subchondral bone plate together with subchondral cyst formation are demonstrable (Figs. 7 and 8).

Results of operation have been good. Follow-up from 3 months to 6 years (mean 11 months) shows all patients to have lost their preoperative pain and to have returned to their former employment. Those taking part in sport have been able to resume. In one patient new bone formation from the cut end of the clavicle required re-excision with complete relief. No case of clavicular instability has occurred, and there have been no other complications.

Discussion

The aetiology of this condition is unknown. Changes in the autonomic nervous system with secondary vascular changes have been postulated [16] particularly since associated homolateral

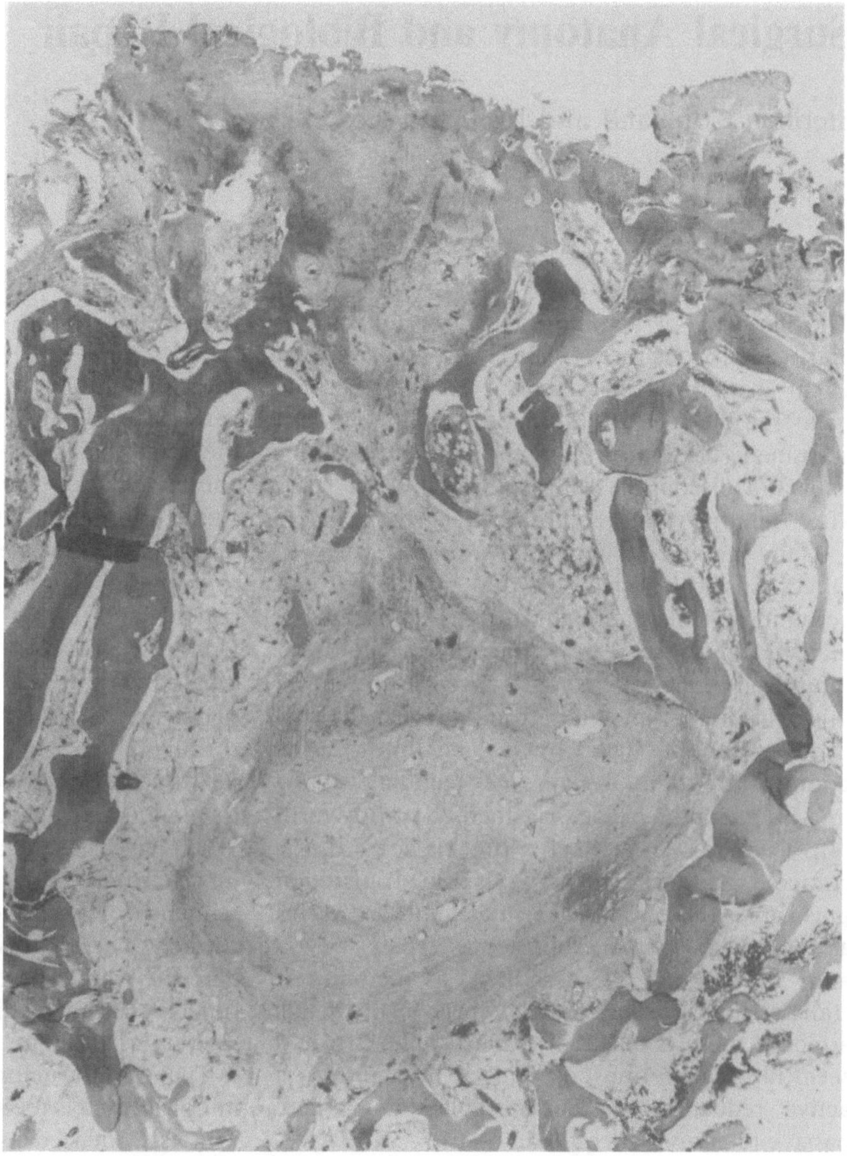

Fig. 8. Section through the outer end of the clavicle showing cartilage destruction, loss of the subchondral bone plate and early cyst formation

pupillary dilatation has been described in some cases [19]. We have not seen this phenomenon in any cases.

Disorder of "bone remodelling units" activated by trauma has been suggested as a cause [18].

We feel this condition to be a *form fruste* of degenerative arthritis resulting from direct trauma or occupational cause, possibly varied by the presence of an intra-articular disc. The disc may be important in absorbing pressure stress across the joint during the rotation of the clavicle that occurs during elevation of the arm [15]. If the disc is damaged, changes may occur in the articular cartilage similar to those seen in the knee following meniscal injury. Whatever the cause of this condition, it appears to be an identifiable condition which can, if recognised, be treated easily and effectively.

VI.3. Disruption of the Acromioclavicular Joint: Surgical Anatomy and Biological Repair

Stephen Copeland and Lipmann Kessel

The majority of acromioclavicular subluxations and dislocations are treated conservatively in Great Britain. Most Patients eventually become pain-free and regain full function but are left with a cosmetic deformity. A minority have persistent pain and discomfort for many months or years after the injury and require further treatment.

Many methods of repair have been advocated. Direct surgical repair of the capsule of the acromioclavicular joint and of the coracoclavicular ligaments may be successful in the fresh injury, but it has poor long-term results in the late injury as disruption and deformity recur. Internal fixation alone as stated by Watson-Jones [29] is doomed to failure because of pain and screw migration and breakage. The method of Bosworth [4], using a screw to fix the clavicle to the coracoid, and of Phemister [21], using transfixion pins across the acromioclavicular joint, are useful as temporary splintage but not as repair. Dewar and Barrington [7] described a method of transferring the tip of the coracoid with its attached muscles to stabilise the clavicle. It would seem illogical to transpose muscle to engineer an active reduction of the unstable joint where passive retention is required.

Anatomy and Function

The topography of the acromioclavicular joint varies considerably from subject to subject, but the relationship of the clavicular and acromial components of each joint is kept remarkably stable throughout its range of movement. The majority of movement taking place at the joint is rotation in the long axis of the clavicle. The conoid and trapezoid ligaments run obliquely from the coracoid to the clavicle in opposing directions and are analagous to the cruciate ligaments of the knee in providing stability throughout the range of movement of the joint.

Horn [11] described the traumatic anatomy of the completely dislocated acromioclavicular joint. We believe that the anatomical findings described in the complete lesions are the end-result of a sequence of events culminating in complete disruption. The progression of these events can elucidate the whole spectrum of injury from subluxation to complete dislocation depending on the severity of trauma.

The first structure to disrupt with relatively minor trauma is the superior joint capsule (Fig. 1). This is evidenced by very localised acute tender-

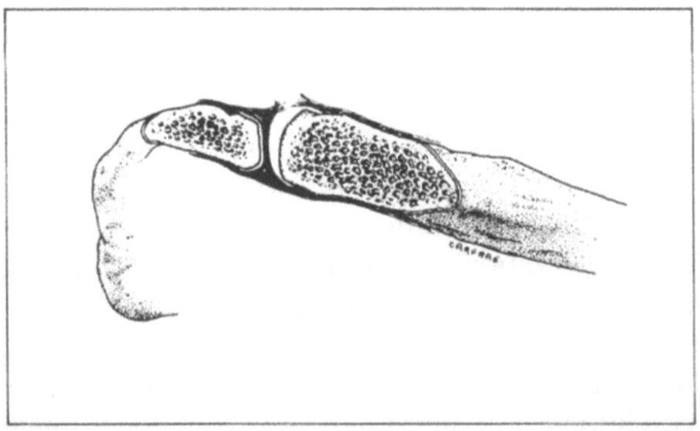

Fig. 1. Rupture of the superior capsule proximal to the intra-articular meniscus

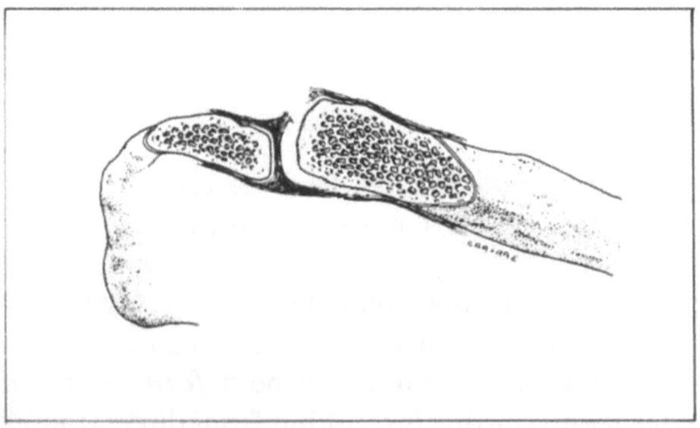

Fig. 2. Detachment of the inferior joint capsule and periosteum from the inferior surface of the clavicle

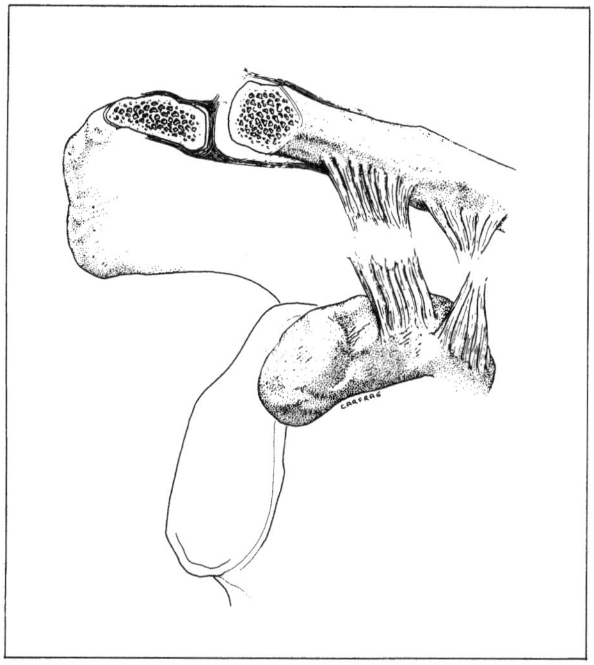

Fig. 3. Rupture of the conoid and trapezoid ligaments

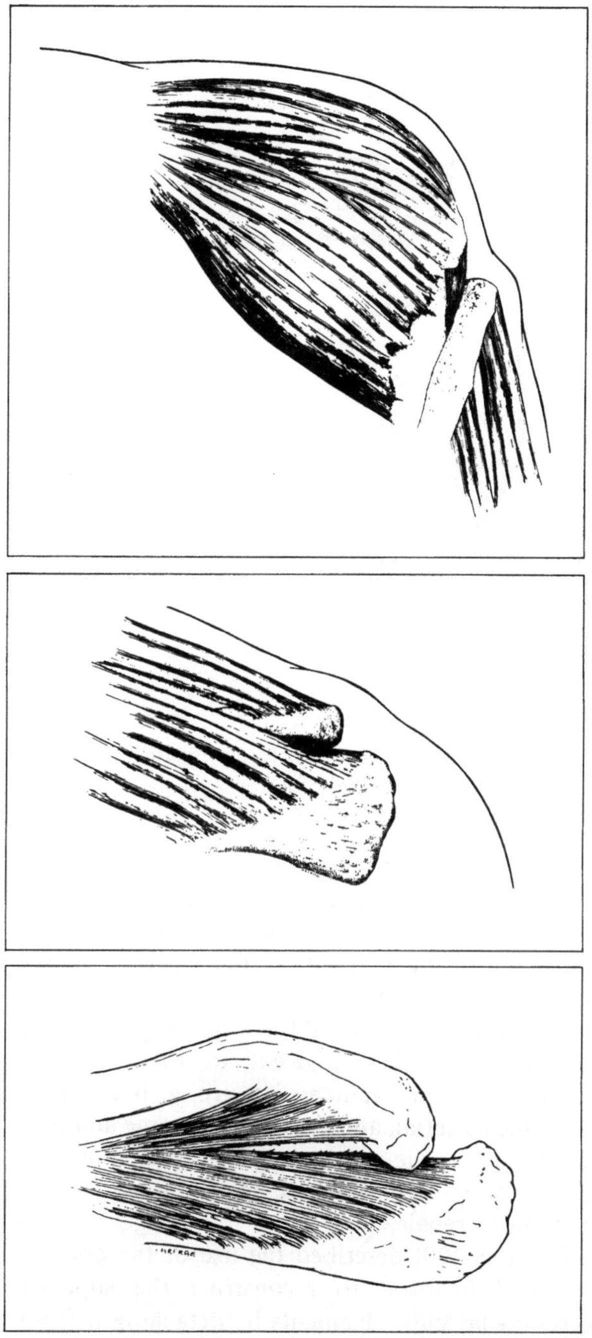

a b c

Fig. 4. a Anterior, **b** Posterior **c** Superior views of the avulsion of the deltoid muscle from the clavicle and horizontal tearing of trapezius

ness related to the superior aspect of the joint. The thickening of the joint capsule ruptures just proximal to the attachment of the intra-articular meniscus. Horn [11] also noted that in complete dislocation the meniscus always maintained its attachment to the acromion.

In a more severe lesion, resulting in subluxation, the periosteum is torn away from its attachment to the inferior surface of the clavicle (Fig. 2). The evidence for this lies in the frequent finding of sub-periosteal new bone formation on the radiograph. With increasing trauma the conoid and trapezoid ligaments, the clavipectoral fascia and its condensations are torn from a lateral to medial direction (Fig. 3). The severest trauma results in complete dislocation and avulsion of deltoid from the outer end of the clavicle, and a horizontal tear in trapezius between the fibres that are attached to the clavicle and those attached to the spine of the scapula (Fig. 4, a,b,c). The scapula is now allowed to fall forwards giving the appearance of posterior subluxation of the clavicle.

At operation in late cases, the end of the clavicle is lying beneath the skin and appears to be buttonholed through trapezius. The acromial fibres of trapezius prevent passive reduction of the dislocation by direct pressure downwards on the clavicle, and these fibres must be divided to allow the joint to be fully reduced.

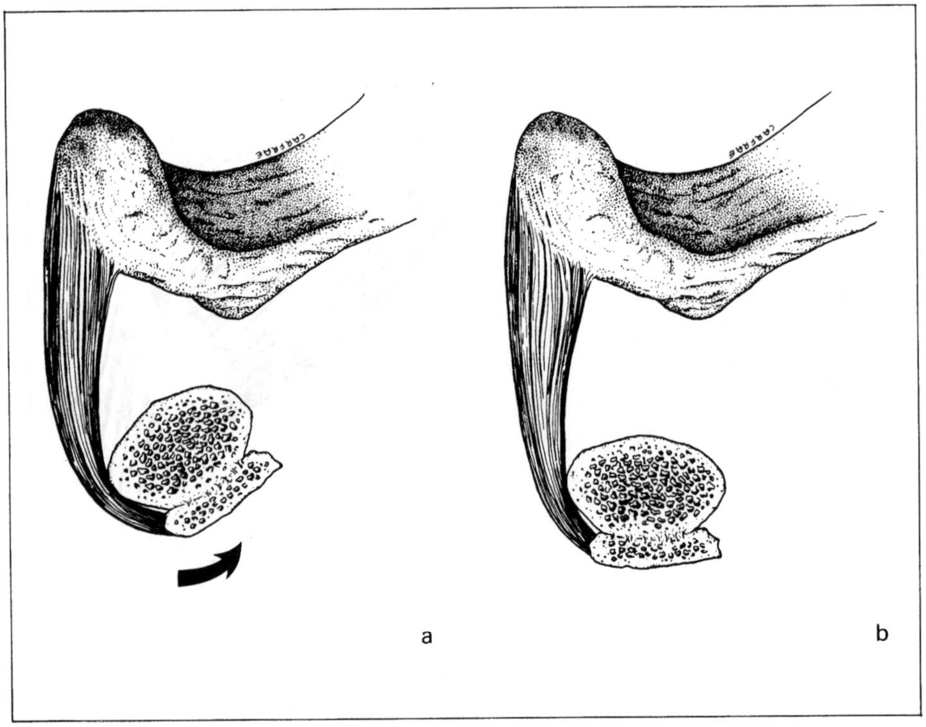

Fig. 5. **a** Lateral view. **b** The clavicle rotates during abduction of the arm tightening the transferred ligament and increasing stability of the acromioclavicular joint

The coracoacromial ligament, passing obliquely between two points on the same bone, the scapula, does not cross the line of separation of the clavicle and scapula and is therefore not stressed. It has always been found to be intact. The coraco-acromial ligament is ideal for stabilising a reduced dislocation. It lies adjacent to the disrupted coracoclavicular ligaments, is strong, is made of the same material, and is part of the same anatomical layer. A true anatomical analogue, replacing ligament by ligament, seems the most logical method of repair.

Neviaser [20] described the use of the coraco-acromial ligament to reconstruct the superior acromioclavicular ligaments by detaching it from the coracoid. Burton [5] has used the ligament detaching it from the acromion and re-attaching it to the undersurface of the clavicle or resecting the outer lip of the clavicle and attaching the coraco-acromial ligament into the divided outer end. The clavicle rotates in a sagittal plane during abduction of the arm, and stability of the joint should be maintained throughout this movement.

We have been using the coracoacromial ligament for repair by detaching it with a sliver of bone from the undersurface of the acromion and re-attaching this to the superior surface of the clavicle. The flake of bone is maintained in position by the use of a temporary Bosworth screw which transfixes the flake and passes through the clavicle and into the coracoid to hold the reduction until the bony fragment has united with the clavicle. The transferred coracoacromial ligament now lies attached to the superior surface of the clavicle and passes over its anterior aspect. As the clavicle rotates, the new ligament becomes tighter and the joint increasingly stable when the arm is abducted (Fig. 5, a,b).

Surgical Technique

The patient lies supine with a sandbag behind the shoulder and head turned to the opposite side. The incision used is shown in Fig. 6. We have found this vertical incision provides the best access to the acromioclavicular joint, acromion, and the clavicle over the coracoid process. Deltoid is split in the line of its fibres and detached from the outer end of the clavicle and acromion. The coraco-acromial ligament is exposed and detached with a large sliver of bone from the full width of the undersurface of the acromion to which it is attached (Fig. 7). The acromioclavicular joint is exposed and the intra-articular meniscus removed – this is usually found to be degenerate. The clavicle is now brought forward and downwards to its normal anatomical position; division of some fibres of trapezius may be necessary to achieve this. The coracoid process is palpated in the wound, and the clavicle drilled vertically, immediately superior to this. The bone immediately adjacent to the hole is scarified. The joint is held reduced by an assistant, and the coracoacromial ligament swung across so that the attached segment of bone lies on the superior surface of the clavicle. With the ligament held taut, a Bosworth screw is passed through the flake of bone, through the clavicle and into the coracoid. The acromioclavicular joint is now stabilised (Fig. 8). The wound is closed, paying great attention to the reattachment of the fibres of deltoid to the acromion and clavicle.

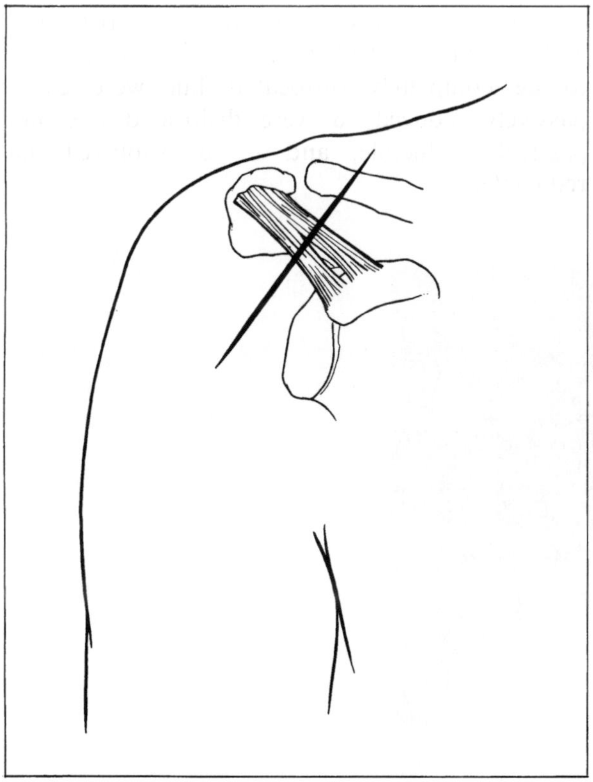

Fig. 6. The incision

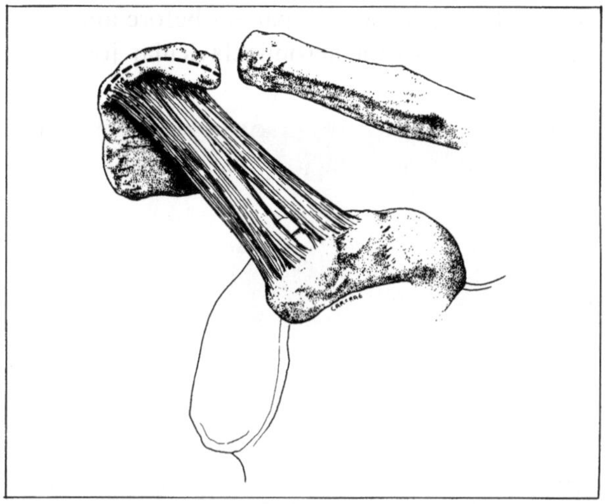

Fig. 7. The coracoacromial ligament is detached with a large sliver of bone from the undersurface of the acromion

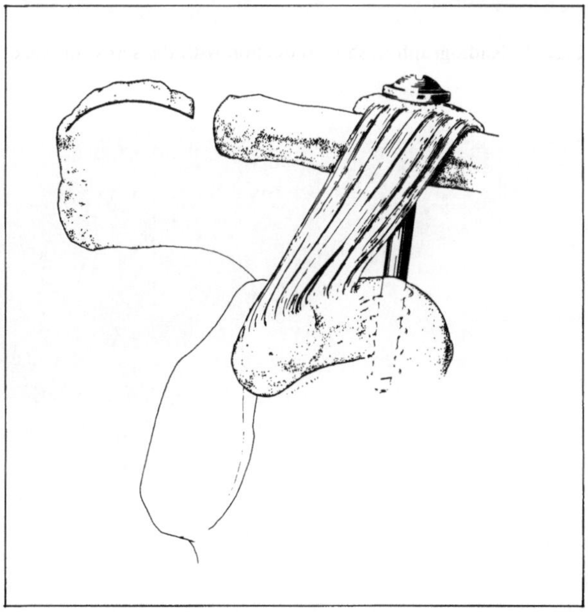

Fig. 8. A Bosworth screw is passed through the flake of bone, the clavicle and into the coracoid for temporary internal splintage

Postoperative Management

The patient is allowed to move his shoulder gently in a sling for three weeks and is then left free with instructions not to abduct the arm beyond 90°. The Bosworth screw is removed about eight weeks after operation. At this time a lucent zone will be seen on the radiograph around the shank of the screw in the clavicle; this is caused by coronal rotation of the clavicle in its own axis. After removal of the screw, full movement is quickly regained and the joint is stable (Figs. 9 and 10). Figures 11 and 12 show a patient before and after reconstruction of the acromioclavicular joint.

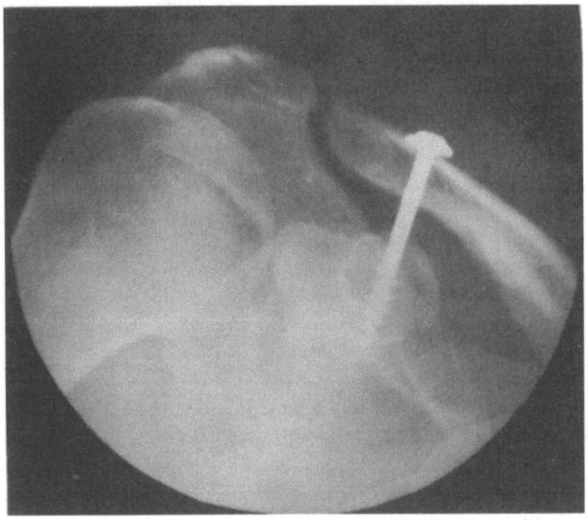

Fig. 9. Radiograph to show reduction with the screw in place

Results

1. Clinical Material

The technique described above has been used in 16 patients (14 males and 2 females) whose average age was 37 years (range 26-60). The average duration of symptoms at the time of operation was 13 months (range 6-34 months). The average length of follow up was 10 months (range 6-20 months).

2. Symptoms and Signs

The main indication for operation was pain, and this was usually related to heavy work; rest pain was not a feature. Eight of the male patients could not work because of pain; 6 young men complained that they could no longer play their favourite games, e.g. squash and tennis; 1 female patient complained of the unattractive appearance and an inabilty to do gardening because of pain. All complained that the shoulder "did not feel right", that "something felt out of place", and that the arm was weak. One patient was a psychiatrist who could not do his work adequately because the perception of his body image was not satisfactory with a joint out of place! Nine joints were found to be completely dislocated but were easily passively reduced, 6 were dislocated and not passively reducible, and 1 was subluxed but reducible.

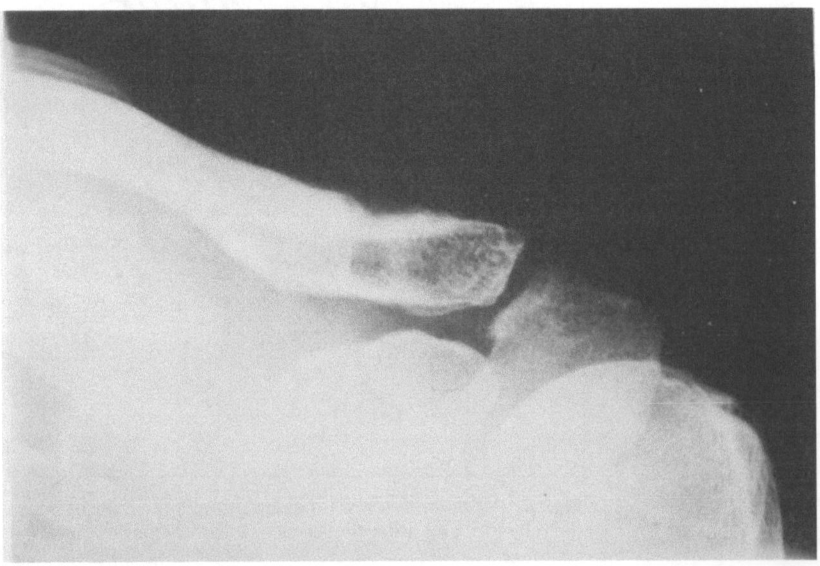

Fig. 10. Stability is maintained after removal of the screw

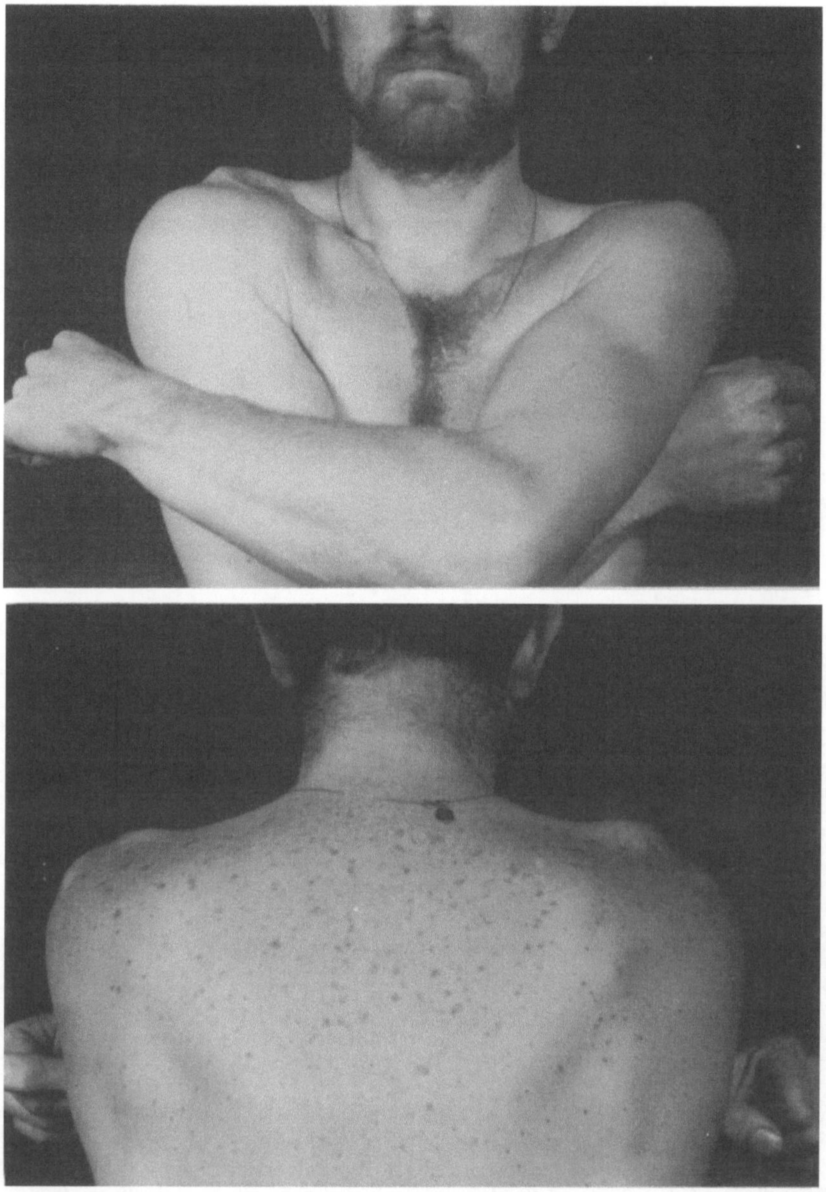

a

b

Fig. 11 a, b. Patient before acromioclavicular joint reconstruction

3. Assessment

Of the 16 patients 14 were satisfied with the result of operation. One patient was dissatisfied because his pain was not relieved, but his arm did feel stronger. This patient had a long-standing subluxation and had severe bony changes in the tip of the clavicle, and in retrospect it would have been wise to excise the tip of the clavicle. This has now been arranged. The other dissatisfied patient still had some discomfort, but this was less than before operation. Six patients who could not work because of the lesion returned to work after operation, and a seventh was unemployed but capable of working. On examination, all the joints were stable and the skyline view of the AC joint was comparable to the opposite side in 13 patients, a prominence of the outer end of the clavicle was seen in 3 patients. The cosmetic appearance of the scar was not ideal: any operation in this area is prone to keloid formation and spreading. In two patients, the deltoid had become detached from its origin on the clavicle and left a depression under the scar, but functionally they were pleased.

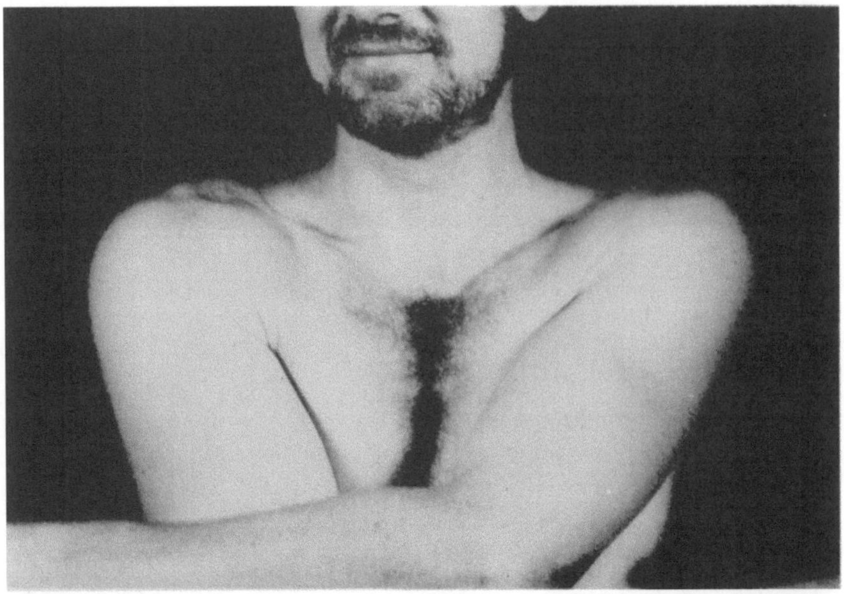

a

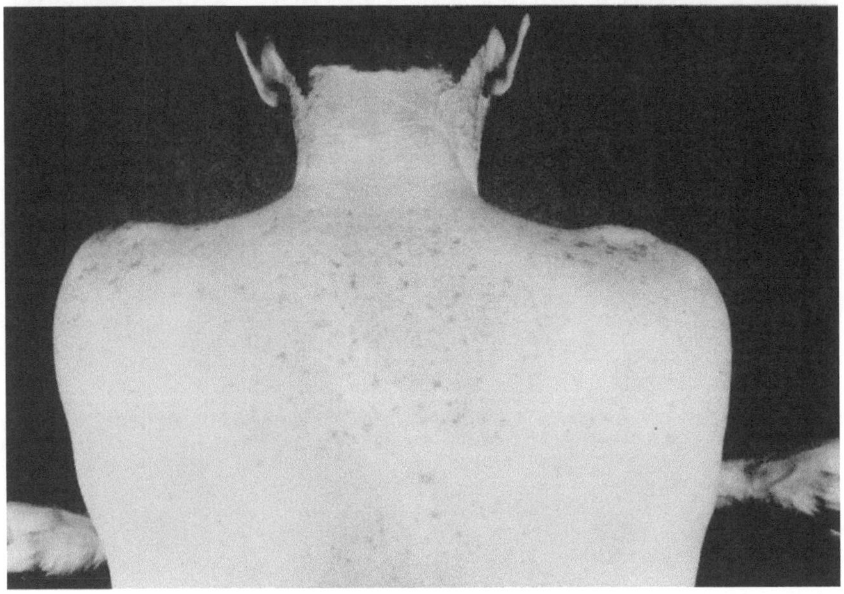

b

Figs. 12 a, b. Patient after removal of the screw

Discussion

No long-term disability results from the loss of the coracoacromial ligament from its normal site. This ligament has been divided as a therapeutic manoeuvre in anterior rotator cuff impingement syndromes without adverse effect. The technique of repair described has been found to be satisfactory for the minority of patients that require treatment for this sometimes disabling lesion.

References

1 Adams JC (1971) Outline of orthopaedics. Churchill Livingstone, Edinburgh London, p 226

2 Alnor P (1951) Die posttraumatische Osteolyse des lateralen Claviculaendes. Fortshritte auf dem Gebiete den Rontgenstrahlen 75: 364-365

3 Alper M, Meyers M (1961) Osteolysis of the acromial end of the clavicles in rheumatoid arthritis. American Journal of Roentgenology, Radium Therapy and Nuclear Medicine 86-2: 251-259

4 Bosworth BM (1941) Acromioclavicular separation; a new method of repair. Gynaecol Obstet. 73: 866

5 Burton ME (1975) Operative treatment of acromioclavicular dislocations. Bull Hosp Joint Dis 36: 109

6 DePalma AJ (1957) Degenerative changes in the sternoclavicular and acromioclavicular joints in various decades. Springfield, Thomas

7 Dewar FP, Barrington TW (1965) The treatment of chronic acromioclavicular dislocation, J Bone Jt Surg 47-B: 32

8 Dvir Z, Berme N (1978) The shoulder complex in elevation of the arm: a mechanistic approach. J Biomechanics 11: 219-226

9 Freedman L, Munro RR (1966) Abduction of the arm in the scapular plane: scapular and gleno-humeral movements. J Bone Jt Surg 48-A: 1503-1510

10 Gorham LW, Stout AP (1955) Massive osteolysis (acute spontaneous absorption of bone, phantom bone, disappearing bone) its relation to hemangiomatosis. J Bone Jt Surg 37-A: 985-1004

11 Horn JS (1954) The traumatic anatomy and treatment of acute acromioclavicular dislocation. J Bone Jt Surg 36-B: 194

12 Kennedy JC, Cameron H (1954) Complete dislocation of the acromioclavicular joint. J Bone Jt Surg 36-B: 202-208

13 Kessel L (1967) In Clinical surgery—orthopaedics, Edited by GC Lloyd-Roberts. Butterworths: London

14 Kessel L, Watson M (1977) The painful arc syndrome. J Bone Jt Surg 59-B: 166-172

15 MacConaill MA (1944) The mechanical anatomy of the acromioclavicular joint of man. Proceedings of the Royal Irish Academy, vol L. Section B, No 7: 159-166

16 Madsen B (1963) Osteolysis of the acromial end of the clavicle following trauma. British Journal of Radiology 36: 822-828

17 Mezaros WT (1958) The regional manifestations of scleroderma. Radiology, 70-3: 313-315

18 Murphy OB, Bellamy R, Wheeler W, Brower TD (1975) Post-traumatic osteolysis of the distal clavicle. Clinical Orthopaedics and Related Research, 109: 108-114

19 Nell W (1953) Die Posttraumatische Osteolyse des Schlusselbeins und ihr Verlauf. Hefte zur Unfallheilunde 44: 151-154

20 Neviaser JS (1952) Acromioclavicular dislocation treated by transference of the coraco-acromial ligament. Arch Surg 64: 292

21 Phemister DB (1942) The treatment of dislocation of the acromioclavicular joint by open reduction and threaded wire fixation. J Bone Jt Surg 24: 166

22 Poirier P, Charpy A (1926) Traité d'Anatomié Humaine. 4th Edition. Masson Ed Paris, pp 126-132

23 Steinbach HL, Gordan GS, Eisenburger E, Crane JT, Silverman S, Goldman L (1961) Primary hyperparathyroidism: A correlation of roentgen, clinical and pathologic features. Amer Journal of Roentgenology, Radium Therapy and Nuclear Medicine 86-2: 329-343

24 Stripp WJ (1979) Special techniques in orthopaedic radiography. Edinburgh, Churchill Livingstone

25 Wallace WA (1980) Shoulder movement studies using the image intensifier, video-recordings, computer analysis and clinical examination. Internal publication, Harlow Wood Orthopaedic Hospital

26 Wallace WA, Johnson F (1) (1980) Dynamic radiography in shoulder kinematics: problems and their solutions. J Bone Jt Surg 62-B: 256

27 Wallace WA, Johnson F (2) (1980) Detection and correction of geometrical distortion in X-ray fluoroscopic images. J Biomechanics—accepted for publication June 1980

28 Watson M (1978) The refractory painful arc syndrome. J Bone Jt Surg 60-B: 544-546

29 Watson-Jones R (1943) Fractures and joint injuries, 3rd ed. Edinburgh, Churchill Livingstone, Vol 2, p 433

30 Werder H (1950) Post-traumatische osteolyse des Schlusselbeinendes. Schweiz Medizinische Wochenschrift, 34: 912-913

31 Zanca P (1971) Shoulder pain: involvement of the acromioclavicular joint. Amer Journal of Roentgenology, Radium Therapy and Nuclear Medicine, 112-3: 493-506

Section VII. Some Fractures of the Proximal Humerus

Moderator—Bo J. Lundberg

VII.1. The Subdeltoid Approach to the Proximal Humerus

Michel Martini

The proximal end of the humerus is well hidden deep to the deltoid muscle and is one of the more difficult regions to expose surgically [11]. The operations commonly used for exposing the shoulder and humerus give a relatively poor view of the proximal shaft of the humerus. To eliminate the obstacle of the deltoid and to gain a good exposure of the whole of the proximal metaphysis of the humerus, we chose to reflect the whole muscle mass upwards after dividing the deltoid tendon at its insertion.

Our early experience with this approach has been previously reported [12,13].

Operative Technique

The patient lies on the operating table in the lateral decubitus position. The incision consists of anterior and posterior arms which meet each other opposite the junction of the middle and upper thirds of the humerus (Figs. 1 and 2). Deltoid and pectoralis major are defined in front. The tendon of insertion of deltoid is elevated and the muscle bulge is separated from long and lateral heads of triceps behind (Fig. 3). When both incisions have been completed, a rubber band is passed beneath the tendon which is then divided (Fig. 4). Deltoid can then be reflected upwards with ease separating it from the deeper structures in a practically bloodless plane. The upper end of the humerus is now widely exposed. The circumflex nerve is usually seen as a large single nerve but may have already divided into two major branches (Fig. 5).

The purpose of the approach has thus been fulfilled: the upper end of the humerus is exposed and the axillary nerve has been preserved. The proposed operative procedure can now be carried out. Closure is affected by reattaching the deltoid to its insertion with a few non-absorbable sutures. Lipmann Kessel has suggested a modification of the approach by elevating a small bone block with the insertion of deltoid, in order to make its reattachment more secure. The average blood loss during operation is in the order of 200 ml. Postoperatively the shoulder is immobilised for at least three weeks, when rehabilitation is commenced.

The advantages of this approach are clear:

It gives wide exposure to the upper quarter of the humerus.

No muscle is divided.

The circumflex nerve is seen and preserved.

The only disadvantage is the size and appearance of the operation scar (Fig. 6).

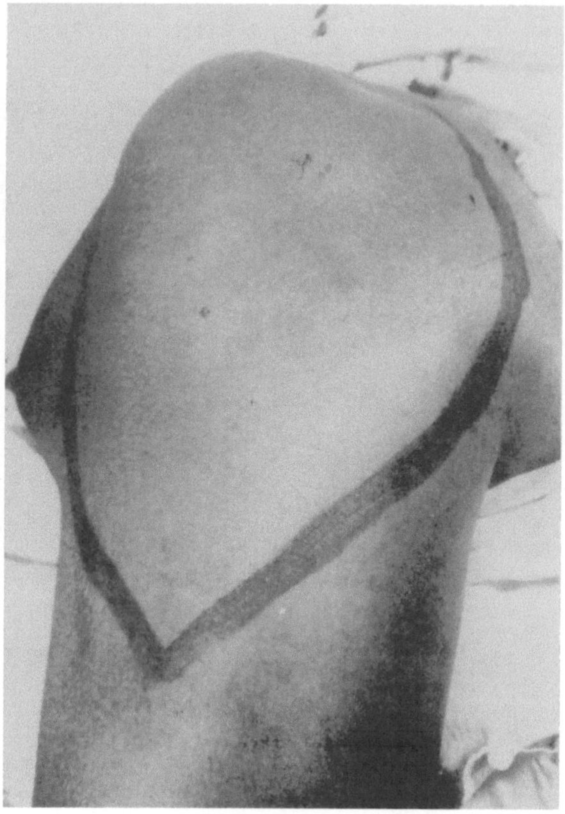

Fig. 1. The incision follows the border of deltoid

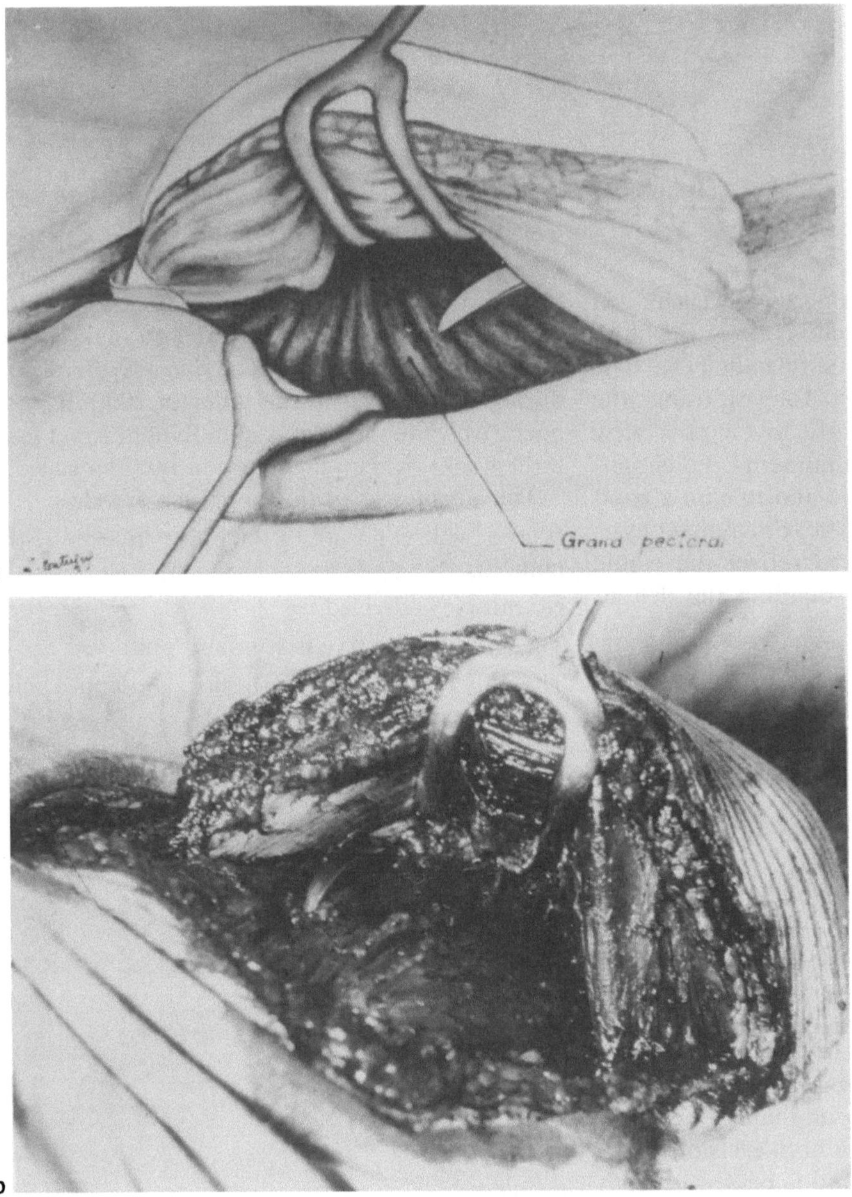

a

b

Fig. 2 a,b Diagram and photograph. The anterior incision is developed in the interval between deltoid and pectoralis major. The scissors have been passed under the tendon of the insertion of deltoid from behind forwards

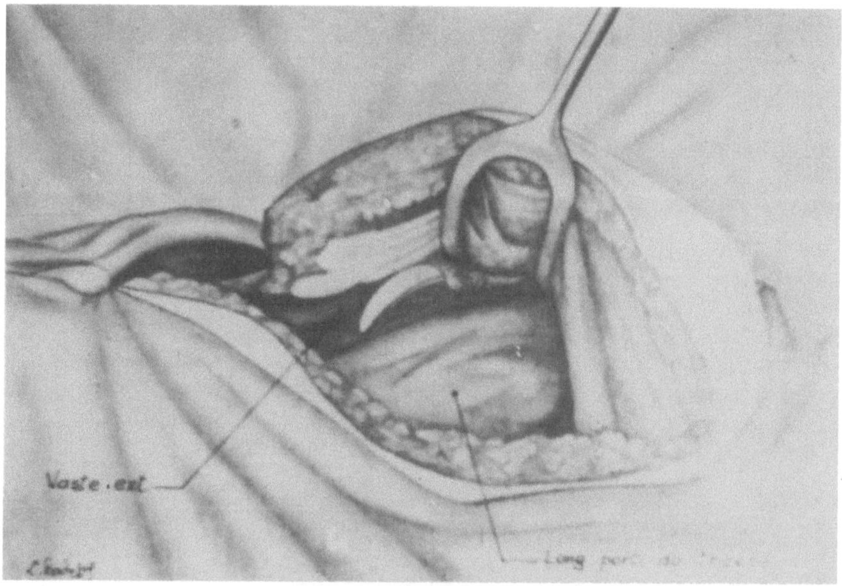

a

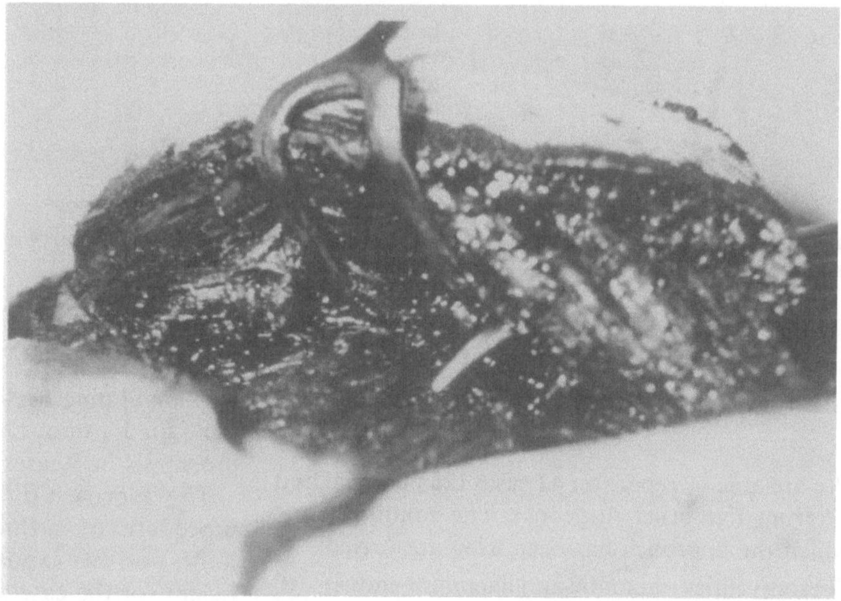

b

Fig 3 a, b Diagram and photograph. The posterior incision is developed in the interval between deltoid and triceps

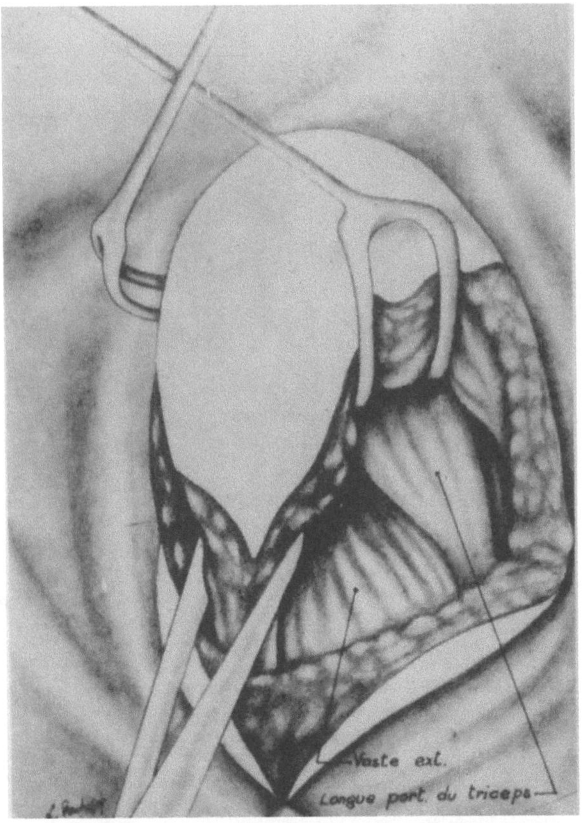

Fig. 4. **When both incisions have been completed**, a rubber band is passed beneath the tendon, which is then divided

Clinical Experience

We are able to report on 42 cases (25 personal and 17 from five other surgeons). The conditions for which the approach has been used are varied:

Osteomyelitis (traumatic and haematogenous)	10
Tumours	8
Arthrodesis of the shoulder	2
Neglected posterior dislocation of the shoulder	1
Non-union of the surgical neck of the humerus	1
Recent fractures of the surgical neck of the humerus, including six fracture dislocations	20
	42

The approach seemed to be excellent in 10 cases of osteomyelitis. It provided a good exposure and allowed a wide sequestrectomy. One complication was noted and that was division of the posterior humeral circumflex artery which had to be ligated. Similarly in the 8 patients with tumours of the proximal humerus, it provided wide exposure and facilitated tumour resection and insertion of a prosthesis in 5 cases.

The approach did not in any way simplify the procedure of arthrodesis of the glenohumeral joint, nor was exposure of the humeral head sufficient for the case of neglected posterior dislocation. Lastly it was judged excellent for fractures of the surgical neck of the humerus. The wide exposure made the reduction and internal fixation of the fragments considerably easier. This was especially true in 6 patients who had fracture-dislocations. In all the operations described, except of course for the two arthrodeses, the functional recovery of the deltoid was good, muscle power being estimated at 4 or 5.

Shoulder function has been assessed in two groups:

a) In the group with non-traumatic conditions of the proximal humerus, 3 patients had normal function of the glenohumeral joint preoperatively

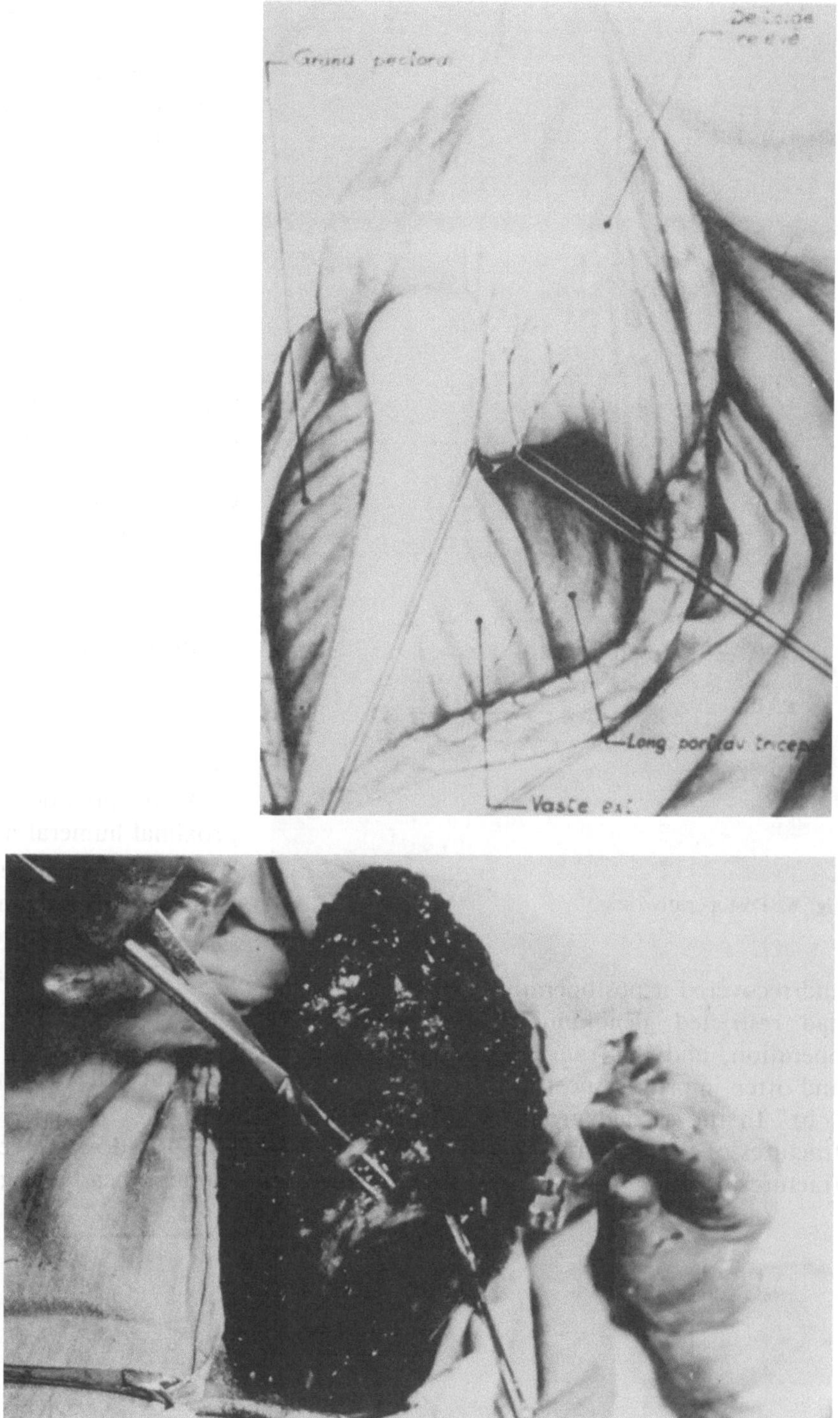

Fig. 5 a, b. In the diagram, the circumflex nerve has already branched into two and threads have been passed around in order to show them more clearly. In the operation photograph the circumflex nerve is seen as a large single trunk

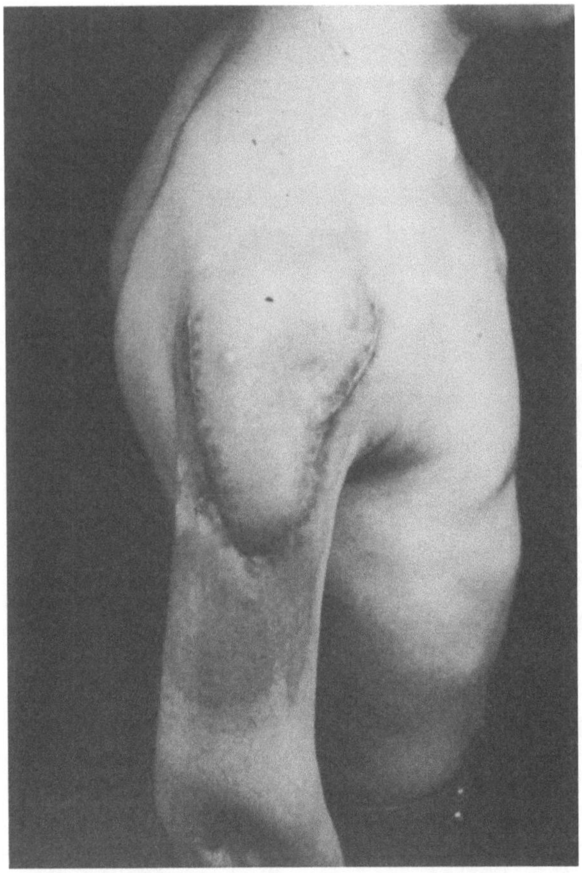

Fig. 6. Postoperative scar

and recovered it postoperatively. Sixteen patients had restricted glenohumeral movement before operation, and this range was always regained, and often improved, postoperatively.

b) In the second group of 20 patients with fractures of the proximal humerus, there were 14 fractures of the surgical neck and 6 fracture-dislocations. The recovery of movement was not as good in this group.

All the patients had a full range of shoulder movement before their fractures occurred, except one who presented with a pathological fracture. However, only 5 patients recovered full active abduction at the shoulder. The reasons for post-operative joint stiffness in the group must be related to their age, the severity of the injury and the duration of immobilisation. In fact, only very displaced and comminuted fractures and fracture-dislocations qualified for the subdeltoid approach. In these severe injuries mediocre results are acceptable, but great caution should be exercised when contemplating this approach in the elderly. Our best results were obtained in the younger patients.

Conclusions

A subdeltoid approach to the upper humerus is desirable:

1) It provides an excellent view of the proximal humeral metaphysis.

2) Its use can be strongly recommended for patients with osteomyelitis, tumours and probably non-union of the proximal humerus.

3) There is a place for it in fractures of the surgical neck and fracture-dislocation.

4) Caution should be exercised when contemplating its application to fractures in the elderly.

5) It does not provide wide exposure of the humeral head and glenoid.

VII.2. Displaced Proximal Humeral Fractures — Results of Non-Prosthetic Treatment

Henrik Svend-Hansen

It has often been claimed that fractures of the neck of the humerus are best treated conservatively and that early mobilisation is essential [9,14]. The aim of this paper is to see whether this applies to displaced proximal humeral fractures.

Material and Method

Patients admitted to the Copenhagen County Hospital with displaced proximal fractures of the humerus were studied over a 5-year period from 1966 to 1971. Only patients older than 20 years of age were included, and the average follow-up time was 4 years. Patients with dislocation of the head fragment were excluded from the study. Of the 55 patients who remained 49 were available for review.

Table 1. Age and sex distribution

Sex	No. of patients	Percentage	Average age
Male	14	29	64
Female	35	71	69

Youngest patient: 29 years; oldest patient: 94 years.

Table 2. Anatomical classification

No. of fragments	No. of patients	Displacement	
2	12	Slight	3
		Moderate	8
		Severe	1
3	22	Slight	1
		Moderate	13
		Severe	8
4	15	Slight	0
		Moderate	4
		Severe	11

Results

Table 1 shows the age and sex distribution of the patients. Table 2 shows the anatomical types of injury, classified according to Neer [16].

- 2 fragments: Fracture of the neck of the humerus
- 3 fragments: Fracture of the neck of the humerus and avulsion of the greater tuberosity
- 4 fragments: Fracture of the neck of the humerus, the greater tuberosity, and the lesser tuberosity.

The results were evaluated in accordance with the criteria proposed by Neer [15]. Maximum score is 100 units, divided as follows:

Pain	35 units
Function	30 units
Motion	25 units
Anatomy	10 units

Table 3. Overall results

Neer classification	No. of patients	Percentage	Percentage
Excellent	12	25	39
Satisfactory	7	14	
Unsatisfactory	7	14	61
Failure	23	47	

Excellent: >89 units
Satisfactory: 80–89 units
Unsatisfactory: 70–79 units
Failure <70 units
Maximum score: 100 units.

Table 4. Average score according to fragmentation

No. of fragments	Average score	Lowest score	Highest score
2	75.5	43	94
3	73.1	36	97
4	63.6	30	98

Table 5. Treatment and result of treatment

Treatment	No. of patients	Average score	Lowest score	Highest score
Sling	12	72	39	95
Hanging cast	21	68	41	92
Reduction	6	89	66	97
Osteosynthesis (Rush)	3	71	50	98
Extirpation of the head	5	47	30	61
Plaster cast	2	75	74	76

Table 3 shows the overall results: 61% were classified as "unsatisfactory" or "failure" so that nearly half the results were failures. The average score as related to fragmentation is shown in Table 4. As expected the score is lower in the more comminuted fractures, but a considerable variation is noted between the highest and lowest scores in all groups.

The results of various forms of treatment are shown in Table 5. As we are dealing with a variety of types of fracture, the numbers are too small to allow for definite conclusions. However, as shown in Table 6, the removal of the humeral head in five cases was disastrous. All were classified as failures with very low scores, the patients complaining of pain, loss of range of motion, and loss of stability. Necrosis of the head fragment was present in four patients, all failures, but no case of pseudarthrosis was observed.

Table 6. Results of the five patients treated by extirpation of the head of the humerus

Age	Sex	No. of fragments	Displacement	Score
66	female	3	moderate	36
74	female	3	severe	61
71	female	3	severe	50
50	female	4	severe	30
67	female	4	severe	60

Discussion

Contrary to the findings of other authors (Moribor and Patterson [14]) the results were not encouraging. The average score was 71, almost half were failures, and only 25% were "excellent". Two- and three-fragment fractures were generally better than four-fragment fractures. The removal of the head fragment invariably resulted in failure. Apart from these patients only three underwent surgery, the remaining 41 patients being treated by closed methods. Einarsson [9] states that 80% of three- and four-fragment fractures treated conservatively obtain a good result. This is in sharp contrast to our findings. Neer [16] treated a consecutive series of 117 patients with three- or four-fragment fractures and compared the results of closed reduction, open reduction and fixation, and prosthetic replacement. In both categories of patients open reduction gave better results, whereas in four-fragment fractures prosthetic replacement seemed preferable. The results of operative treatment are a good deal better than in our series treated conservatively, and we believe that at least half of our patients would have done better by open reduction and stable internal fixation, or prosthetic replacement especially in four fragment fractures and fracture-dislocations.

VII.3. Prosthetic Replacement in the Treatment of Serious Fractures of the Proximal Humerus

Carlos E. de Anquin and Carlos Alberto de Anquin

The great majority of fractures of the proximal humerus can be successfully treated conservatively; some require surgical reduction and internal fixation; prosthetic replacement is rarely indicated and should be employed in a very few cases with definite indications, when the blood supply of the head has been compromised or articular congruity has been lost.

Since 1950 [3,4] we have employed a classification based on the division of the proximal humerus into three zones, each with very different biomechanical features. Only a few fractures of the head, chiefly the complicated fractures in Group 4, have required prosthetic replacement because of the risk of avascular necrosis or the impossibility of satisfactory replacement of the articular surface. Prosthetic replacement may be indicated for post-traumatic arthritis, avascular necrosis, non-union, or a flail shoulder following excision of the humeral head.

In 1965 [5] we presented to the 6th Latin American Congress of Orthopaedics and Traumatology in Lima, a classification of complicated fractures in Group 4, based on the number of fragments into which the upper humerus has been divided (Table 2) [7]. This classification is similar to that published by Neer in 1970 [16]. Table 3 shows the indications for prosthetic replacement, based on our classification.

Prosthetic replacement is not indicated in comminuted fractures limited to the tuberosity zone, without damage to the articular surface, nor in three-fragment fractures of any type in which the blood supply to the head is usually preserved, except fracture-dislocation through the anatomical neck [6,8,1,2].

General Policy of Treatment

1) An attempt is made at manipulative reduction in every case. An incomplete reposition may be accepted as satisfactory.

Table 1. Classification of Fractures of the Proximal Humerus

1) Intracapsular Fractures
   a) Fracture of the head
   b) Fracture of the anatomical neck
2) Tuberosity Zone Fractures
   a) Transtuberosity fracture
   b) Fracture of the greater tuberosity
   c) Fracture of the lesser tuberosity
3) Surgical Neck Fractures
   a) Subtuberosity
   b) Metaphyseal
4) Complex Fractures
   a) Comminuted fracture
   b) Fracture-dislocation

Table 2. Classification of Complex Fractures

A) Comminuted Fractures
   i) Three-fragment fracture: (a) free, (b) impacted
   ii) Four-fragment fracture: (a) free, (b) impacted
B) Fracture Dislocation
   I) Anterior II Posterior
   i) Two-fragment: (a) anatomical neck, (b) surgical neck
   ii) Three-fragment fracture-dislocation
   iii) Four-fragment fracture-dislocation

Table 3. Indications for prosthetic replacement in serious fractures

1) Fracture of the head with severe incongruity or detached major fragment
2) Four-fragment comminuted fracture (or more) with or without impaction
3) Fracture-dislocation of the anatomical neck, with or without associated fracture of the greater tuberosity
4) Four-fragment anterior fracture-dislocation
5) Posterior fracture-dislocation of the anatomical neck (with or without fracture of the lesser tuberosity)
6) Four-fragment posterior fracture-dislocation

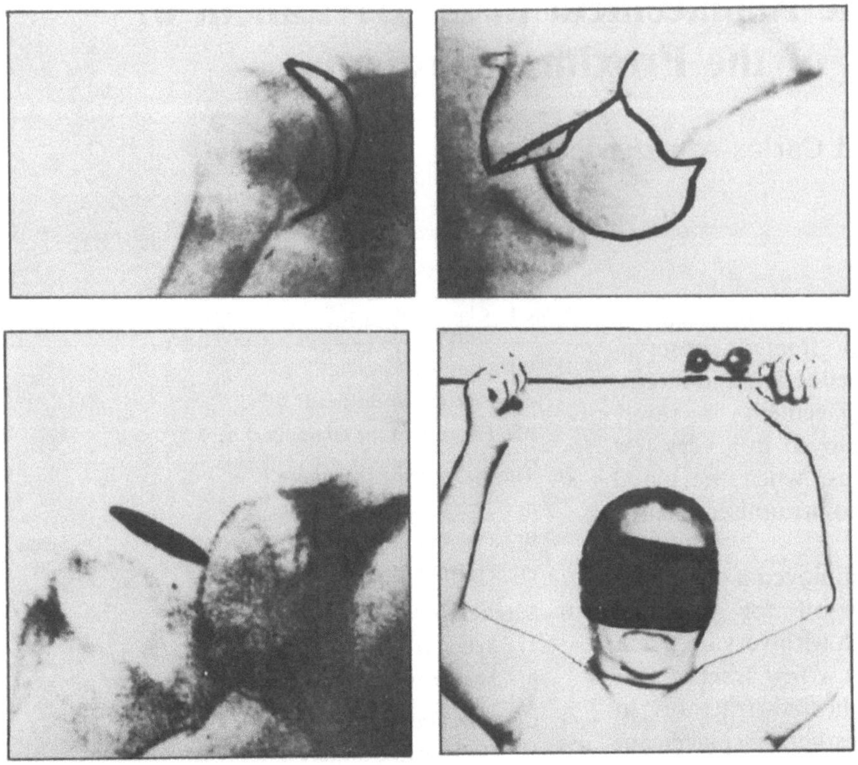

Fig. 1. Impacted fracture of head of humerus. Posterior half of the head deeply impacted; no blood supply following disimpaction. Prosthetic replacement (acrylic 1953). Excellent result three years following surgery

2) After the initial manipulation, the fracture is re-appraised, with particular reference to the number of fragments, the articular congruity, and the damage to the greater tuberosity.

3) Operation is elected when the fragments are markedly displaced especially if joint congruity is disturbed and in four-fragment fractures.

4) If operation is performed we prefer the superior approach. In the past, the majority of our patients had partial acromionectomy for access, now however, a simple transverse osteotomy of the acromial process is performed, sometimes with arthroplasty of the acromioclavicular joint by removing 15 mm of the anterior portion of the acromial process. We believe that such a transacromial approach is preferable in traumatic cases, because it provides an ample operative field and diminishes the risks of devascularisation of the head by dividing the tendons which could be carrying the sole remaining vascular supply to the head. This problem mainly arises in relation to the division of subscapularis when the usual anterior approach is used. In non-traumatic cases this does not matter, but in severe trauma it carries significant hazards.

5) Once the fragments have been replaced, the articular surface is carefully inspected for important incongruity which might justify the use of a prosthesis.

6) An appraisal of the blood supply of any major fragment is carefully carried out in order to determine whether there is an indication for prosthetic replacement.

7) If the head of the humerus has to be removed, prosthetic replacement offers the prospect of a better functional result than simple excision of the head.

Fractures of the Head of the Humerus

Head cleavage fractures and impaction fractures sometimes maintain sufficient connection with soft tissues to enable the surgeon to reduce and secure both fragments with one screw introduced from behind. If one of the fragments is completely detached, as commonly occurs, it is better to proceed to prosthetic replacement.

Figure 1 shows an impacted posterior fragment, detached from soft tissues. Twenty-seven years ago a prosthetic replacement was performed using an acrylic device. Until she died some three years following operation the result was excellent.

Comminuted Fractures

When fragmentation is limited to the tuberosity zone, the treatment of choice is conservative (Fig. 2). When complete comminution including the articular surface has occurred, a prosthetic replacement is recommended. This severely comminuted fracture offers the worst prognosis because it involves damage to the tendinous insertions which carry the blood supply to the head of the humerus.

Impacted Fractures with Inferior Subluxation

The shaft is deeply impacted into the epiphysis, and the upper humerus explodes into three, four or more fragments. The impacted head rotates laterally, so that the articular surface comes to look outwards. In three-fragment impacted fractures in which the lesser tuberosity has not been detached, the treatment of choice is by open reduction with disimpaction of the head and fixation of the greater tuberosity (Fig. 3). In four-fragment impacted fractures, operation is advised to disimpact the head, thereafter to re-appraise its blood supply which usually is insufficient so that a prosthetic replacement becomes necessary. The tuberosities must be repaired with their attached tendons (Fig. 4).

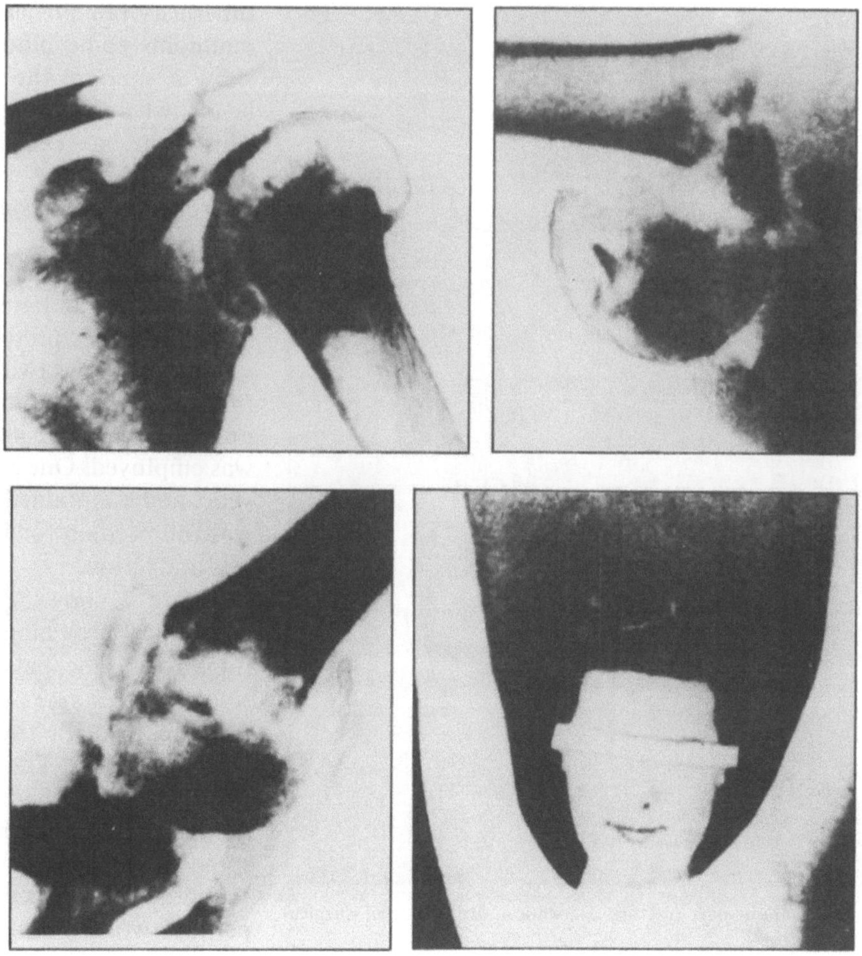

Fig. 2. Comminuted three-part fracture involving the tuberosities. The comminution is better appreciated in an axiliary lateral view. Satisfactory closed reduction. Excellent result

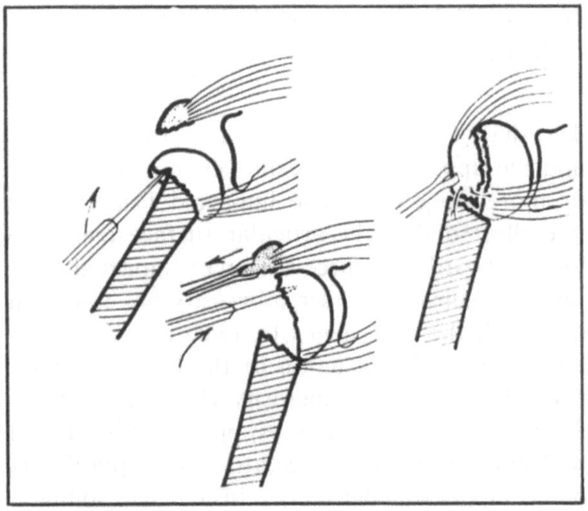

Fig. 3. Three-fragment impacted fracture. Disimpaction and reposition of greater tuberosity. The circulation is maintained through the lesser tuberosity; prosthetic replacement not indicated

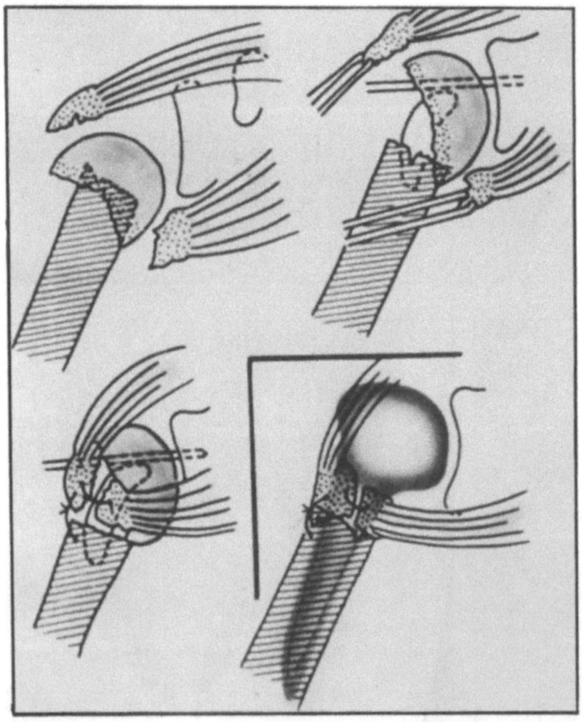

Fig. 4. Four-part fracture-dislocation. Principles of surgical reconstruction

Anterior Fracture-Dislocation

In addition to the dislocation there is a fracture through the anatomical or surgical neck of the humerus. In fracture-dislocation of the surgical neck, open reduction is generally required with appropriate internal fixation. Prosthetic replacement is not indicated because the blood supply to the head is maintained (Fig. 5).

In fracture-dislocation of the anatomical neck, either a simple two-fragment injury or one associated with a fracture of the greater tuberosity, which in both cases deprives the head of its blood supply, prosthetic replacement is indicated and gives the best results [10,15]. In our series, the best results have been obtained in this type of lesion. The anatomical neck fracture-dislocation associated with fracture of the greater tuberosity is not the usual type of three-fragment injury, because the lesser tuberosity remains attached to the shaft. It is important to differentiate this from a three-fragment fracture-dislocation, in which the lesser tuberosity remains attached to the head and thus maintains some blood supply. Radiographs will show a spur on the infero-internal angle of the head, where subscapularis tendon is attached. This is the best example of how the head may be devascularised by using a standard anterior approach in which subscapularis is divided. In the former condition, with the lesser tuberosity attached to the shaft, prosthetic replacement is indicated; in the latter it is not necessary because subscapularis is preserved on the head fragment.

Figure 6 shows two cases of fracture-dislocation through the anatomical neck, taken from amongst our earliest cases, in which an acrylic prosthesis was employed. One patient was followed up for 20 years and maintained an excellent result; the other was followed up for 15 years and had 60° of painless abduction.

Figure 7 shows a fracture-dislocation of the anatomical neck alone without fracture of greater tuberosity. The patient maintained an excellent result for 15 years when he suffered a further fracture through the surgical neck in an automobile accident. The stem of the acrylic prosthesis was broken and had to be replaced by a metallic non-cemented prosthesis. At the present time, some 13 years after the second operation, the function is rated as good and he has no pain. It is perhaps worth noting that when it was taken out

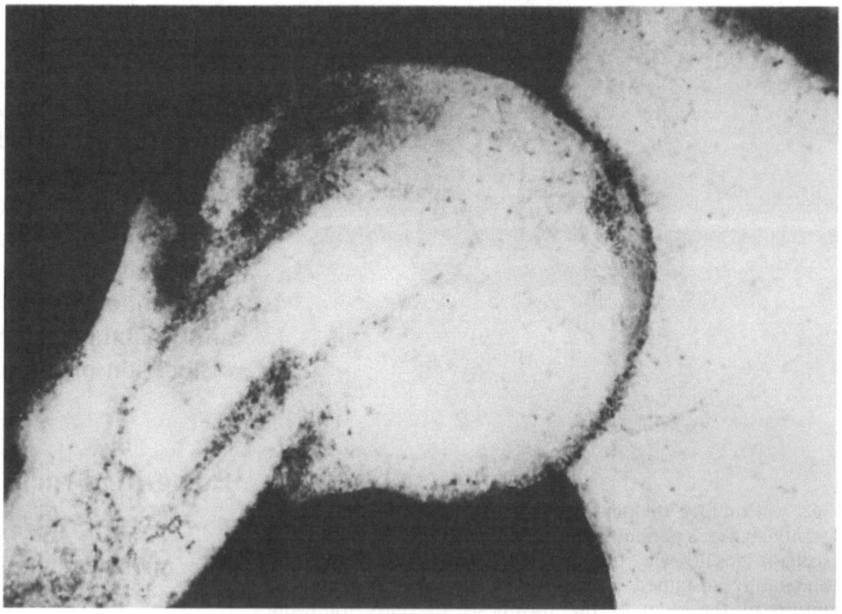

Fig. 5. Fracture-dislocation of the surgical neck after operative reduction. The head has a good blood supply and prosthetic replacement is not required. Operation was by a transacromial approach, the acromial process being used as a graft for internal fixation

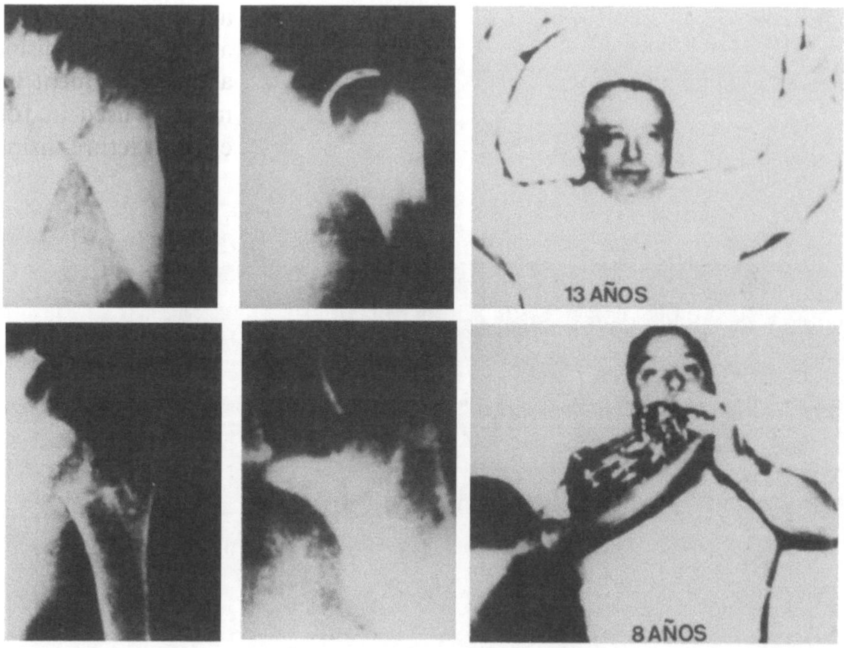

Fig. 6. Fracture-dislocation of anatomical neck. Two cases, both associated with non-displacement of greater tuberosity. Acrylic prosthetic replacement in both cases. (*Above*) A dentist who continued to work for 20 years without shoulder disability. (*Below*) A musician who continued playing a heavy instrument without pain

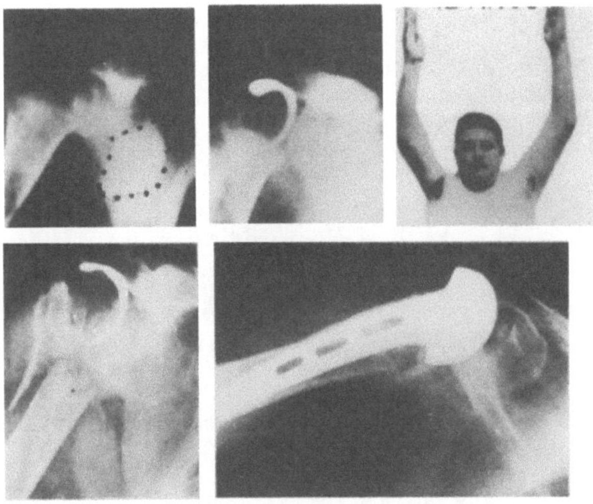

Fig. 7. Fracture-dislocation of the anatomical neck. Twenty-six years previously an acrylic prosthesis was used. An excellent result was obtained for many years until he accidentally sustained a fracture of the surgical neck and rupture of the stem of the prosthesis 15 years following operation. It was replaced by a non-cemented metallic prosthesis with a good end-result

the acrylic prosthesis showed marked resorption but without any soft-tissue reaction around it.

One of the first patients on whom we operated is shown in Fig. 8. Although the result was good, it was the wrong indication for prosthetic replacement, as the radiograph on review showed the telltale spur on the inferior angle of the head indicating retention of intact subscapularis attachment. This was a case of three-fragment fracture-dislocation in which the head should be reduced and maintained in position, as for fracture-dislocation of the surgical neck.

Posterior Fracture-Dislocation

The management is similar to that for anterior fracture-dislocation, but we have been more successful in closed reduction of posterior than of anterior fracture-dislocations. If closed reposition fails, operation is performed by a posterior transacromial approach, and proceeds in the same way as for anterior dislocation: no prosthesis is used in a three-fragment injury but a prosthetic replacement is used in four-fragment injuries. In posterior fracture-dislocation the fourth fragment is

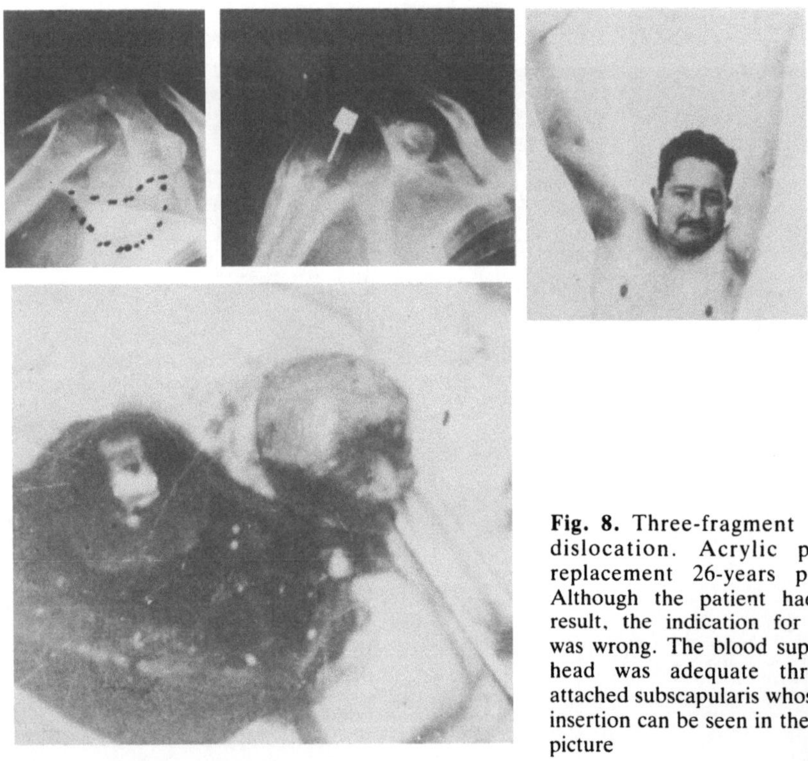

Fig. 8. Three-fragment fracture-dislocation. Acrylic prosthetic replacement 26-years previously. Although the patient had a good result, the indication for operation was wrong. The blood supply to the head was adequate through the attached subscapularis whose point of insertion can be seen in the operative picture

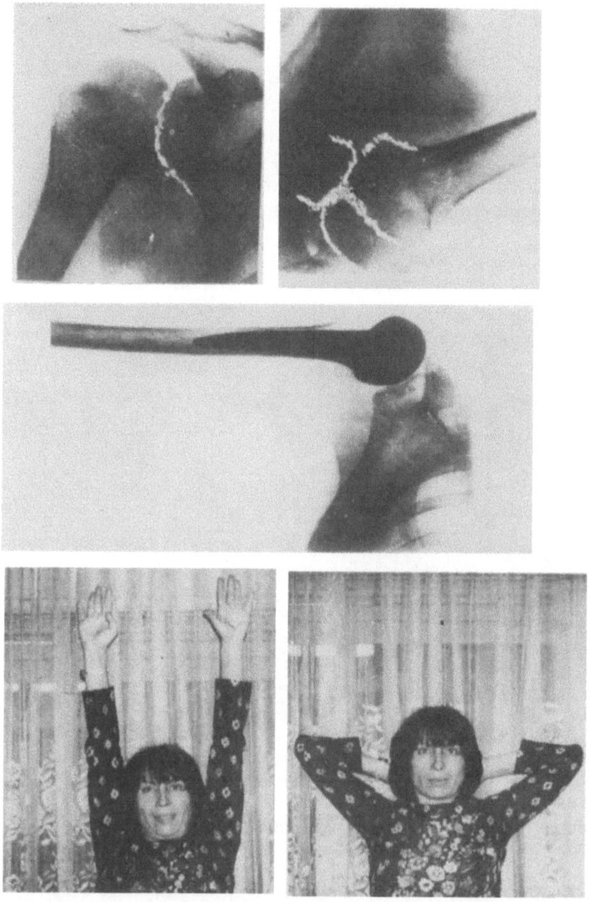

Fig. 9. Posterior fracture-dislocation of the anatomical neck. Non-cemented metallic prosthesis. Excellent result 8 years after surgery. She had complete movement and no pain

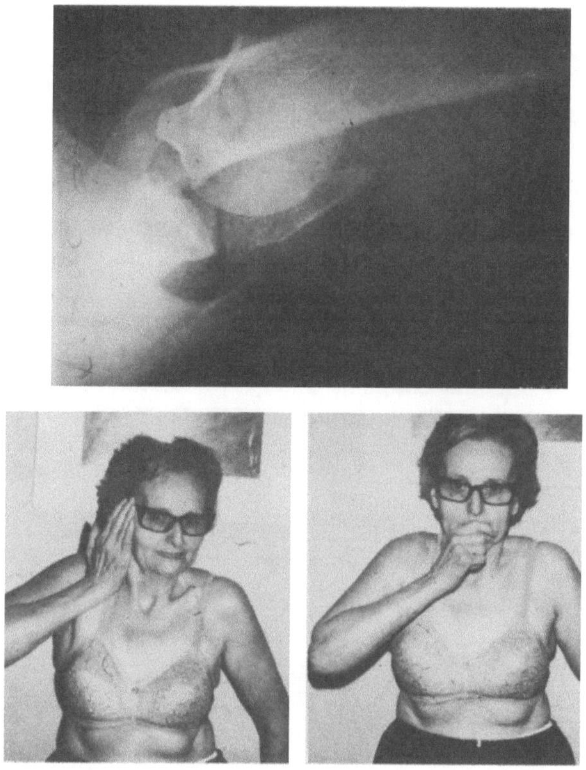

Fig. 10. Four-fragment posterior fracture-dislocation treated with metallic prosthetic replacement. One year after surgery there was no pain but only 25° of abduction due to myosytis ossificans. Poor result compared to the patient shown in Fig. 9

the greater tuberosity and preserves the circulation to the head of the humerus.

Figure 9 shows a woman with posterior fracture-dislocation, treated by a non-cemented metallic prosthesis. Eight years following operation she had no pain and full function. Figure 10, on the other hand, shows a similar injury with a poor result of limited motion and some pain. Figure 11 shows a bilateral posterior fracture-dislocation produced by convulsion. On the left shoulder closed reduction was obtained; the right shoulder required a prosthetic replacement. Functional result was good and very similar on both sides.

Post-traumatic Necrosis

This is not a common condition in the shoulder, but occasionally does follow trauma in which the head of the humerus has become devascularised. Figure 12 shows a three-fragment fracture-dislocation treated by reposition of the fragments and wire fixation. Four months later the head was necrotic. An inadequate acrylic prosthesis was used, with a poor result.

Figure 13 shows a woman with avascular necrosis of the head of the humerus 18 months after a fall. She complained of unbearable pain and a totally stiff joint. Two years ago she underwent prosthetic replacement which has resulted in a painless shoulder of good function.

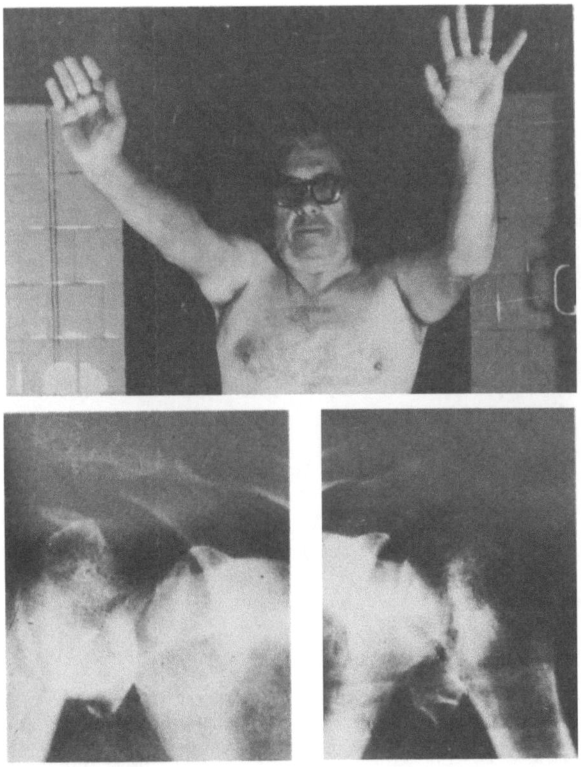

Fig. 11. Bilateral posterior fracture-dislocation. Closed reduction on the left side; prosthetic replacement on the right. Similar results in both shoulders

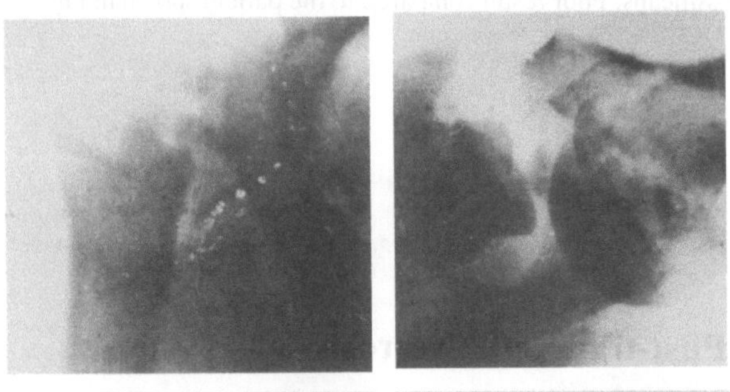

Fig. 12. Three-fragment posterior fracture-dislocation. Six months after open reduction avascular necrosis was evident. Prosthetic replacement of the present design was used. One year after operation there was good function and no pain

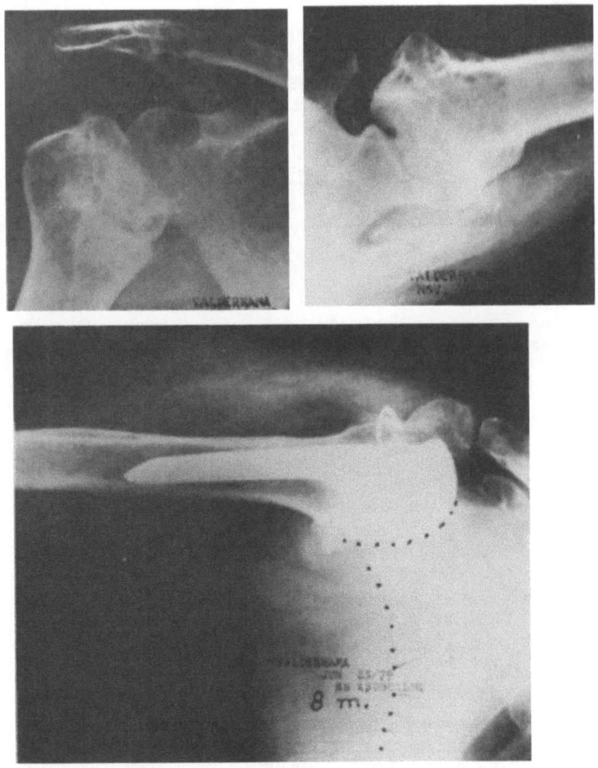

Fig. 13. Resorption of the head 18 months after trauma. A prosthetic replacement of the present design was used. One year after operation there was good function and no pain

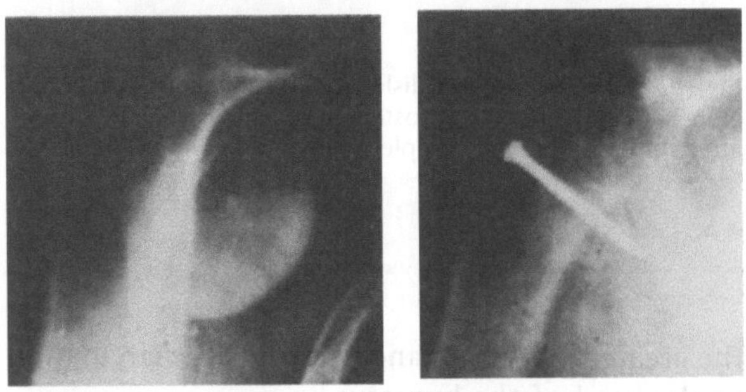

Fig. 14. Fracture-dislocation of the anatomical neck treated elsewhere by removal of the head and fixation of the greater tuberosity. Two years later the shoulder was stiff and painful. Prosthetic replacement with satisfactory movement and no pain

Sequelae of Excision of the Humeral Head

Simple removal of the head of the humerus is still performed in severe traumatic cases, and we have indeed seen satisfactory results with this operation. Many cases, however, are left with flail shoulders or very painful and stiff joints. We have operated on three such patients, and Fig. 14 shows one of them with a poor functional result but with no pain.

Prosthetic Replacement of Humeral Head

Since 1953 we have developed several modifications of our original design, which was made of acrylic material, as was usual at the time. It was discontinued after eleven such devices had been used. Some of these cases are shown in this paper, (despite the risk of our being judged surgically primitive), because they are very good examples of particular problems and have been followed for many years. The original device is shown also, because we believe that the prosthesis is one of the first conceived with the object of replacing the upper end of the humerus and allowing tendinous re-attachment around the prosthesis (Fig. 15).

The second model of a similar design was made in metal and used without cement, like the Moore prosthesis for the hip; it gave some of the best results. With the introduction of surgical bone cement the stem has been modified.

To obtain more outward rotation we tried to imitate the Weber hip prosthesis with a third design using polyethylene. All three operations

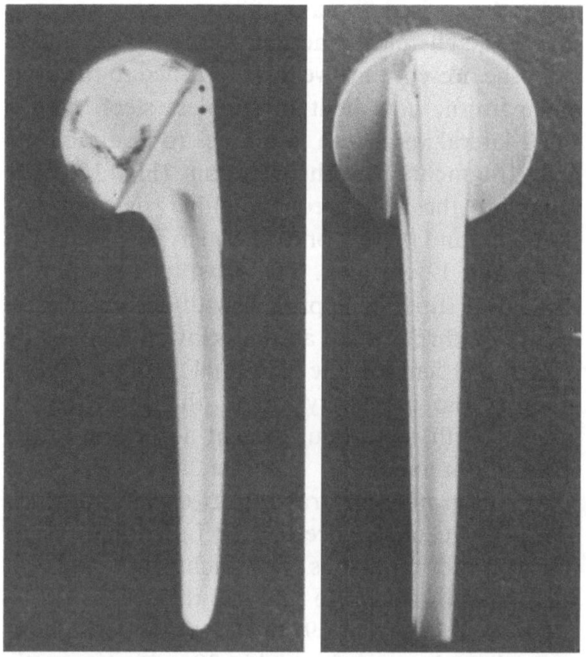

Fig. 16. Prosthesis in use at present. Metallic; with or without cementation, according to the quality of fixation obtained. Same design as the first acrylic model with two lateral holes to attach the tuberosities

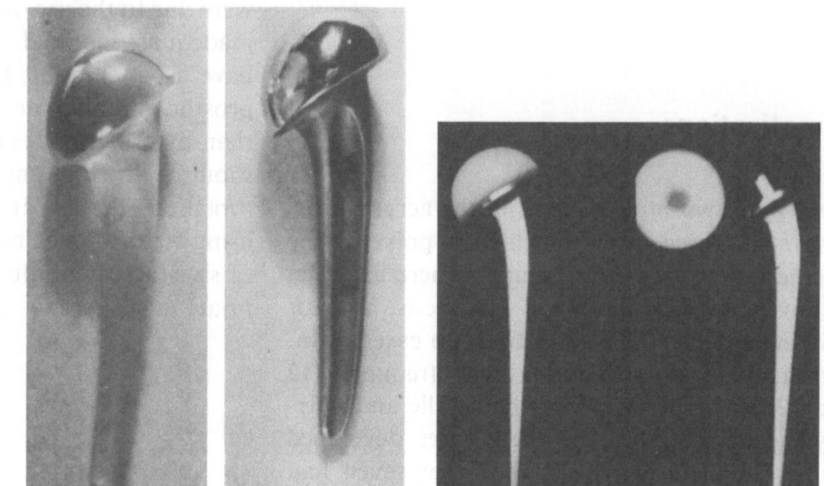

Fig. 15. Obsolete designs of prostheses. **a** Acrylic (1952) conceived with the intention of replacing only the articular portion; similar to the present models for hemi-arthroplasty. **b** Metallic non-cemented (1956) of the same design. **c** Imitation of Weber hip prosthesis. All the cases on whom this device was used required revision

a b c

had to be revised because of serious abrasion and soft-tissue chemical reaction.

At the present time we have returned to the original pattern, now built in stainless steel, with a small lateral wing with two holes to re-attach the bone fragments with their tendons (Fig. 16). The same prosthesis is used for either right or left shoulder, and there is only one stem size, 10 mm in width and 12 cm long. The prosthesis is inserted through a superior approach with acromial osteotomy or through the acromioclavicular joint by resecting 1 cm of the acromial process. After reaming the medullary canal, the prosthesis is inserted with or without cement according to the fixation obtained.

Attention must be drawn to two matters which are of great importance for the functional result: (i) accurate tendinous re-attachment, and (ii) adequate postoperative physical therapy.

Between 1953 and 1979, 36 prosthetic replacements have been performed in 30 acute traumatic cases and 6 post-traumatic sequelae (Table 4). Only 6 prostheses have been cemented (3 polyethylene and 3 of the present design).

Table 4. Prosthetic replacement

Anterior fracture-dislocations	8	(22%)
Posterior fracture-dislocations	13	(36%)
Four-fragment comminuted fractures	9	(25%)
Avascular necrosis (postraumatic)	2	(5.5%)
Sequelae of head ablation	3	(8.3%)
Surgical neck non-union	1	(2.7%)
Total	36	cases

Complications

There were two broken stems in the acrylic prostheses. All three cases in which a polyethylene prosthesis was used were failures. There has been no loosening with the metal prosthesis, with or without cement. There have been no cases of infection. Ectopic ossification was frequent (12 cases, 33%), especially with the acrylic and polyethylene devices. Five of these cases developed almost complete ankylosis; the other seven had relatively minor symptoms.

Results

We were able to evaluate 36 shoulders from 1 to 25 years following operation with an average duration of follow-up of 7.5 years. Six shoulders have been evaluated from 10-25 years following operation. The follow-up consisted of clinical and radiological examination or a questionnaire. The three most recent cases operated upon during 1980 have not been taken into account, but their progress is satisfactory to date. The classification has been based on functional criteria which take the normal daily movements and the level of pain into account:

Excellent: 5 cases (14%). Complete overhead motion or abduction above 120° (Fig. 9).

Good: 9 cases (25%). The patient can touch his opposite ear, which is equivalent to 90° of abduction and 30° of outward rotation.

Poor: 17 cases (47%). The patient can easily reach his mouth with his hand, without pain or with insignificant pain.

Failure: 5 cases (14%). Complete stiffness or significant pain.

Approximately 80% of patients declared themselves satisfied with the operation. Nearly 50% of the "poor" results are considered satisfactory by us in view of the functional problems that the shoulder joint presents. Failures, in great part, were due to the use of the early prostheses made of inadequate material. At least 40% of patients will have a better result following the use of modern prosthetic replacement when it is indicated, rather than by other modes of treatment, and this figure should be further improved by an improvement in prosthetic design. It is possible to conceive that using an adequate device and technique some 90% of satisfactory results could be obtained in appropriate cases.

Conclusions

In properly selected cases prosthetic replacement offers a better functional result than simple excision of the head of the humerus.

i) The functional result is unpredictable. In general the best results were obtained in cases with little damage to tendinous insertions, such as in cases of fracture-dislocation of the anatomical neck.

ii) The prognosis with regard to pain is better than that for movement. The majority of patients were relieved of pain; the majority of patients had some restriction of motion.

iii) The results of prosthetic replacement of the humeral are less good for traumatic than non-traumatic conditions [17].

Although indications for prosthetic replacement of the proximal humerus following trauma are rare, when properly indicated it can be performed with an expectation of acceptably good results.

References

1 de Anquin CA, de Anquin CE (1974) Fracturas Graves de la Extremidad Superior del Húmero. Clasificación de las Fracturas Multifragmentarias. Actas y Trabajos IX° Congreso Latinoamericano de Ortopedia y Traumatologia. 359. (Buenos Aires)

2 de Anquin CA, de Anquin CE (1974) Fracturas Graves de la Extremidad Superior del Húmero. Clasificación de las Fracturas Luxaciones. Actas y Trabajos del IX° Congreso de Ortop. y Traumatol 359 (Buenos Aires)

3 de Anquin CE (1953) Fracturas de la Extremidad Superior del Húmero. Symposium 2° Congreso Latinoamericano de Ortopedia y Traumatologia (Rio de Janeiro, San Pablo)

4 de Anquin CE (1953) Fracturas de la Extremidad Superior del Húmero. Edin "El Ateneo", Buenos Aires

5 de Anquin CE (1965) Clasificación de las fracturas graves de la extremidad superior del húmero. 5° Congreso Latinoamericano de Ortopedia y Traumatologia. (Lima, Peru)

6 de Anquin CE (1966) Substitution par prothése de la tête humérale. Acta X° Congres SICOT 731-738 (Paris)

7 de Anquin CE (1972) Fracture-dislocation of the shoulder. Classification and plan of treatment. Proceedings of the 12th Congress SICOT 932 (Tel Aviv)

8 de Anquin CE (1974) Fracturas Graves de la Extremidad Superior del Húmero. Tratamiento. Actas y Trabajos del IX° Congreso de Ortop. y Traumatol 367 (Buenos Aires)

9 Einarsson F (1958) Fracture of the upper end of the humerus. Acta Orthop Scand Suppl XXXII

10 Kraulis J and Hunter G (1976) The results of prosthetic replacement in fracture-dislocation of the upper end of the humerus. Injury 8: 129

11 Lecène P (1929) Chirurg des os et des articulations (p 591) Masson et Cie, Paris

12 Martini M (1976) Journal of Bone and Joint Surgery 58A: 377

13 Martini M (1973) Revue de Chirurgie Orthopédique 59: 615-622

14 Moribor L, Patterson RL (1967) Fractures of the proximal end of the humerus. J Bone Jt Surg 49-A: 1018

15 Neer CS (1955) Articular replacement of the humeral head. J Bone Joint Surg 37-A: 215-228

16 Neer CS (1970) Displaced proximal humeral fractures. Part I and II. J Bone Joint Surg 52-A: 1077-1103

17 Neer CS (1974) Replacement arthroplasty for glenohumeral osteoarthritis. J Bone Joint Surg 56-A: 1-13

Subject Index

Progress in Orthopaedic Surgery

Progress inn Orthopaedic Surgery was created to provide acommon ground for communication between English-speaking and non English-speaking European orthopaedic surgeons and to satisfy their need for information on the most recent developments in the field. Each volume is devoted to one or two themes in orthopaedic surgery and closely related fields and presents a broad overview of the current state of knowledge. The major emphasis of this series on diagnosis, prevention, and therapy of orthopaedic disorders.

Volume 1

Leg Length Discrepancy The Injured Knee

Editor: D. S. Hungerford
With contributions by numerous experts
1977. 100 figures. X, 160 pages
ISBN 3-540-08037-6

Contents: Leg Length Discrepancy: Basic Rehabilitation Principles of Persons with Leg Length Discrepancy: An Overview. Etiology and Pathophysiology of Leg Length Discrepancies. Measurement of Leg Length. Methodological Errors in Documenting Leg Length and Leg Length Discrepancies. Equalitzation of Leg Length with Orthopaedic Shoe Measures. Subtrochanteric Shortening and Lengthening Osteotomy. Sugical Lenghtening or Shortening of Femur und Tibia. Technique and Indications. - The Injured Knee: The Importance of Arthography Following Trauma to the Knee Joint. The Knee Joint of the Soccer Player(Its Stresses and Damages). Trauma-Induced Chondromalacia Patellea. Injuries to the Articular Cartilage of the Knee.

Volume 2

Acetabilar Dysplasia - Skeletal Dysplasia in Childhood

Editor: U. H. Weil
With contributions by numerous experts
1978. 133 figures, 20 tables. IX, 200 pages
ISBN 3-540-08400-2

Contents: Acetabular Dysplasia: Pathologic Anatomy of Congenital Hip Disease. Development and Clinical Importance of the Dysplastic Acetabulum. Radiologic Interpretation of Dysplasia of the Acetabulum. Femoral Osteotomies for Congenital Hip Dislocation. Our Experience with Salter's Innominate Osteotomy in the Treatment of Hip Dysplasia. Chiari Pelvic Osteotomy for Hip Dysplasia in Patients Below the Age of 20. Experience with Spherical Acetabular Osteotomy for the Correction of the Dysplastic Acetabulum. Comparison of Pelvic Osteotomies in the Treatment of Congenital Hip Dislocation. - Skeletal Dysplasias in Childhood: Constitutional Disorders of Skeletal Development: The Skeletal Dysplasias Orthopaedic Corrections in Patients with Vitamin D-Resistant Rickets.

Volume 3

The Knee: Ligament and Articular Cartilage Injuries

Guesteditor: D. E. Hastings
With contributions by numerous experts
1978. 139 figures, 20 tables. X, 191 pages
ISBN 3-540-08679-X

Contents: Biomechanics and Pathophysiology. - The Acute Knee Ligament Injury. - Chronic Knee Ligament Instability. - The Acute Cartilage Injury. - The Old Cartilage Injury. - Retropatellar Cartilage Degeneration.

Volume 4

Joint Preserving Procedures of the Lower Extremity

Editor: U. H. Weil
With contribution by numerous experts
1980. 87 figures, 9 tables. VIII, 121 pages
ISBN 3-540-09856-9

Contents: Resurfacing of the Hip Jount. - Long Term Results of Chiari Pelvic Osteotomies. - Results of Intertrochanteric Osteotomies in Patients with Coxarthrosis 12–15 Years After Surgery. - Long Term Results of Acetabular Shelf Arthroplasty. - Treatment of Osteoarthritis of the Knee by Osteotomy. - Principles of Corrective Osteotomies in Osteoarthrosis of the Knee. - Gait Analysis and its Benefit to the Patient. - Conservative Orthopaedic Management of Children with Myelomeningoceles. Subject Index. - List of Contributors.

Volume 5

Segmental Idiopathic Necrosis of the Femoral Head

Editor: U.H. Weil
With contributions by numerous experts
1981. 68 figures. Approx. 128 pages
ISBN 3-540-10718-5

Contents: The Question of Posture. - Early Diagnosis of Osteonecrosis by Functional Bone Investigation. - Early Diagnosis and Treatment of Ischemic Necrosis of the Femoral Head. - Revitalization of the Osteonecrotic Femoral Head by Vascular Bundle Transplantation. - Transtrochanteric Ventral Rotation Osteotomy After Sugioka for Treatment of Femoral Head Necrosis. - Results of Flexion Osteotomy on Segmental Femoral Head Necrosis in Adults. - Treatment of Idiopathic Necrosis of the Femoral Head by Modified Cup Arthroplasty. - Idiopathic Necrosis of the Femoral Head. Results of Intertrochanteric Osteotomy and Joint Resurfacing. - Subject Index. - List of Contributors.

Springer-Verlag
Berlin
Heidelberg
New York

MIX
Papier aus verantwortungsvollen Quellen
Paper from responsible sources
FSC® C105338
FSC
www.fsc.org

If you have any concerns about our products,
you can contact us on
ProductSafety@springernature.com

In case Publisher is established outside the EU,
the EU authorized representative is:
Springer Nature Customer Service Center GmbH
Europaplatz 3, 69115 Heidelberg, Germany

Printed by Libri Plureos GmbH
in Hamburg, Germany